High-Yield Histopathology

SECOND EDITION

High-Yield Histopathology

SECOND EDITION

Ronald W. Dudek, PhD

Professor
Department of Anatomy and Cell Biology
Brody School of Medicine
East Carolina University
Greenville, North Carolina

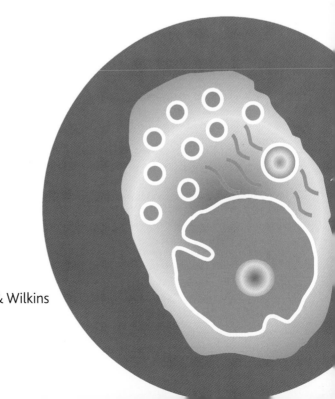

Wolters Kluwer | Lippincott Williams & Wilkins
Health

Philadelphia · Baltimore · New York · London
Buenos Aires · Hong Kong · Sydney · Tokyo

Acquisitions Editor: Crystal Taylor
Product Manager: Catherine Noonan
Manufacturing Manager: Margie Orzech
Designer: Terry Mallon
Vendor Manager: Bridgett Dougherty
Compositor: Aptara, Inc.

Second Edition

9 8 7 6 5 4 3 2 1

Library of Congress Cataloging-in-Publication Data

Dudek, Ronald W., 1950–
  High-yield histopathology / Ronald W. Dudek.—2nd ed.
    p. ; cm.
  Includes bibliographical references and index.
  ISBN 978-1-60913-015-2
1. Histology, Pathological—Outlines, syllabi, etc. I. Title.
[DNLM: 1. Histology—Outlines. 2. Pathology—Outlines. QS 518.2
D845ha 2011]
  RB32.D83 2011
  611′.018—dc22

                                    2010025885

DISCLAIMER

   Care has been taken to confirm the accuracy of the information present and to describe generally accepted practices. However, the authors, editors, and publisher are not responsible for errors or omissions or for any consequences from application of the information in this book and make no warranty, expressed or implied, with respect to the currency, completeness, or accuracy of the contents of the publication. Application of this information in a particular situation remains the professional responsibility of the practitioner; the clinical treatments described and recommended may not be considered absolute and universal recommendations.

   The authors, editors, and publisher have exerted every effort to ensure that drug selection and dosage set forth in this text are in accordance with the current recommendations and practice at the time of publication. However, in view of ongoing research, changes in government regulations, and the constant flow of information relating to drug therapy and drug reactions, the reader is urged to check the package insert for each drug for any change in indications and dosage and for added warnings and precautions. This is particularly important when the recommended agent is a new or infrequently employed drug.

   Some drugs and medical devices presented in this publication have Food and Drug Administration (FDA) clearance for limited use in restricted research settings. It is the responsibility of the health care provider to ascertain the FDA status of each drug or device planned for use in their clinical practice.

To purchase additional copies of this book, call our customer service department at **(800) 638-3030** or fax orders to **(301) 223-2320**. International customers should call **(301) 223-2300**.

Visit Lippincott Williams & Wilkins on the Internet: http://www.lww.com. Lippincott Williams & Wilkins customer service representatives are available from 8:30 am to 6:00 pm, EST.

I would like to dedicate this book to my mother, Lottie Dudek, who was born on November 11, 1918. Through the years my mother raised her children, maintained a loving marriage, and worked 40 hours per week. In the year 2004, society would describe such a person as a "liberated woman" or "supermom." I would like to acknowledge that my mother was a "supermom" 20 years before the word was fashionable. A son cannot repay a mother. My hope is that "I love you and thank you" will suffice.

Preface

High-Yield Histopathology does more than just review histology. The questions on the USMLE Step 1 cross traditional course boundaries, making it difficult to identify a question that is "strictly histology." Many USMLE Step 1 questions fall into the categories such as histopathology, histophysiology, histomicrobiology, and histopharmacology. To write a review book on basic, traditional histology would not be helpful to the student preparing for the USMLE Step 1 since there are no basic traditional histology questions on the exam. In this regard, *High-Yield Histopathology* reviews important histology concepts as a gateway to the pathology, physiology, microbiology, and pharmacology of clinically relevant topics.

In addition, many students have commented that cell biology topics have been well represented on the USMLE Step 1. To this end, I have included Chapter 1 (Nucleus), Chapter 2 (Cytoplasm and Organelles), and Chapter 3 (Cell Membrane) with up-to-date and clinically relevant information.

I would appreciate any comments or suggestions concerning *High-Yield Histopathology,* especially after you have taken the USMLE Step 1 exam, that you think might improve the book. You may contact me at dudekr@ecu.edu.

Contents

Chapter 1

Nucleus

I **Nuclear Envelope.** The nuclear envelope is a two-membrane structure. The **inner membrane** is associated with a network of **intermediate filaments (lamins A, B, C)** called the **nuclear lamina,** which plays a role in the disassembly of the nuclear envelope during prometaphase of mitosis by phosphorylation of the lamins by **lamin kinase** and in the reassembly of the nuclear envelope during telophase. The **outer membrane** is studded with ribosomes and is continuous with the rough endoplasmic reticulum (rER). The inner and outer membranes are separated by a **perinuclear cisterna.** The nuclear envelope contains many pores that allow passage of molecules between the nucleus and cytoplasm (e.g., ions, messenger RNA (mRNA), transfer RNA (tRNA), ribosomal RNA (rRNA), gene regulatory proteins, DNA polymerases, RNA polymerases). The pores are associated with a **nuclear pore complex** that consists of many different proteins arranged in octagonal symmetry with a central channel.

II **Apoptosis.** Apoptosis is a **noninflammatory programmed cell death ("cell suicide")** that is characterized by **DNA fragmentation, a decrease in cell volume, loss of mitochondrial function, cell membrane blebbing,** and **formation of apoptotic bodies,** which are rapidly phagocytosed without an inflammatory response.

A. The chromatin is eventually cleaved by a specific endonuclease into DNA fragments that generate a distinctive **180-bp ladder** that is pathognomonic of apoptotic cell death.

B. Apoptosis is related to a family of proteases called **caspases,** which are found in all cells.

C. Caspases are activated by either extracellular death signals (e.g., killer lymphocytes produce **Fas ligand,** which binds to the **Fas death receptor** on the target cell; **tumor necrosis factor [TNF]** binds to the **TNF death receptor** on the target cell) or intracellular death signals (e.g., mitochondria release **cytochrome c** into the cytoplasm where it activates **Apaf-1 adaptor protein,** which in turn activates caspases).

D. The **Bcl-2** and the **IAP (inhibitor of apoptosis) family of proteins** are the main regulators of apoptosis.

E. Apoptosis occurs in hormone-dependent involution of cells during the menstrual cycle, embryogenesis, toxin-induced injury (e.g., diphtheria), viral cell death (e.g., Councilman bodies in yellow fever), and cell death via cytotoxic T cells or other immune cells.

III **Nucleolus**

A. The nucleolus consists of portions of five pairs of chromosomes (i.e., 13, 14, 15, 21, and 22) that contain about **200 copies of rRNA** genes per haploid genome that code for **rRNA.**

B. In humans, **RNA polymerase I** catalyzes the formation of **45S rRNA** and **RNA polymerase III** catalyzes the formation of **5S RNA**.

 Chromatin. Chromatin is double-helical DNA associated with histones and nonhistone proteins.

A. HETEROCHROMATIN is condensed chromatin and is **transcriptionally inactive.** In electron micrographs, heterochromatin is electron dense (i.e., very black). An example of heterochromatin is the **Barr body**, which is found in female cells and represents the inactive X chromosome. Heterochromatin makes up ~10% of the total chromatin.
   1. **Constitutive heterochromatin** is always condensed (i.e., transcriptionally inactive) and consists of repetitive DNA found near the centromere and other regions.
   2. **Facultative heterochromatin** can be either condensed (i.e., transcriptionally inactive) or dispersed (i.e., transcriptionally active). An example of facultative heterochromatin is the **XY body**, which forms when both the X and Y chromosome are inactivated for ~15 days during male meiosis.

B. EUCHROMATIN is dispersed chromatin and makes up ∼90% of the total chromatin. Of this 90%, 10% is transcriptionally active and 80% is transcriptionally inactive. When chromatin is transcriptionally active, there is weak binding to the H1 histone protein and **acetylation** of the H2A, H2B, H3, and H4 histone proteins.

C. NUCLEOSOME
   1. The most fundamental unit of packaging of DNA is the nucleosome.
   2. A nucleosome consists of a histone protein octamer (two each of **H2A, H2B, H3, and H4 histone proteins**) around which 146 bp of DNA is coiled in 1.75 turns. The nucleosomes are connected by spacer DNA, which results in 10-nm-diameter fiber that resembles a "beads on a string" appearance by electron microscopy.
   3. Histones are small proteins containing a high proportion of **lysine** and **arginine** that impart a positive charge to the proteins that enhances their binding to negatively charged DNA. Histones bind to DNA in A-T–rich regions of DNA.
   4. Histone proteins have exposed N-terminal amino acid tails that are subject to modification and are crucial in regulating nucleosome structure.
   5. **Histone acetylation** reduces the affinity between histones and DNA. An increased acetylation of histone proteins will make a DNA segment more likely to be transcribed into RNA and hence any genes in that DNA segment will be expressed (i.e., ↑ acetylation of histones = expressed genes).

D. 30-nm CHROMATIN FIBER. The 10-nm nucleosome fiber is joined by **H1 histone protein** to form a **30-nm chromatin fiber.** When the general term "chromatin" is used, it refers specifically to the 30-nm chromatin fiber.

 Chromosomes. The human genome refers to the total DNA content in the cell, which is divided into two genomes: the very complex **nuclear genome** and the relatively simple **mitochondrial genome.** The human nuclear genome consists of 24 different chromosomes (22 autosomes; X and Y sex chromosomes). The human nuclear genome codes for ≈30,000 **genes** (precise number is uncertain), which make up ≈2% of the human nuclear genome. There are ≈27,000 protein-coding genes and ≈3000 RNA-coding genes. The fact that the ≈30,000 genes make up only ≈2% of the human nuclear genome means that **≈2% of the human nuclear genome consists of coding DNA and ≈98% of the human nuclear genome consists of noncoding DNA.**

A. CENTROMERE
   1. A centromere is a specialized nucleotide DNA sequence that binds to the mitotic spindle during cell division.

2. Chromosomes have a single centromere that is observed microscopically as a **primary constriction**, which is the region where sister chromatids are joined.

3. During prometaphase, a pair of protein complexes called **kinetochores** forms at the centromere where one kinetochore is attached to each sister chromatid.

4. Microtubules produced by the **centrosome** of the cell attach to the kinetochore (called **kinetochore microtubules**) and pull the two sister chromatids toward opposite poles of the mitotic cell.

B. THE TELOMERE

1. The human telomere is a 3- to 20-kb repeating nucleotide sequence (**TTAGGG**) located at the end of a chromosome.

2. The telomere allows replication of linear DNA to its full length. Since DNA polymerases *cannot* synthesize in the 3′ → 5′ direction or start synthesis de novo, removal of the RNA primers will always leave the 5′ end of the newly synthesized lagging strand shorter than the lagging strand template. If the 5′ end of the newly synthesized lagging strand is not lengthened, a chromosome would get progressively shorter as the cell goes through a number of cell divisions. This would lead to cell death, which some investigators believe may be related to the aging process in humans.

3. This problem is solved by a special **RNA-directed DNA polymerase or reverse transcriptase** called **telomerase**, which adds many repeats of TTAGGG to the newly synthesized lagging strand.

4. Telomerase is present in **human germline cells** (i.e., spermatogonia, oogonia) and **stem cells** (e.g., in skin, bone marrow, and gut), but is absent from most other somatic cells.

VI Types of DNA Damage and DNA Repair. Chromosomal breakage refers to breaks in chromosomes due to sunlight (or ultraviolet [UV]) irradiation, ionizing irradiation, DNA cross-linking agents, or DNA-damaging agents. These insults may cause **depurination of DNA, deamination of cytosine to uracil,** or **pyrimidine dimerization,** which must be repaired by **DNA repair enzymes.** The system that detects and signals DNA damage is a multiprotein complex called **BASC (BRCA1-associated genome surveillance complex).**

A. DEPURINATION. About 5000 purines (As or Gs) per day are lost from DNA of each human cell when the N-glycosyl bond between the purine and deoxyribose sugar phosphate is broken. This is the most frequent type of lesion and leaves the deoxyribose sugar phosphate with a missing purine base.

B. DEAMINATION OF CYTOSINE TO URACIL. About 100 cytosines (C) per day are spontaneously deaminated to uracil (U). If the U is not corrected back to a C, then upon replication, instead of the occurrence of a correct C-G base pairing, a U-A base pairing will occur instead.

C. PYRIMIDINE DIMERIZATION. Sunlight (UV radiation) can cause covalent linkage of adjacent pyrimidines forming, for example, **thymine dimers.**

VII Clinical Importance of DNA Repair (Table 1-1). The clinical importance of DNA repair enzymes is illustrated by some rare inherited diseases that involve genetic defects in DNA repair enzymes such as xeroderma pigmentosa (XP), ataxia-telangiectasia (AT), Fanconi anemia (FA), and Bloom syndrome (BS), as indicated in Table 1-1.

TABLE 1-1	DNA REPAIR ENZYME PATHOLOGY	
Genetic Disorder	Gene Gene Product Chromosome	Clinical Features
Xeroderma pigmentosum (XP) is an autosomal recessive genetic disorder caused by mutations in nucleotide **excision repair enzymes** that results in the inability to remove pyrimidine dimers and individuals who are hypersensitive to **sunlight (ultraviolet [UV] radiation)**	*XPA* gene DNA repair enzyme 9q22.3 *XPC* gene DNA repair enzyme 3p25	Sunlight (UV radiation) hypersensitivity with sunburnlike reaction, severe skin lesions around the eyes and eyelids, and malignant skin cancers (basal and squamous cell carcinomas and melanomas) whereby most individuals die by 30 years of age
Ataxia-telangiectasia (AT) is an autosomal recessive genetic disorder caused by mutations in **DNA recombination repair enzymes** that results in individuals who are hypersensitive to **ionizing radiation**	*ATM* gene PI-3 kinase and a DNA repair enzyme/cell cycle checkpoint protein 11q22-q23	Ionizing radiation hypersensitivity; cerebellar ataxia with depletion of Purkinje cells; progressive nystagmus; slurred speech; oculocutaneous telangiectasia initially in the bulbar conjunctiva followed by ear, eyelid, cheeks, and neck; immunodeficiency; and death in the second decade of life. A high frequency of structural rearrangements of chromosomes 7 and 14 is the cytogenetic observation with this disease.
Fanconi anemia (FA) is an autosomal recessive genetic disorder caused by mutations in **DNA recombination repair** that results in individuals who are hypersensitive to **DNA cross-linking agents**	*FA-A* gene A protein that normalizes cell growth, corrects sensitivity to chromosomal breakage in the presence of mitomycin C, and generally promotes genomic stability 16q24	DNA cross-linking agent hypersensitivity, short stature, hypopigmented spots, café-au-lait spots, hypogonadism, microcephaly, hypoplastic or aplastic thumbs, renal malformation including unilateral aplasia or horseshoe kidney, acute leukemia, progressive aplastic anemia, head and neck tumors, and medulloblastoma; is the most common form of congenital aplastic anemia
Bloom syndrome (BS) is an autosomal recessive genetic disorder caused by mutations in **DNA repair enzymes** that results in individuals who are hypersensitive to **DNA-damaging agents**	*BLM* gene RecQ helicase 15q26	Hypersensitivity to DNA-damaging agents; long, narrow face; erythema with telangiectasias in butterfly distribution over the nose and cheeks; high-pitched voice; small stature; small mandible; protuberant ears; absence of upper lateral incisors; well-demarcated patches of hypopigmentation and hyperpigmentation; immunodeficiency with decreased immunoglobulin A (IgA), IgM, and IgG levels; and predisposition to several types of cancers

VIII   Cell Cycle

A. PHASES OF THE CELL CYCLE (TABLE 1-2)

1. **G_0 (Gap) Phase.** The G_0 phase is the resting phase of the cell where the cell cycle is suspended.

TABLE 1-2   **PHASES OF CELL CYCLE**

G₀ Phase

Resting phase
Cell cycle suspended

G₁ Phase

Lasts 5 hours
RNA, protein, and organelle synthesis
Cdk2-cyclin D and Cdk2-cyclin E synthesis

p53
⊖

Cdk2-cyclin D
Cdk2-cyclin E ⊕ →G₁ checkpoint

S Phase

Lasts 7 hours
DNA synthesis
RNA and histone synthesis
Centrosome (MTOC) duplicates but remains together as a complex on one side of the nucleus
Methotrexate (Folex), 5-fluorouracil (Adrucil), Cytarabine (cytosine arabinoside), 6-mercaptopurine, Doxorubicin (Adriamycin), Daunorubicin (Cerubidine) are S phase specific

←——Etoposide prevents entry into G₂ phase

G₂ Phase

Lasts 3 hours
ATP synthesis
Cdk1-cyclin A and Cdk1-cyclin B synthesis
Bleomycin (Blenoxane) is G₂ phase specific

Cdk1-cyclin A
Cdk1-cyclin B ⊕ →G₂ checkpoint

PROPHASE

Chromatin condenses to form well-defined chromosomes
Centrosomes (MTOC) move to opposite poles
Mitotic spindle (microtubules) forms between the centrosomes

PROMETAPHASE

Nuclear envelope dis-assembles
Nucleolus disappears
Kinetochores assemble at each centromere
Kinetochore, polar, and astral microtubules are apparent

METAPHASE

Chromosomes align at the metaphase plate
Cells can be arrested in this phase by microtubule inhibitors (e.g., colchicine)
Cells can be isolated for karyotype analysis

ANAPHASE

Cyclins are inactivated by polyubiquitination
Kinetochores separate and chromosomes move to opposite poles

TELOPHASE

Chromosomes decondense to form chromatin
Nuclear envelope re-assembles
Nucleolus reappears

CYTOKINESIS

Cytoplasm divides by a process called cleavage
A cleavage furrow forms around the middle of the cell
A contractile ring (actin and myosin) forms at the cleavage furrow

Interphase Lasts 15 hours

M Phase Lasts 1 hour
Vinblastin (Velban), Vincristine (Oncovin), and Paclitaxel (Taxol) are M phase specific

2. **G₁ (Gap) Phase.** The G_1 phase is the gap of time between mitosis (M phase) and DNA synthesis (S phase). The G_1 phase is the phase where **RNA, protein, and organelle synthesis** occurs. The G_1 phase lasts about **5 hours** in a typical mammalian cell with a 16-hour cell cycle.

3. **S (Synthesis) Phase.** The S phase is the phase where **DNA synthesis** occurs. The S phase lasts about **7 hours** in a typical mammalian cell with a 16-hour cell cycle.

4. **G₂ (Gap) Phase.** The G_2 phase is the gap of time between DNA synthesis (S phase) and mitosis (M phase). The G_2 phase is the phase where **adenosine triphosphate (ATP) synthesis** occurs. The G_2 phase lasts about **3 hours** in a typical mammalian cell with a 16-hour cell cycle.

5. **M (Mitosis) Phase.** The M phase is the phase where **cell division** occurs. The M phase is divided into six stages called **prophase, prometaphase, metaphase, anaphase, telophase,** and **cytokinesis.** The M phase lasts about **1 hour** in a typical mammalian cell with a 16-hour cell cycle.

B. CONTROL OF THE CELL CYCLE (FIGURE 1-1)

1. **Cdk–Cyclin Complexes.** The two main protein families that control the cell cycle are **cyclins** and the **cyclin-dependent protein kinases (Cdks).** A cyclin is a protein that regulates the activity of Cdks and is named because cyclins undergo a cycle of synthesis and degradation during the cell cycle. The cyclins and Cdks form complexes called **Cdk–cyclin complexes.** The ability of Cdks to phosphorylate target proteins is dependent on the particular cyclin that complexes with it.

    a. **Cdk2–cyclin D and Cdk2–cyclin E** mediate the $G_1 \rightarrow$ **S phase** transition at the G_1 checkpoint.

    b. **Cdk1–cyclin A and Cdk1–cyclin B** mediate the $G_2 \rightarrow$ **M phase** transition at the G_2 checkpoint.

2. **Checkpoints.** The checkpoints in the cell cycle are specialized signaling mechanisms that regulate and coordinate the cell response to **DNA damage** and **replication fork blockage.** When the extent of DNA damage or replication fork blockage is beyond the steady-state threshold of DNA repair pathways, a checkpoint signal is produced and a checkpoint is activated. The activation of a checkpoint slows down the cell cycle so that DNA repair may occur and/or blocked replication forks can be recovered. This prevents DNA damage from being converted into inheritable mutations producing highly transformed, metastatic cells.

3. **ATR Kinase.** ATR kinase responds to the **sustained presence of single-stranded DNA (ssDNA).** ATR kinase activates (i.e., phosphorylates) Chk1 **kinase and p53.**

4. **ATM Kinase.** ATM kinase responds to **double-stranded DNA breaks.** ATM kinase activates (i.e., phosphorylates) Chk2 **kinase and p53.**

5. **Control of the G₁ Checkpoint.** There are three pathways that control the G_1 checkpoint.

    a. Depending on the type of the DNA damage, **ATR kinase** and **ATM kinase** will activate (i.e., phosphorylate) **Chk1 kinase** or **Chk2 kinase,** respectively. The activation of Chk1 kinase or Chk2 kinase causes the inactivation of **CDC25A phosphatase.** The inactivation of CDC25A phosphatase causes the downstream stoppage at the G_1 checkpoint.

    b. Depending on the type of the DNA damage, **ATR kinase** and **ATM kinase** will activate (i.e., phosphorylate) p53, which allows p53 to disassociate from **Mdm2.** The activation of p53 causes the transcriptional upregulation of **p21.** The binding of p21 to Cdk2–cyclin D and Cdk2–cyclin E inhibits their action and causes downstream stoppage at the G_1 checkpoint.

    c. Depending on the type of the DNA damage, **ATR kinase** and **ATM kinase** will activate (i.e., phosphorylate) **p16,** which inactivates **Cdk4/6–cyclin D** and thereby causes downstream stoppage at the G_1 checkpoint.

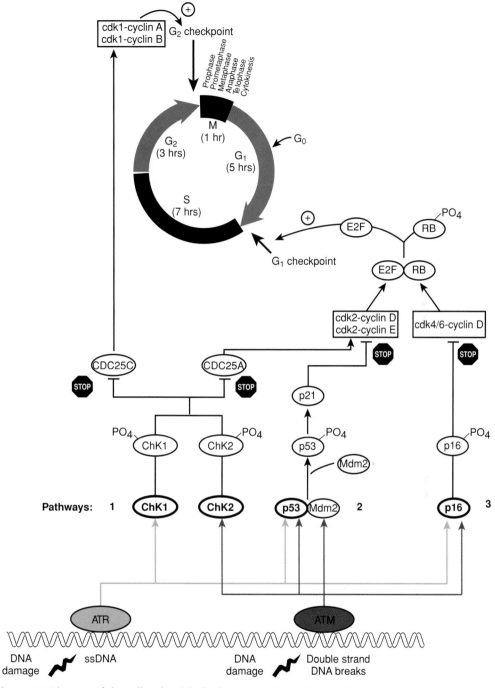

● **Figure 1-1 Diagram of the cell cycle with checkpoints and signaling mechanisms.** ATR kinase responds to the sustained presence of single-stranded DNA (ssDNA) because ssDNA is generated in virtually all types of DNA damage and replication fork blockage by activation (i.e., phosphorylation) of **Chk1 kinase, p53,** and **p16.** ATM kinase responds particularly to **double-stranded DNA breaks** by activation (i.e., phosphorylation) of **Chk2 kinase, p53,** and **p16.** The downstream pathway past the STOP sign is as follows: Cdk2–cyclin D, Cdk2–cyclin E, and Cdk4/6–cyclin D phosphory-late the E2F–RB complex, which causes phosphorylated RB to disassociate from E2F. E2F is a transcription factor that causes the expression of gene products that stimulate the cell cycle. Note the location of the four stop signs. →, activation; ⊤, inactivation.

6. **Control of the G_2 Checkpoint.** Depending on the type of the DNA damage, **ATR kinase** and **ATM kinase** will activate (i.e., phosphorylate) **Chk1 kinase** or **Chk2 kinase**, respectively. The activation of Chk1 kinase or Chk2 kinase causes the inactivation of **CDC25C phosphatase**. The inactivation of CDC25C phosphatase will cause the downstream stoppage at the G_2 checkpoint.

7. **Inactivation of Cyclins.** Cyclins are inactivated by **protein degradation** during **anaphase of the M phase**. **Ubiquitin** (a 76-amino-acid protein) is covalently attached to lysine residues of cyclin by the enzyme **ubiquitin ligase**. This process is called **poly-ubiquitination**. Poly-ubiquitinated cyclins are rapidly degraded by proteolytic enzyme complexes called **proteosomes**.

IX Proto-Oncogenes and Oncogenes

A. DEFINITIONS

1. A **proto-oncogene** is a normal gene that encodes a protein involved in **stimulation of the cell cycle**.

2. An **oncogene** is a mutated proto-oncogene that encodes for an **oncoprotein** that is involved in the **hyperstimulation of the cell cycle**, leading to oncogenesis.

B. ALTERATION OF A PROTO-ONCOGENE TO AN ONCOGENE. The majority of human cancers are not caused by viruses. Instead, the majority of human cancers are caused by the alteration of proto-oncogenes so that oncogenes are formed, producing an oncoprotein.

1. **Point Mutation.** A point mutation (i.e., a **gain-of-function mutation**) of a proto-oncogene leads to the formation of an oncogene. A **single mutant allele** is sufficient to change the phenotype of a cell from normal to cancerous (i.e., a **dominant mutation**). This results in a hyperactive oncoprotein that hyperstimulates the cell cycle, leading to oncogenesis. Note: Proto-oncogenes only require a mutation in one allele for the cell to become oncogenic, whereas, tumor suppressor genes require a mutation in both alleles for the cell to become oncogenic.

2. **Translocation** (see Chapter 11). A translocation results from breakage and exchange of segments between chromosomes. This may result in the formation of an oncogene (also called a fusion gene or chimeric gene), which encodes for an oncoprotein (also called a fusion protein or chimeric protein). A good example is seen in chronic myeloid leukemia (CML). CML t(9;22)(q34;q11) is caused by a reciprocal translocation between chromosomes 9 and 22 with breakpoints at q34 and q11, respectively. The resulting der(22) is referred to as the **Philadelphia chromosome**. This results in a hyperactive oncoprotein that hyperstimulates the cell cycle, leading to oncogenesis.

3. **Amplification**. Cancer cells may contain hundreds of extra copies of proto-oncogenes. These extra copies are found as either small paired chromatin bodies separated from the chromosomes (double minutes) or as insertions within normal chromosomes. This results in increased amounts of normal protein that hyperstimulate the cell cycle, leading to oncogenesis.

4. **Translocation into a Transcriptionally Active Region.** A translocation results from breakage and exchange of segments between chromosomes. This may result in the formation of an oncogene by placing a gene in a transcriptionally active region. A good example is seen in Burkitt lymphoma. **Burkitt lymphoma t(8;14)(q24;q32)** is caused by a reciprocal translocation between band q24 on chromosome 8 and band q32 on chromosome 14. This results in placing the *MYC* gene on chromosome 8q24 in close proximity to the *IGH* gene locus (i.e., an immunoglobulin gene locus) on chromosome 14q32, thereby putting the *MYC* gene in a transcriptionally active area in B lymphocytes (or antibody-producing plasma

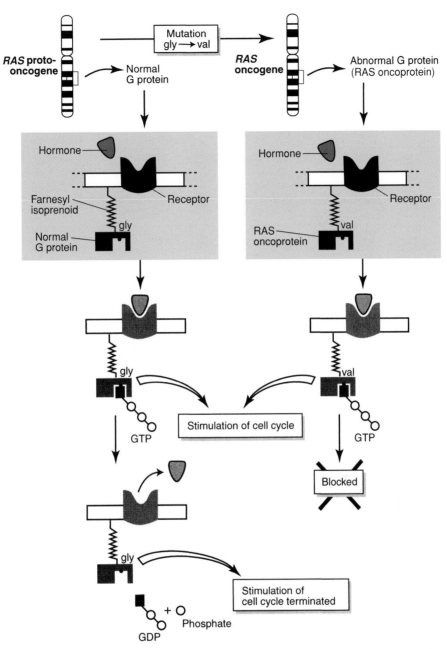

● **Figure 1-2 Diagram of *RAS* proto-oncogene and oncogene action.** The *RAS* proto-oncogene encodes a normal G protein with guanosine triphosphatase (GTPase) activity. The G protein is attached to the cytoplasmic face of the cell membrane by a lipid called farnesyl isoprenoid. When a hormone binds to its receptor, the G protein is activated. The activated G protein binds guanosine triphosphate (GTP), which stimulates the cell cycle. After a brief period, the activated G protein splits GTP into guanosine diphosphate (GDP) and phosphate such that the stimulation of the cell cycle is terminated. If the *RAS* proto-oncogene undergoes a mutation, it forms the *RAS* oncogene. The *RAS* oncogene encodes an abnormal G protein (RAS oncoprotein) where a glycine is changed to a valine at position 12. The RAS oncoprotein binds GTP, which stimulates the cell cycle. However, the RAS oncoprotein **cannot** split GTP into GDP and phosphate so that the stimulation of the cell cycle is never terminated.

cells). This results in increased amounts of normal protein that hyperstimulate the cell cycle, leading to oncogenesis.

C. MECHANISM OF ACTION OF THE *RAS* GENE: A PROTO-ONCOGENE (FIGURE 1-2)

D. A LIST OF PROTO-ONCOGENES (TABLE 1-3)

TABLE 1-3			A LIST OF PROTO-ONCOGENES
Class	Protein Encoded by Proto-oncogene	Gene	Cancer Associated with Mutations of the Proto-oncogene
Growth factors	Platelet-derived growth factor (PDGF)	PDGFB	Astrocytoma, osteosarcoma
	Fibroblast growth factor	FGF4	Stomach carcinoma
	Epidermal growth factor receptor (EGFR)	EGFR	Squamous cell carcinoma of lung; breast, ovarian, and stomach cancers
Receptors	Receptor tyrosine kinase	RET	Multiple endocrine adenomatosis 2
	Receptor tyrosine kinase	MET	Hereditary papillary renal carcinoma, hepatocellular carcinoma
	Receptor tyrosine kinase	KIT	Gastrointestinal stromal tumors
	Receptor tyrosine kinase	ERBB2	Neuroblastoma, breast cancer
Signal transducers	Tyrosine kinase	ABL/BCR	CML t(9;22)(q34;q11)
	Serine/threonine kinase	BRAF	Melanoma, colorectal cancer
	G protein	KRAS	Lung, colon, and pancreas cancers
	Leucine zipper protein	FOS	Finkel-Biskes-Jinkins osteosarcoma
	Helix-loop-helix protein	N-MYC	Neuroblastoma, lung carcinoma
	Helix-loop-helix protein	MYC	Burkitt's lymphoma t(8;14)(q24;q32)
Transcription factors	Retinoic acid receptor (zinc finger protein)	PML/RARα	APL t(15;17)(q22;q12)
	Transcription factor	FUS/ERG	AML t(16;21)(p11;q22)
	Transcription factor	PBX/TCF3	Pre–B-cell ALL t(1;19)(q21;p13.3)
	Transcription factor	FOXO4/MLL	ALL t(X;11)(q13;q23)
	Transcription factor	AFF1/MLL	ALL t(4;11)(q21;q23)
	Transcription factor	MLLT3/MLL	ALL t(9;11)(q21;q23)
	Transcription factor	MLL/MLLT1	ALL t(11;19)(q23;p13)
	Transcription factor	FLI1/EWSR1	Ewing sarcoma t(11;22)(q24;q12)

PDGFB, platelet-derived growth factor beta gene; FGF4, fibroblast growth factor 4 gene; EGFR, epidermal growth factor receptor gene; RET, rearranged during transfection gene; MET, met proto-oncogene (hepatocyte growth factor receptor); KIT, v-kit Hardy-Zuckerman 4 feline sarcoma viral oncogene homolog; ERBB2, v-erb-b2 erythroblastic leukemia viral oncogene homolog 2; ABL/BCR, Abelson murine leukemia/breakpoint cluster region oncogene; BRAF, v-raf murine sarcoma viral oncogene homolog B1; KRAS, Kirsten rat sarcoma 2 viral oncogene homolog; FOS, Finkel-Binkes-Jinkins osteosarcoma; N-MYC, neuroblastoma v-myc myelocytomatosis viral oncogene homolog; MYC, v-myc myelocytomatosis viral oncogene homolog; PML/RARα, promyelocytic leukemia/retinoic acid receptor alpha; FUS/ERG, fusion [involved in t(12;16) in malignant liposarcoma]/v-ets erythroblastosis virus E26 oncogene homolog; PBX/TCF3, pre–B-cell leukemia homeobox/transcription factor 3 (E2A immunoglobulin enhancer binding factors E12/E47); FOXO4/MLL, forkhead box O4/myeloid/lymphoid or mixed-lineage leukemia; AFF1/MLL, AF4/FMR2 family, member 1/myeloid/lymphoid or mixed-lineage leukemia; MLLT3/MLL, myeloid/lymphoid or mixed-lineage leukemia translocated to 3/myeloid/lymphoid or mixed-lineage leukemia; MLL/MLLT1, myeloid/lymphoid or mixed-lineage leukemia/myeloid/lymphoid or mixed-lineage leukemia translocated to 1; FLI1/EWSR1, Friend leukemia virus integration 1/Ewing sarcoma breakpoint region 1; CML, chronic myeloid leukemia; APL, acute promyelocytic leukemia; AML, acute myelogenous leukemia; ALL, acute lymphoblastoid leukemia.

Ⓧ Tumor Suppressor Genes

A. DEFINITION. A **tumor suppressor gene** is a normal gene that encodes a protein involved in **suppression of the cell cycle.** Many human cancers are caused by **loss-of-function mutations** of tumor suppressor genes. Note: Tumor suppressor genes require a mutation in both alleles for a cell to become oncogenic, whereas proto-oncogenes only require a mutation in one allele for a cell to become oncogenic. Tumor suppressor genes can be either "gatekeepers" or "caretakers."

B. GATEKEEPER TUMOR SUPPRESSOR GENES. These genes encode for proteins that either regulate the transition of cells through the checkpoints ("gates") of the cell cycle or promote apoptosis. This prevents oncogenesis. Loss-of-function mutations in gatekeeper tumor suppressor genes lead to oncogenesis.

C. **CARETAKER TUMOR SUPPRESSOR GENES.** These genes encode for proteins that either detect/repair DNA mutations or promote normal chromosomal disjunction during mitosis. This prevents oncogenesis by maintaining the integrity of the genome. Loss-of-function mutations in caretaker tumor suppressor genes lead to oncogenesis.

D. **MECHANISM OF ACTION OF THE *RB1* GENE: A TUMOR SUPPRESSOR GENE (RETINOBLASTOMA; FIGURE 1-3)**

E. **MECHANISM OF ACTION OF THE *TP53* GENE: A TUMOR SUPPRESSOR GENE ("GUARDIAN OF THE GENOME") (FIGURE 1-4)**

F. **A LIST OF TUMOR SUPPRESSOR GENES (TABLE 1-4)**

XI Oncofetal Antigens and Tumor Markers (Table 1-5)

XII Transcription in Protein Synthesis

A. During the process of transcription, RNA polymerase II produces an RNA transcript by a complex process that involves a number of **general transcription factors** called **TFIIs** (transcription factors for RNA polymerase II).

B. **TFIID** binds to the TATA box, which then allows the adjacent binding of **TFIIB**.

C. The next step involves **TFIIA, TFIIE, TFIIF, TFIIH,** and RNA **polymerase II** engaged to the promoter forming a **transcription initiation (TI) complex.**

D. The TI complex must gain access to the DNA template strand at the transcription start site. This is accomplished by TFIIH, which contains a **DNA helicase.**

E. TFIIH also contains a **protein kinase** that phosphorylates RNA polymerase II so that RNA polymerase II is released from the TI complex after transcription is completed.

F. However, the TI complex will produce only a **basal level of transcription** or **constitutive expression.** Other factors called **cis-acting DNA sequences** and **trans-acting proteins** are necessary to increase transcription higher than the basal level.

XIII Processing the RNA Transcript into mRNA (Figure 1-5). A cell involved in protein synthesis will use RNA polymerase II to transcribe a protein-coding gene into an **RNA transcript** that must be further processed into mRNA. This processing involves:

A. **RNA Capping** is the addition of a **7-methylguanosine** to the first nucleotide at the **5′ end** of the RNA transcript. RNA capping functions to protect the RNA transcript from exonuclease attack, to facilitate transport from the nucleus to the cytoplasm, to facilitate RNA splicing, and to attach the mRNA to the 40S subunit of the ribosome.

B. **RNA Polyadenylation** is the addition of a **poly-A tail** (about 200 repeated adenosine monophosphates [AMPs]) to the **3′ end** of the RNA transcript. The **AAUAAA sequence** is a **polyadenylation signal sequence,** which signals the 3′ cleavage of the RNA transcript. After 3′ cleavage, polyadenylation occurs. RNA polyadenylation functions to protect against degradation, to facilitate transport from the nucleus to the cytoplasm, and to enhance recognition of the mRNA by the ribosomes.

C. **RNA Splicing** is a process whereby all **introns (noncoding regions; intervening sequences)** are removed from the RNA transcript and all **exons (coding regions; expression sequences)** are joined together within the RNA transcript. RNA splicing requires that the intron/exon boundaries (or **splice junctions**) be recognized. In most cases, introns start with a GT sequence and end with an AG sequence (called the **GT-AG rule**). RNA splicing is carried out by a large RNA–protein complex called the **spliceosome,**

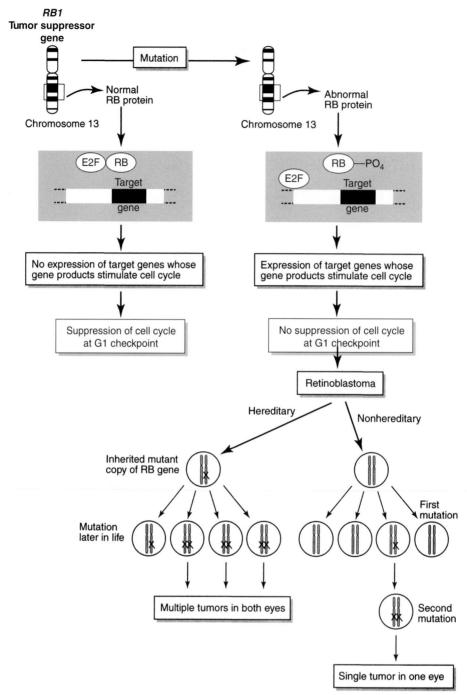

● **Figure 1-3 Diagram of *RB1* tumor suppressor action.** The *RB1* tumor suppressor gene is located on chromosome 13q14.1 and encodes for **normal RB protein** that will bind to E2F (a gene regulatory protein) such that there will be no expression of target genes whose gene products stimulate the cell cycle. Therefore, there is suppression of the cell cycle at the G_1 checkpoint. A mutation of the *RB1* tumor suppressor gene will encode an **abnormal RB protein** that cannot bind E2F (a gene regulatory protein) such that there will be expression of target genes whose gene products stimulate the cell cycle. Therefore, there is no suppression of the cell cycle at the G_1 checkpoint. This leads to the formation of a **retinoblastoma** tumor. There are two types of retinoblastomas. In **hereditary retinoblastoma,** the individual inherits one mutant copy of the *RB1* gene from his or her parents (an inherited germline mutation). A somatic mutation of the second copy of the *RB1* gene may occur later in life within many cells of the retina, leading to **multiple tumors in both eyes.** In **nonhereditary retinoblastoma,** the individual does **not** inherit a mutant copy of the *RB1* gene from his or her parents. Instead, two subsequent somatic mutations of both copies of the *RB1* gene may occur within one cell of the retina, leading to **one tumor in one eye.** This has become known as Knudson's two-hit hypothesis and serves as a model for cancers involving tumor suppressor genes.

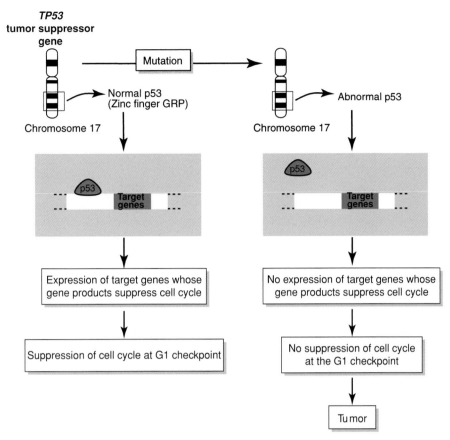

● **Figure 1-4 Diagram of TP53 tumor suppressor action.** The TP53 tumor suppressor gene is located on chromosome 17p13 and encodes for **normal p53 protein (a zinc finger gene regulatory protein)** that will cause the expression of target genes whose gene products suppress the cell cycle at **G₁** by inhibiting **Cdk–cyclin D** and **Cdk–cyclin E**. Therefore, there is suppression of the cell cycle at the G₁ checkpoint. A mutation of *TP53* tumor suppressor gene will encode an **abnormal p53 protein** that will cause no expression of target genes whose gene products suppress the cell cycle. Therefore, there is no suppression of the cell cycle at the G₁ checkpoint. The *TP53* tumor suppressor gene is the **most common target** for mutation in human cancers. The *TP53* tumor suppressor gene plays a role in **Li-Fraumeni syndrome.**

which consists of **small nuclear RNA (snRNA)** and more than **50 different proteins.** Each snRNA is complexed to specific proteins to form **small nuclear ribonucleoprotein particles (snRNPs).**

ⓍⅣ Selected Photomicrographs

A. Nucleus, nuclear envelope, nuclear pore complex, and apoptosis (Figure 1-6)

B. Chromatin, nucleosome, and metaphase chromosome (Figure 1-7).

TABLE 1-4	A LIST OF TUMOR SUPPRESSOR GENES		
Class	Protein Encoded by Tumor Suppressor Gene	Gene	Cancer Associated with Mutations of the Tumor Suppressor Gene
Gatekeeper	Retinoblastoma-associated protein p110^{RB}	RB1	Retinoblastoma; carcinomas of the breast, prostate, bladder, and lung
	Tumor protein 53	TP53	Li-Fraumeni syndrome; most human cancers
	Neurofibromin protein	NF1	Neurofibromatosis type 1, schwannoma
	Adenomatous polyposis coli protein	APC	Familial adenomatous polyposis coli, carcinomas of the colon
	Wilms tumor protein 2	WT2	Wilms tumor (most common renal malignancy of childhood)
	Von Hippel-Lindau disease tumor suppressor protein	VHL	Von Hippel-Lindau disease, retinal and cerebellar hemangioblastomas
Caretaker	Breast cancer type 1 susceptibility protein	BRCA1	Breast and ovarian cancer
	Breast cancer type 2 susceptibility protein	BRCA2	Breast cancer
	DNA mismatch repair protein MLH1	MLH1	Hereditary nonpolyposis colon cancer
	DNA mismatch repair protein MSH2	MSH2	Hereditary nonpolyposis colon cancer

APC, familial adenomatous polyposis coli; *VHL*, von Hippel-Lindau disease; *WT*, Wilms tumor; *NF-1*, neurofibromatosis; *BRCA*, breast cancer; *RB*, retinoblastoma; *TP53*, tumor protein; *MLH1*, mut L homolog 1; *MSH2*, mut S homolog 2.

TABLE 1-5	ONCOFETAL ANTIGENS AND TUMOR MARKERS
Antigen	Associated Tumor
α-Fetoprotein (AFP)	Hepatocellular carcinoma, germ cell neoplasms, yolk sac or endodermal sinus tumors of the testicle or ovary
AAT	Hepatocellular carcinoma, yolk sac or endodermal sinus tumors of the testicle or ovary
Carcinoembryonic antigen (CEA)	Colorectal cancer, pancreatic cancer, breast cancer, and small cell cancer of the lung; bad prognostic sign if elevated preoperatively
β_2-Microglobulin	Multiple myeloma (excellent prognostic factor), light chains in urine (Bence Jones protein)
CA 125	Surface-derived ovarian cancer
CA 15-3	Breast cancer
CA 19-9	Pancreatic cancer (excellent marker)
Neuron-specific enolase (NSE)	Small cell carcinoma of the lung, seminoma, neuroblastoma
Prostate-specific antigen (PSA)	Prostate cancer
hCG	Trophoblastic tumors; hydatidiform mole (benign); choriocarcinoma (malignant)
Bombesin	Small cell carcinoma of the lung, neuroblastoma
LDH	Hodgkin disease
S-100	Melanoma
Placental alkaline phosphatase	Seminoma
CD1	Histiocytosis
Synaptophysin	Carcinoid tumors
Calcitonin	Medullary carcinoma of the thyroid
Catecholamines	Pheochromocytoma, neuroblastoma

AAT, α_1-antitrypsin; CA, cancer antigen; hCG, human chorionic gonadotropin; LDH, lactate dehydrogenase.

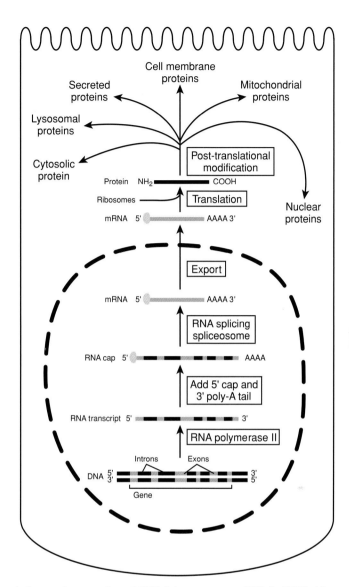

● **Figure 1-5 Transcription and processing of RNA into messenger RNA (mRNA).** All eucaryotic genes contain noncoding regions (introns) separated by coding regions (exons). During transcription, RNA polymerase II transcribes both intron and exon sequences into an RNA transcript. A 5'-cap and a 3'-polyA tail are added. The introns are spliced out of the RNA transcript by a spliceosome so that all the exons are joined in sequence. The mRNA with the 5'-cap and 3'-polyA tail is then able to exit the nucleus through the nuclear pore complex into the cytoplasm for subsequent translation into protein. Proteins then undergo posttranslational modifications and are directed to various regions of the cell.

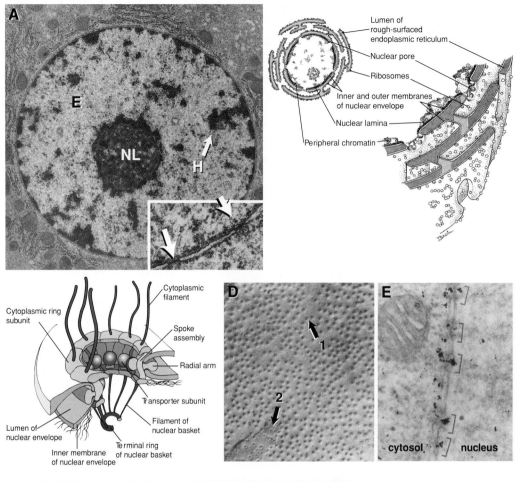

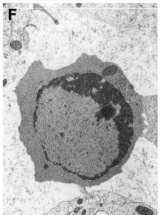

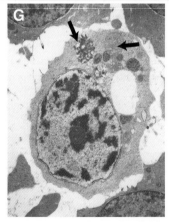

● **Figure 1-6 A:** Electron micrograph (EM) of a nucleus shows predominately euchromatin (E), peripherally located heterochromatin (H), and a conspicuous nucleolus (NL). *Inset:* Nuclear envelope with nuclear pores (*large arrows*) is shown. **B:** Diagram shows the interconnections between the nuclear envelope and the rough endoplasmic reticulum. **C:** Diagram of a model of the nuclear pore complex. **D:** A freeze-fracture replica of the nuclear envelope shows a nuclear pore complex (*arrow 1*) and the outer membrane of the nuclear envelope that has been stripped away (*arrow 2*), exposing the perinuclear cisterna. **E:** EM of nucleoplasmin labeled with colloidal gold particles. Nucleoplasmin is a large protein synthesized in the cytoplasm and transported into the nucleus. *Brackets* denote a nuclear pore complex. Note that the gold particles are localized specifically at the nuclear pore complex as nucleoplasmin moves from the cytoplasm to nucleus. **F–H:** Apoptosis. Human T cells treated with a lipid hydroperoxide that is toxic to cells and induces apoptosis. **F:** EM shows the chromatin of an apoptotic cell condensed into a distinctive crescent-shaped pattern along the inner margins of the nuclear envelope. **G:** EM shows chromatin clumping and mitochondrial changes (*arrows*).

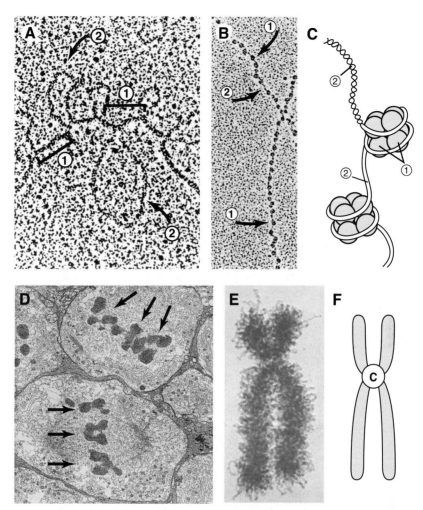

● **Figure 1-7 A: Electron micrograph of DNA containing the gene for ovalbumin hybridized with ovalbumin messenger RNA (mRNA).** Linear regions of the gene (*bracket 1*) that hybridize to mRNA are called **exons** because the processed mRNA "exits" the nucleus into the cytoplasm to participate in translation. Looped regions of the gene (*arrow 2*) that do *not* hybridize to mRNA are called **introns. B:** Electron micrograph of DNA isolated and subjected to treatments that unfold its native structure. This "beads on a string" appearance is the basic unit of chromatin packing called a **nucleosome.** The globular structure ("bead") (*arrow 1*) is a histone octamer that is composed of specific proteins (H2A, H2B, H3, and H4). The linear structure ("string") (*arrow 2*) is DNA. **C:** A diagram of a nucleosome demonstrating the histone octamer (*arrow 1*) and DNA (*arrow 2*). **D:** Electron micrograph of a mitotic cell in metaphase showing the metaphase chromosomes (*arrows*) aligned at the metaphase plate. **E:** Electron micrograph of an isolated metaphase chromosome. **F:** Diagram of a metaphase chromosome showing the centromere (C).

Chapter 2

Cytoplasm and Organelles

Ⅰ **Cytoplasm.** The cytoplasm has a wide composition, which includes:

A. ENZYMES involved in various biochemical pathways: **glycolysis** (e.g., hexokinase, phosphofructokinase), **fatty acid synthesis** (e.g., fatty acid synthase), three reactions of the **urea cycle (using argininosuccinate synthetase, argininosuccinate lyase, and arginase), glycogen synthesis** (e.g., glycogen synthase), **glycogen degradation** (e.g., glycogen phosphorylase), and **protein synthesis** (e.g., aminoacyl-transfer RNA [tRNA] synthetase, peptidyl transferase).

B. PROTEOSOMES are proteolytic enzyme complexes that are involved in the rapid degradation of a **ubiquitinylated protein** (i.e., addition of **ubiquitin** to the lysine amino acid of a protein by **ubiquitin ligase**). For example, **cyclins** are inactivated by this process during anaphase of mitosis. In addition, **endogenous antigens** (produced by intracellular viruses or bacteria) undergo proteosomal degradation by proteosomes to form antigen peptide fragments that become associated with class **I major histocompatibility complex (MHC)** and are transported and exposed on the cell surface of the infected cell.

C. INTERMEDIATES OF METABOLISM

D. COFACTORS (e.g., nicotinamide adenine dinucleotide [NAD], reduced nicotinamide adenine dinucleotide [NADH])

E. STEROID HORMONE RECEPTORS (FIGURE 2-1). Steroid hormone receptors are composed structurally of a polypeptide with a zinc atom that is bound to four cysteine amino acids, which falls into the classification of a **zinc finger protein.** A zinc finger protein has a **hormone-binding** region and a **DNA-binding region** that activates gene transcription. Steroid hormone receptors include the **estrogen receptor, glucocorticoid receptor, progesterone receptor, thyroid hormone** (triiodothyronine [T_3] and thyroxine [T_4]) **receptor, retinoic acid receptor,** and **1,25-dihydroxyvitamin D_3 receptor.**

Ⅱ **Ribosomes**

A. Ribosomes are large RNA–protein complexes that consist of a **40S (small) subunit** and a **60S (large) subunit**, both of which contain rRNA and various proteins.

B. The 40S subunit **binds to messenger RNA (mRNA) and tRNA and finds the start codon AUG.**

C. The 60S subunit **binds to the 40S subunit** after it finds the start codon and has **peptidyl transferase activity.**

D. Ribosomes provide the structural framework for the **translation of mRNA** into an amino acid sequence (i.e., **protein synthesis**) to occur.

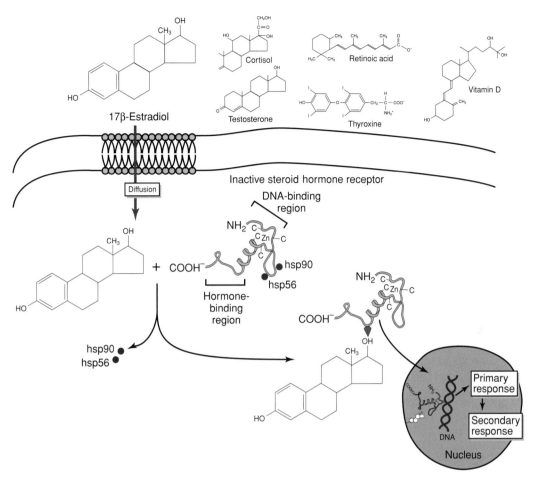

● **Figure 2-1 Mechanism of steroid hormone action.** An inactive steroid hormone receptor is found in the cytoplasm where it is bound to **heat shock proteins (hsp 90 and hsp 56).** When a steroid hormone (e.g., 17β-estradiol) diffuses across the cell membrane and binds to the hormone-binding regions of the receptor, hsp 90 and hsp 56 are released and the DNA-binding region is exposed. Subsequently, the steroid hormone–receptor complex is transported into the nucleus where it binds to DNA and activates the transcription of a small number of specific genes within approximately 30 minutes **(primary response).** The gene products of the primary response activate other genes to produce a **secondary response.** Steroid hormone receptors are actually gene regulatory proteins.

    E.   Ribosomes may cluster along a strand of mRNA to form a **polyribosome (or polysome)** that is involved in the **synthesis of cytoplasmic proteins** (e.g., actin, hemoglobulin).

    F.   Ribosomes may also be directed to the endoplasmic reticulum to form rough endoplasmic reticulum (rER) if the nascent protein contains a hydrophobic **signal sequence** at its amino terminal end.

III **Rough Endoplasmic Reticulum (rER).** This membranous organelle contains ribosomes attached to its cytoplasmic surface by the binding of **ribophorins I and II** to the **60S subunit** of the ribosome. The rER is the site of **synthesis of secretory proteins** (e.g., insulin), **cell membrane proteins** (e.g., receptors), and **lysosomal enzymes**. The rER is the site of **cotranslational modification** of proteins, which includes:

    A.   ***N*-LINKED GLYCOSYLATION** (addition of sugars to asparagine begins in the rER and is completed in the Golgi complex)

    B.   **HYDROXYLATION OF PROLINE AND LYSINE** during collagen synthesis

C. **CLEAVAGE** of the signal sequence

D. **FOLDING** of the nascent protein into three-dimensional configuration

E. **ASSOCIATION** of protein subunits into a multimeric complex

 Translation (Figure 2-2) is the mechanism by which only the centrally located **nucleotide sequence of mRNA** is translated into the **amino acid sequence of a protein** and occurs in the **cytoplasm**. The end or flanking sequences of the mRNA (called the **5′ and 3′ untranslated regions; 5′UTR and 3′UTR**) are not translated. Translation decodes a set of **three** nucleotides (called a **codon**) into **one** amino acid (e.g., GCA codes for alanine, UAC codes for tyrosine, etc.). The code is said to be **redundant**, which means that more than one codon specifies a particular amino acid (e.g., GCA, GCC, GCG, and GCU all specify alanine, and UAC and UAU both specify tyrosine).

A. Translation uses **tRNA**, which has two important binding sites. The first site of tRNA, called the **anticodon**, binds to the complementary codon on the mRNA and demonstrates **tRNA wobble**, whereby the normal A-U and G-C pairing is required only in the first two base positions of the codon but variability or wobble occurs at the third position. The second site of tRNA is the **amino acid–binding site** on the acceptor arm, which covalently binds the amino acid to the 3′ end of tRNA.

B. Translation uses the enzyme **aminoacyl-tRNA synthetase**, which links an amino acid to tRNA. **tRNA charging** refers to the fact that the amino acid–tRNA bond contains the energy for the formation of the peptide bond between amino acids. There is a specific aminoacyl-tRNA synthetase for each amino acid. Since there are 20 different amino acids, there are 20 different aminoacyl-tRNA synthetase enzymes.

C. Translation uses the enzyme **peptidyl transferase**, which participates in forming the peptide bond between amino acids of the growing protein.

D. Translation requires the use of ribosomes, which are large RNA–protein complexes that consist of a 40S subunit and a 60S subunit. The ribosome moves along the mRNA in a **5′ → 3′ direction** such that the **NH2-terminal end** of a protein is synthesized **first** and the **COOH-terminal end** of a protein is synthesized **last**.

E. Translation begins with the start **codon AUG** that codes for **methionine** (the optimal initiation codon recognition sequence is **GCACCAUGG**) so that all newly synthesized proteins have methionine as their first (or NH2-terminal) amino acid, which is usually removed later by a protease.

F. Translation terminates at the **stop codon (UAA, UAG, UGA)**. The stop codon binds **release factors** that cause the protein to be released from the ribosome into the cytoplasm.

G. **CLINICAL CONSIDERATION: β-THALASSEMIA**

1. β-Thalassemia is an autosomal recessive genetic disorder caused by more than 200 missense or frameshift mutations in the *HBB* gene on **chromosome 11p15.5** for the **β-globin subunit of hemoglobin**.

2. β-Thalassemia is defined by the absence or reduced synthesis of β-globin subunits of hemoglobin. A **β^0 mutation** refers to a mutation that causes the absence of β-globin subunits. A **β^+ mutation** refers to a mutation that causes the reduced synthesis of β-globin subunits.

3. The mutations in the *HBB* gene result in the **reduced amounts of HbA (Hb $\alpha_2\beta_2$)** since there is reduced synthesis of β-globin subunits, which are found only in HbA.

4. There are two clinically significant forms of β-thalassemia:

    a. **Thalassemia Major.** Thalassemia major results from the inheritance of a β^0 mutation of both β-globin alleles (β^0/β^0) and is the most severe form of β-thalassemia. **Clinical features include:** microcytic hypochromatic hemolytic anemia, abnormal peripheral blood smear with nucleated red blood cells, reduced amounts of HbA, severe anemia, hepatosplenomegaly, and failure to thrive; regular blood transfusions are necessary, and the patient becomes progressively pale and usually comes to medical attention between 6 months and 2 years of age.

    b. **Thalassemia Intermedia.** Thalassemia intermedia results from the inheritance of a β^0 mutation of one β-globin allele (β^0/normal β) and is a less severe form of β-thalassemia. **Clinical features include:** a mild hemolytic anemia; individuals are at risk for iron overload, regular blood transfusions are rarely necessary, and patients usually come to medical attention when they are older than 2 years of age.

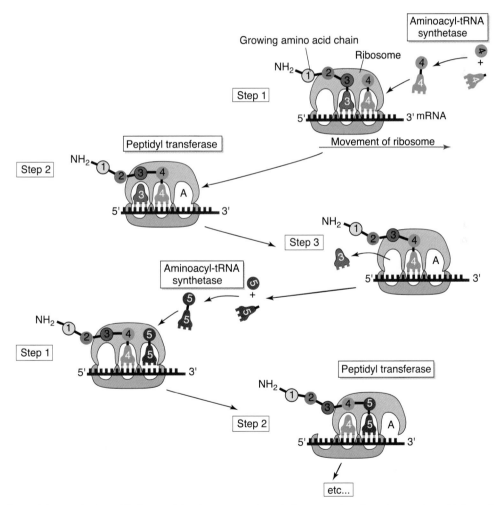

● **Figure 2-2 Translation.** This diagram joins the process of translation at a point where three amino acids have already been linked together (amino acids 1, 2, and 3). The process of translation is basically a three-step process that is repeated over and over during the synthesis of a protein. The enzyme aminoacyl-tRNA synthetase links a specific amino acid with its specific tRNA. In step 1, the tRNA and amino acid complex 4 binds to the A site on the ribosome. Note that the direction of movement of the ribosome along the mRNA is in a 5' → 3' direction. In step 2, the enzyme peptidyl transferase forms a peptide bond between amino acid 3 and amino acid 4 and the small subunit of the ribosome reconfigures so that the A site is vacant. In step 3, the used tRNA 3 is ejected and the ribosome is ready for tRNA and amino acid complex 5.

Golgi Complex. The Golgi complex is a stack of membranous cisternae with a *cis*-face (**convex**) that receives vesicles of newly synthesized proteins from the rER and a *trans*-face (**concave**) that releases condensing vacuoles of posttranslationally modified proteins. The functions of the Golgi complex include:

A. POSTTRANSLATIONAL MODIFICATION of proteins, which includes **completion of N-linked glycosylation** that began in the rER, **O-linked glycosylation** (addition of sugars to serine, threonine, or hydroxylysine by glycosyltransferase), **sulfation, phosphorylation** (of tyrosine, serine, or threonine by kinases/phosphatases), **methylation** (of lysine by methylases/demethylases), **acetylation** (of lysine by acetylases/deacetylases), **carboxylation** (of glutamate by γ-carboxylase); **addition of glycosyl-phosphatidylinositol** (GPI, a glycolipid added to aspartate), **myristoylation** (addition of a C_{14} fatty acyl group to glycine), **palmitoylation** (addition of a C_{16} fatty acyl group to cysteine), **farnesylation** (addition of a C_{15} prenyl group to cysteine), and **granylgeranylation** (addition of a C_{20} prenyl group to cysteine).

B. PROTEIN SORTING AND PACKAGING. Secretory proteins (e.g., insulin) are packaged into **clathrin-coated vesicles.** Cell membrane proteins (e.g., receptors) are packaged into **non–clathrin-coated vesicles. Lysosomal enzymes** are packaged into **clathrin-coated vesicles** after phosphorylation of mannose to form **mannose-6-phosphate.**

C. MEMBRANE RECYCLING

VI Smooth Endoplasmic Reticulum (sER). This membranous organelle contains no ribosomes and is involved in:

A. SYNTHESIS OF MEMBRANE PHOSPHOLIPIDS (phosphatidylcholine, sphingomyelin, phosphatidylserine, phosphatidylethanolamine), **cholesterol, and ceramide**

B. SYNTHESIS OF STEROID HORMONES in testes, ovary, adrenal cortex, and placenta

C. DRUG DETOXIFICATION USING CYTOCHROME P_{450} MONOOXYGENASE, which is a family of heme proteins (also called **mixed function oxidase system**) that catalyzes (**phase I reactions**) the biotransformation of drugs by hydroxylation, dealkylation, oxidation, and reduction reactions.

D. DRUG DETOXIFICATION USING GLUCURONYL TRANSFERASE that catalyzes (**phase II reactions**) the conjugation of glucuronic acid to a variety of drugs using **UDP-glucuronic acid** as the glucuronide donor.

E. GLYCOGEN DEGRADATION. The enzyme glucose-6-phosphatase is an integral membrane protein of the sER.

F. FATTY ACID ELONGATION

G. LIPOLYSIS begins in the sER with the release of a fatty acid from triacylglyceride.

H. LIPOPROTEIN ASSEMBLY

I. CALCIUM FLUXES associated with muscle contraction

VII Mitochondria

A. FUNCTION. Mitochondria are involved in the production of acetyl coenzyme A (CoA), the tricarboxylic acid cycle, fatty acid β-oxidation, amino acid oxidation, and oxidative phosphorylation (which causes the **synthesis of adenosine triphosphate [ATP]** driven by electron transfer to oxygen).

1. Substrates are metabolized in the mitochondrial matrix to produce **acetyl CoA**, which is oxidized by the tricarboxylic acid cycle to carbon dioxide.
2. The energy released by this oxidation is captured by NADH and flavin adenine dinucleotide ($FADH_2$). NADH and $FADH_2$ are further oxidized, producing **hydrogen ions** and **electrons**.
3. The electrons are transferred along the **electron transport chain**, which is accompanied by the outward pumping of hydrogen ions into the intermembrane space (**chemiosmotic theory**).
4. The F_0 **subunit of ATP synthase** forms a transmembrane hydrogen ion pore so that hydrogen ions can flow from the intermembrane space into the matrix, where the F_1 **subunit of ATP synthase** catalyzes the reaction $ADP + P_i \rightarrow ATP$.

B. **COMPONENTS AND CONTENTS** are listed in Table 2-1.

C. **CLINICAL CONSIDERATIONS**
   1. **Myoclonic epilepsy with ragged red fibers syndrome (MERRF)**
      a. MERRF is a mitochondrial genetic disorder caused by a mutation in the $tRNA^{Lys}$ gene whereby a A$\rightarrow$G transition occurs at **nucleotide position 8344 (A8344G)**.
      b. The mutated $tRNA^{Lys}$ causes a **premature termination of translation** of the amino acid chain (the amount and the aminoacylation activity of the mutated $tRNA^{Lys}$ are not affected).
      c. Mitochondrial enzymes with a large number of lysine residues will have a low probability of being completely synthesized. In this regard, **NADH dehydrogenase (complex I)** and **cytochrome oxidase (complex IV)**, both of which have a large number of lysine residues, have been shown to be synthesized at very low rates.
      d. **Clinical features include:** myoclonus (muscle twitching), seizures, cerebellar ataxia, dementia, mitochondrial myopathy (abnormal mitochondria within skeletal muscle that impart an irregular shape and blotchy red appearance to the muscle cells, hence the term ragged red fibers).
   2. **Leber's Hereditary Optic Neuropathy (LHON)**
      a. LHON is a mitochondrial genetic disorder caused by three mitochondrial DNA (mtDNA) missense mutations that account for 90% of all cases worldwide and are therefore designated as **primary LHON mutations**.
      b. The primary LHON mutations include the following:
         i. A mutation in the *ND4* gene (which encodes for subunit 4 of NADH dehydrogenase; complex I) whereby an A$\rightarrow$G transition occurs at **nucleotide position 11778 (A11778G)**. This is the most common cause ($\approx$50% of all LHON cases) of LHON.
         ii. A mutation in the *ND1* gene (which encodes for subunit 1 of NADH dehydrogenase; complex I) whereby a G$\rightarrow$A transition occurs at **nucleotide position 3460 (G3460A)**
         iii. A mutation in the *ND6* gene (which encodes for subunit 6 of NADH dehydrogenase; complex I) whereby a T$\rightarrow$C transition occurs at **nucleotide position 14484 (T14484C)**
      c. All three primary LHON mutations **decrease production of ATP** such that the demands of a very active neuronal metabolism cannot be met and suggest a common disease-causing mechanism.
      d. **Clinical features include:** progressive optic nerve degeneration that results clinically in blindness, blurred vision, or loss of central vision; telangiectatic microangiopathy; disk pseudoedema; and vascular tortuosity. Onset occurs at $\approx$20 years of age with precipitous vision loss; males are affected far more often than females for some unknown reason.

3. **Kearns-Sayre Syndrome (KS)**

   a. KS is a mitochondrial genetic disorder caused by **partial deletions of mtDNA** (delta-mtDNA) and **duplication of mtDNA** (dup-mtDNA). The partial deletions of mtDNA have been associated with a marked reduction in the enzymatic activity of NADH dehydrogenase (complex I), succinate dehydrogenase (complex II), ubiquinone-cytochrome c oxidoreductase (complex III), and cytochrome oxidase (complex IV).

   b. **Clinical features include:** chronic progressive external ophthalmoplegia (CPEO; degeneration of the motor nerves of the eye), pigmentary degeneration of the retina ("salt and pepper" appearance), heart block, short stature, gonadal failure, diabetes mellitus, thyroid disease, deafness, vestibular dysfunction, and cerebellar ataxia; onset occurs at ≈ 20 years of age.

4. **Cyanide, carbon monoxide,** and **antimycin A** inhibit the electron transport chain and thus block ATP synthesis.

5. **Oligomycin** and **venturicidin** are antibiotics that bind to ATP synthase and thus block ATP synthesis.

6. **Isocarboxazid (Marplan), Phenelzine (Nardil),** and **Tranylcypromine (Parnate)** are monamine oxidase (MAO) inhibitors used in the treatment of depression. MAO is a mitochondrial enzyme that oxidatively deaminates catecholamines (i.e., epinephrine, norepinephrine, and serotonin). MAO inhibitors reversibly or irreversibly inhibit MAO, which results in the accumulation of catecholamines in the presynaptic neuron and synaptic cleft. A side effect of these drugs is a hypertensive crisis that can be eliminated by avoiding foods (e.g., cheese and wine) that contain tyramine.

TABLE 2-1	COMPONENTS AND CONTENTS OF MITOCHONDRIA
Components	**Contents**
Outer membrane	**Porin** (a transport protein that increases permeability to metabolic substrates)
Intermembrane space	H^+ ions
Inner membrane (folded into cristae)	Electron transport chain (NADH dehydrogenase, succinate dehydrogenase, ubiquinone-cytochrome c oxidoreductase, cytochrome oxidase) ATP synthase (found on elementary particles) ATP-ADP translocator (moves ADP into the matrix and ATP out of the matrix) Various transporters or translocators
Matrix compartment	TCA cycle enzymes (except succinate dehydrogenase) Fatty acid β-oxidation enzymes Amino acid oxidation enzymes Pyruvate dehydrogenase complex Carbamoylphosphate synthetase I[a] Ornithine transcarbamoylase[a] Monoamine oxidase (MAO; oxidation of catecholamines) Desmolase, 18-methyloxidase, 11β-hydroxylase[b] DNA, mRNA, tRNA, rRNA Granules containing Ca^{2+} and Mg^{2+}

NADH, reduced nicotinamide adenine dinucleotide; ATP, adenosine triphosphate; ADP, adenosine diphosphate; TCA, tricarboxylic acid cycle (Krebs cycle).
[a]Part of the urea cycle; other enzymes of urea cycle are located in the cytoplasm.
[b]Involved in steroid hormone synthesis.

Lysosomes. Lysosomes are membrane-bound organelles that contain lysosomal enzymes (also called **acid hydrolase enzymes**) that function at **pH 5**. Most lysosomes function intracellularly; however, some cells (e.g., neutrophils, osteoclasts) release their lysosomal contents extracellularly.

A. LYSOSOMAL ACTION occurs as follows:

1. **Golgi hydrolase vesicles** bud from the Golgi complex and contain inactive acid hydrolase enzymes. The Golgi hydrolase vesicles fuse with an **endosome**, which contains an H^+-adenosine triphosphatase (ATPase) in its membrane that produces a pH 5 environment and activates the acid hydrolases. This forms an **endolysosome**.

2. An endolysosome may fuse with a **phagocytic vacuole**, forming a **phagolysosome**, which degrades material phagocytosed by the cell.

3. An endolysosome may also fuse with an **autophagic vacuole**, forming an **autophagolysosome**, which degrades cell organelles.

4. **Residual bodies** contain undigestible material and may accumulate within a cell as **lipofuscin pigment.**

5. In addition, **exogenous protein antigens** are phagocytosed by antigen-presenting cells (APCs or macrophages) and undergo lysosomal degradation in endolysosomes to form antigen peptide fragments that become associated with **class II MHC** and are transported and exposed on the cell surface of the APC.

B. CLINICAL CONSIDERATIONS. There are a number of genetic diseases that involve mutations of genes for various lysosomal enzymes (acid hydrolases; Table 2-2).

 Peroxisomes are membrane-bound organelles.

A. CONTENTS OF PEROXISOMES INCLUDE:

1. **Amino acid oxidase** and **hydroxyacid oxidase** that use molecular (O_2) to oxidize organic substances, producing hydrogen peroxide ($R-H_2 + O_2 \rightarrow R + H_2O_2$). About 25% of all ethanol we drink is oxidized in peroxisomes (sometimes called the **microsomal ethanol oxidizing system**) to **acetaldehyde** by this reaction. The remaining 75% of ethanol is handled outside the peroxisomes by being converted to acetaldehyde by alcohol dehydrogenase, which is then converted to either **acetate** (which enters the tricarboxylic acid [TCA] cycle to be converted to $CO_2 + H_2O$) or **acetyl CoA** (which enters fatty acid synthesis and the TCA cycle).

2. **Catalase** and **other peroxidases** that decompose hydrogen peroxide to water and oxygen ($H_2O_2 \rightarrow H_2O + O_2$)

3. **Fatty acid β-oxidation enzymes** that oxidize long-chain fatty acids (>20 carbons) to short-chain fatty acids, which are transferred to mitochondria for complete oxidation

4. **Enzymes for bile acid synthesis**

5. **Urate oxidase** that breaks down purines

B. CLINICAL CONSIDERATION: ADRENOLEUKODYSTROPHY (ALD)

1. ALD is an X-linked genetic disorder caused by mutations in the *ABCD1* **gene** on chromosome Xq28 for an **A**TP-**b**inding **c**assette transporter (**ABC transporter**), which transports very long-chain fatty acids (VLCFAs) into peroxisomes.

2. This results in a disorder of β-oxidation of VLCFAs and the accumulation of VLCFAs in the adrenal cortex, central nervous system, and Leydig cell of testes.

3. **Clinical features include:** adrenocortical failure and inflammatory demyelination in the cerebral and cerebellar white matter leading to dementia.

TABLE 2-2		LYSOSOMAL STORAGE DISEASES	
Genetic Disorder	**Gene** **Gene Product** **Chromosome**	**Accumulation** **Product**	**Clinical Features**
Mucopolysac-charidosis type I (Hurler, Hurler-Scheie, or Scheie syndromes)	*IDUA* gene a-L-iduronidase 4p16.3	Heparan sulfate Dermatan sulfate	Infants initially appear normal up to ≈9 mo of age but then develop symptoms; coarsening of facial features; thickening of alae nasi, lips, ear lobules, and tongue; corneal clouding; severe visual impairment; progressive thickening of heart valves leading to mitral and aortic regurgitation; dorsolumbar kyphosis; skeletal dysplasia involving all the bones; linear growth ceases by 3 y of age; hearing loss; chronic recurrent rhinitis; severe mental retardation; and zebra bodies within neurons
Gaucher disease (GD)	*GBA* gene β-Glucosylceramidase 1p21	Glucosylceramide Other glycolipids	Bone disease (e.g., focal lytic lesions, sclerotic lesions, osteonecrosis) is the most debilitating pathology of type I GD; hepatomegaly; splenomegaly; cytopenia and anemia due to hypersplenism, splenic sequestration, and decreased erythropoiesis; and pulmonary disease (e.g., interstitial lung disease, alveolar/lobar consolidation; pulmonary hypertension); no primary central nervous system (CNS) involvement
Hexosaminidase A deficiency (Tay-Sachs)	*HEXA* gene Hexosaminidase α-subunit 15q23-q24	GM2 ganglioside	Infants initially appear normal up to 3–6 mo of age but then develop symptoms; progressive weakness and loss of motor skills; decreased attentiveness; increased startle response; a cherry red spot in the fovea centralis of the retina; generalized muscular hypotonia; later, progressive neurodegeneration, seizures, blindness, and spasticity occur followed by death at ≈2–4 y of age
Mucopolysac-charidosis type III A (Sanfilippo A syndrome)	*SGSH* gene Sulfamidase 17q25.3	Heparan sulfate	Dysostosis multiplex (thickened skull, anterior thickening of ribs, vertebral abnormalities, and short/thick long bones), mental retardation, and behavioral problems (aggressive behavior followed by progressive neurologic decline)
Niemann-Pick type 1A disorder	*SMPD1* gene Acid sphingomyelinase 11p15	Sphingomyelin	Hepatosplenomegaly, feeding difficulties, and loss of motor skills are seen within 1–3 mo of age; a cherry red spot in the fovea centralis of the retina; later, a rapid, profound, and progressive neurodegeneration occurs followed by death at ≈2–3 y of age
Krabbe disorder	*GALC* gene Galactocerebrosidase 14q31	Galactosylce-ramide	Developmental delay, limb stiffness, hypotonia, absent reflexes, optic atrophy, microcephaly, and extreme irritability within 1–6 mo of age; later, seizures and tonic extensor spasms associated with light, sound, or touch stimulation occur; a rapid regression to the decerebrate condition followed by death at ≈2 y of age

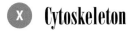 **Cytoskeleton**

A. **FILAMENTOUS ACTIN (F-ACTIN) is a 6-nm-diameter microfilament** arranged in a helix of polymerized **globular monomers of actin (G-actin)**. F-actin is in dynamic equilibrium with a cytoplasmic pool of G-actin such that a polymerization end (plus end) and a depolymerization end (minus end) are present on each actin filament. The functions of F-actin include exocytosis, endocytosis, cytokinesis, locomotion of cells forming lamellipodia, and movement of cell membrane proteins. **Cytochalasin** is a toxic fungal alkaloid that causes F-actin to depolymerize. **Phalloidin** is a toxic substance derived from the *Amanita* mushroom that binds to F-actin, thereby inhibiting polymerization/depolymerization.

B. **INTERMEDIATE FILAMENTS** are 10- to 12-nm-diameter filaments. Intermediate filament function as a cytoplasmic link between the extracellular matrix, cytoplasm, and nucleus. Intermediate filaments demonstrate specificity for certain cell types/tumors, and therefore can be used as markers for pathologic analysis (Table 2-3).

TABLE 2-3	SPECIFICITY OF INTERMEDIATE FILAMENTS FOR CELL TYPES OR TUMORS
Cytokeratin	Epithelial cells Epithelial tumors (e.g., squamous carcinoma, adenocarcinoma)
Vimentin	Endothelial cells, vascular smooth muscle, fibroblasts, chondroblasts, and macrophages Mesenchymal tumors (e.g., fibrosarcoma, liposarcoma, angiosarcoma, chondrosarcoma, osteosarcoma)
Desmin	Skeletal muscle, nonvascular smooth muscle Muscle tumors (e.g., rhabdomyosarcoma)
Neurofilament	Neurons Neuronal tumors
Glial fibrillar acidic protein (GFAP)	Astrocytes, oligodendroglia, microglia, Schwann cells, ependymal cells, and pituicytes Gliomatous tumors
Lamins A, B, C	Inner membrane of nuclear envelope

C. **MICROTUBULES are 25-nm-diameter tubules** that consist of 13 circularly arranged proteins called α- and β-tubulin.
1. Microtubules are in dynamic equilibrium with a cytoplasmic pool of α- and β-tubulin such that a polymerization end (plus end) and a depolymerization end (minus end) are present on each microtubule.
2. Microtubules are always associated with **microtubule-associated proteins (MAPs)**. MAPs include:
    a. **Kinesin** has ATPase activity for movement of vesicles along microtubules toward the plus end (**anterograde transport**).
    b. **Dynein** has ATPase activity for movement of vesicles along microtubules toward the minus end (**retrograde transport**).
    c. **Dynamin** has ATPase activity for elongation of nerve axons.
3. Microtubule functions include maintenance of cell shape (polarity), movement of chromosomes (karyokinesis), movement of secretory granules and neurosecretory vesicles, beating of cilia and flagella, and phagocytosis/lysosomal function.

4. The **microtubular organizing center (MTOC)** of the cell for the assembly of microtubules is called the **centrosome**. At the center of the centrosome are two **centrioles** that are oriented perpendicular to each other. During mitosis, each centriole duplicates by tubulin polymerization and the parent and daughter centrioles move to opposite poles of the cell.

5. **Clinical considerations**
   a. **Colchicine** is an M phase–specific drug (antimitotic) that inhibits microtubule assembly (i.e., polymerization). It is used in the treatment of acute and chronic gout by reducing the motility, phagocytosis, and secretion in inflammatory leukocytes (i.e., anti-inflammatory effect).
   b. **Vinblastine (Velban)** and **Vincristine (Oncovin)** are M phase–specific drugs (antimitotic) that bind tubulin and inhibit microtubule assembly (i.e., polymerization).
   c. **Paclitaxel (Taxol)** is an M phase–specific drug (antimitotic) that binds tubulin and inhibits microtubule disassembly (i.e., depolymerization).

XI Lipofuscin.
Lipofuscin is a mixture of **phospholipids complexed with proteins** along with a **yellow-brown "wear and tear"** pigment called **ceroid**. Lipofuscin is found predominately in **residual bodies** and is probably derived as an end point of lysosomal digestion of cellular membranes. Lipofuscin is a telltale sign of **free radical damage** and is found prominently within hepatocytes, skeletal muscle cells, cardiac myocytes, and nerve cells of elderly people or patients with severe malnutrition.

XII Hemosiderin.
Hemosiderin is a golden brown hemoglobin-derived pigment consisting of iron.

A. Iron is absorbed mainly by surface absorptive cells within the duodenum, transported in the plasma by a protein called **transferrin**, and normally stored in cells as **ferritin**, which is a protein–iron complex.

B. Small amounts of ferritin normally circulate in the plasma, making plasma ferritin a good indicator of the adequacy of body iron stores.

C. In iron deficiency, serum ferritin is less than 12 mg/L.

D. In iron overload, serum ferritin approaches 5000 mg/L. Also during iron overload, intracellular ferritin undergoes lysosomal degradation, in which the ferritin protein is degraded and the iron aggregates within the cell as hemosiderin in a condition called **hemosiderosis**.

E. CLINICAL CONSIDERATION: HFE-ASSOCIATED HEREDITARY HEMOCHROMATOSIS (HH)
1. HH is an autosomal recessive genetic disorder caused by ≈ 28 different mutations in the *HFE* gene on **chromosome 6p21.3** for **hereditary hemochromatosis protein**, which is a cell surface protein expressed as a heterodimer with β_2-microglobulin, binds the transferrin receptor 1, and reduces cellular iron uptake.
2. Due to the reduced iron uptake, surface absorptive cells of the duodenum up-regulate **divalent metal transporter (DMT-1)** expression, which then increases absorption of dietary iron. This leads to an increased concentration of non–transferrin-bound iron and its subsequent accumulation in organs. These mutations

result in elevated transferrin–iron saturation, elevated serum ferritin concentration, and hepatic iron overload assessed by **Prussian blue** staining of a liver biopsy.

3. **Clinical features include:** excessive storage of iron in the liver, heart, skin, pancreas, joints, and testes; abdominal pain; weakness; lethargy; weight loss; and hepatic fibrosis. Without therapy, symptoms appear in males at 40 to 60 years of age and in females after menopause.

 Glycogen. Glycogen is the **storage form of glucose** and is composed of glucose units linked by **α-1,4-glycosidic bonds.** Glycogen synthesis is catalyzed by **glycogen synthase.** Glycogen degradation is catalyzed by **glycogen phosphorylase.** Liver hepatocytes and skeletal muscle cells contain the largest glycogen stores, but the function of glycogen differs widely.

A. **LIVER GLYCOGEN** functions in the **maintenance of blood glucose levels.**
   1. Liver glycogen is synthesized (using glycogen synthase) during a high-carbohydrate meal due to **hyperglycemia** and an **increase in the insulin:glucagon ratio.**
   2. Liver glycogen is degraded (using liver glycogen phosphorylase isoenzyme) during **hypoglycemia** (e.g., fasting), **exercise,** or other **stressful situations** because of a **decrease in the insulin:glucagon ratio** or the **secretion of epinephrine.**
   3. Liver glycogen is degraded to **glucose-6-phosphate,** which is catalyzed to free glucose by the enzyme glucose-6-phosphatase. **Glucose-6-phosphatase** is found only in the liver and kidney.

B. **SKELETAL MUSCLE GLYCOGEN** functions in the **formation of ATP** through glycolysis.
   1. Skeletal muscle glycogen is synthesized (using glycogen synthase) during a high-carbohydrate meal due to **hyperglycemia** and an **increase in the insulin:glucagon ratio.**
   2. Skeletal muscle glycogen is degraded (using muscle glycogen phosphorylase isoenzyme) during **exercise** or other **stressful situations,** when **calcium is released during contraction,** and during **secretion of epinephrine.**
   3. Skeletal muscle glycogen is degraded to **glucose-6-phosphate,** which enters glycolysis to produce ATP. The **absence of glucose-6-phosphatase** enzyme in skeletal muscle prevents the degradation of glycogen to free glucose.

C. **CLINICAL CONSIDERATIONS: GLYCOGEN STORAGE DISEASES (TABLE 2-4)** are genetic diseases that involve mutations in one of the enzymes of glycogen synthesis or degradation.

TABLE 2-4	GLYCOGEN STORAGE DISEASES (GSDs)	
Genetic Disorder	**Gene** **Gene Product** **Chromosome**	**Clinical Features**
GSD type Ia von Gierke disease	*G6PC* gene Glucose-6-phosphatase catalytic subunit 17q21	Accumulation of glycogen and fat in the liver and kidney resulting in hepatomegaly and renomegaly, severe hypoglycemia, lactic acidosis, hyperuricemia, hyperlipidemia, hypoglycemic seizures, doll-like faces with fat cheeks, relatively thin extremities, short stature, protuberant abdomen, and neutropenia with recurrent bacterial infections Glucose-6-phosphatase catalyzes the reaction glucose-6-phosphate → glucose + phosphate
GSD type V McArdle disease	*PYGM* gene Muscle glycogen phosphorylase 11q13	Exercise-induced muscle cramps and pain, "second wind" phenomenon with relief of myalgia and fatigue after a few minutes of rest, episodes of myoglobinuria, increased resting basal serum creatine kinase (CK) activity, onset typically occurs around 20–30 y of age; clumsiness, lethargy, slow movement, and laziness in preadolescents Muscle glycogen phosphorylase initiates glycogen breakdown by removing α-1, 4-glucosyl residues from the outer branches of glycogen with liberation of glucose-1-phosphate
GSD type II Pompe disease	*GAA* gene Lysosomal acid α-glucosidase 17q25.2-q25.3	Muscle and heart are affected

GSD type IIIa
Cori disease
	AGL gene
	Amylo-1,6-glucosidase,
	  4-α-glucanotransferase
	  (or glycogen branching
	  enzyme)
	1p21
		Muscle and liver are affected

ⓧⓘⓥ Selected Photomicrographs

A. Electron micrographs of cytoplasmic organelles (Figure 2-3)

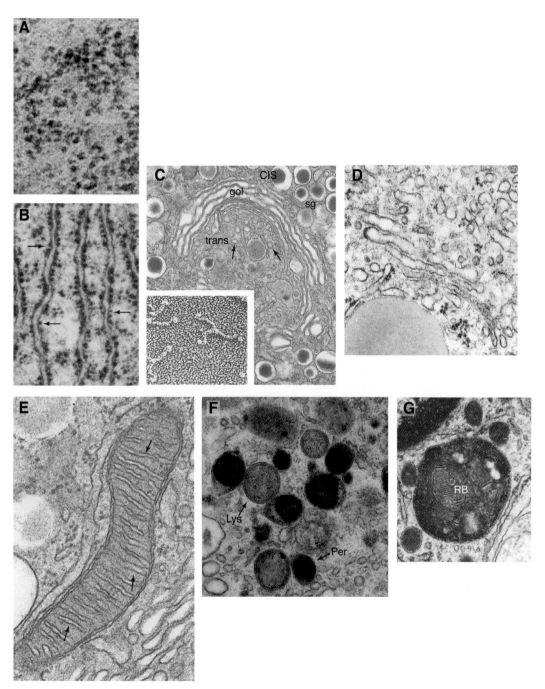

● **Figure 2-3 Cytoplasmic organelles. A:** Polyribosomes or polysomes are arranged in a spiral or rosette pattern. **B:** Rough endoplasmic reticulum (rER) shows membranous cisterna covered with ribosomes (*arrows*). **C:** Golgi complex (gol) shows *cis*-face and *trans*-face. Note the clathrin-coated vesicles budding from the *trans*-face (*arrows*). Sg, secretory granules. Inset: Isolated clathrin protein showing a distinctive three-legged structure called a triskelion. **D:** Smooth endoplasmic reticulum (sER) shows membranous cisternae with no ribosomes. **E:** Mitochondria and cristae (*arrows*). **F:** Lysosome (Lys) and peroxisome (Per). **G:** Residual body (RB).

B. Electron micrographs of the cytoskeleton and light micrograph of cytokeratin immunocytochemical localization (Figure 2-4)

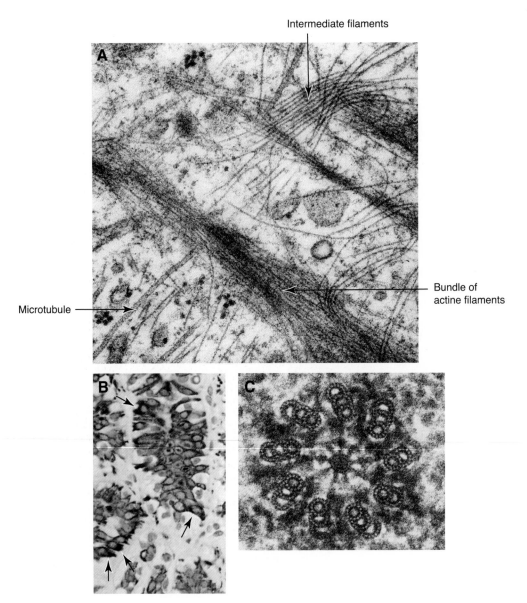

● **Figure 2-4 Cytoskeleton. A:** Electron micrograph shows a bundle of actin filaments, intermediate filaments, and microtubules of a negatively stained actin filament. Note the plus end and the minus end. **B:** Immunocytochemical staining for the intermediate filament (cytokeratin) in breast carcinoma. Note the localization of cytokeratin within the cytoplasm of the malignant epithelial cells (*arrows*). **C:** Electron micrograph shows a centriole composed of microtubules arranged in bundles of three (triplets; 9+0 arrangment) around an axial structure.

C. Electron micrographs of cell inclusions (Figure 2-5)

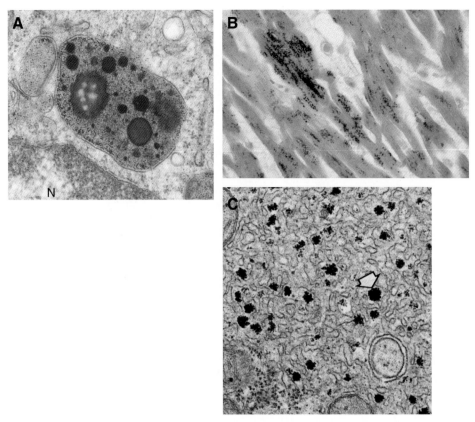

● **Figure 2-5 Cell inclusions. A:** Electron micrograph of lipofuscin pigment, which is the "wear and tear" pigment generally found in residual bodies. **B:** Light micrograph of hemosiderin within cardiac myocytes (hemosiderosis). The cardiac myocytes were stained with Prussian blue, which is specific for iron. **C:** Electron micrograph of glycogen particles within a hepatocyte (*arrow*).

D. Electron micrographs of a protein-secreting cell and steroid-secreting cell (Figure 2-6)

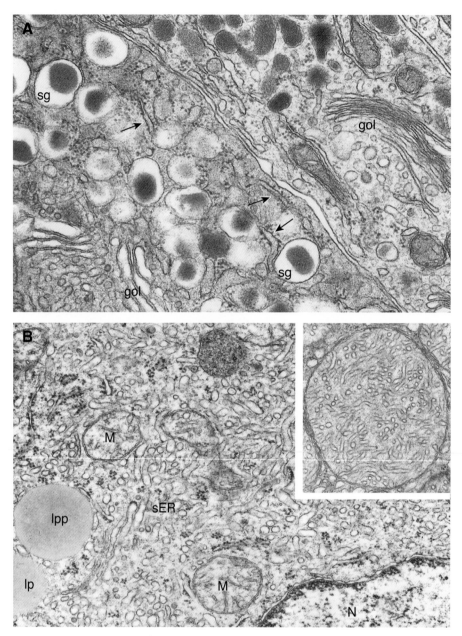

● **Figure 2-6 Protein- versus steroid-secreting cell. A:** Electron micrograph demonstrates the hallmarks of a protein-secreting cell: rough endoplasmic reticulum (rER, *arrows*), Gogli (gol), and secretory granules (sg). **B:** Electron micrograph demonstrates the hallmarks of a steroid-secreting cell: smooth endoplasmic reticulum (sER), mitochondria with tubular cristae (m), and lipid droplets (lp). N, nucleus. *Inset:* High magnification of mitochondria with tubular cristae.

Case Study 2-1

A 25-year-old man comes to your office complaining that "I feel weak when I do my exercise routine in the morning. I like to work out hard like a Navy Seal." He also tells you that "sometimes my urine is red and it scares me." After some discussion, he informs you that he takes a rest period when the weakness occurs and the symptoms resolve. But, the symptoms reappear when he resumes exercise. The man is obviously frustrated and says, "Doc, I can't stay in shape if this keeps happening." What is the most likely diagnosis?

Differentials

- Anemia, muscular dystrophy, myasthenia gravis, polymyositis

Relevant Physical Examination Findings

- Burning pain, cramping, and exhaustion in legs and arms during strenuous exercise
- Normal muscle tone and strength bilaterally
- No enlargement of the liver or spleen

Relevant Lab Findings

- Blood chemistry: creatine phosphokinase (CPK) = 100 U/L (high); hematocrit (Hct) = 45% (normal); hemoglobin (Hgb) = 15.2 g/dL (normal); blood urea nitrogen (BUN) = 15 mg/dL (normal)
- Urinalysis: red blood cells (RBCs) = 20–30 (high); glucose = high
- Diagnostic anaerobic exercise test showed muscle pain, cramping, and exhaustion; increase in CPK; and no increase in blood lactate.
- Muscle biopsy showed elevated glycogen content and low phosphorylase activity.

Diagnosis: McArdle Disease

- **McArdle Disease**. McArdle disease (type V glycogenosis) is an autosomal recessive disease and results from a deficiency in muscle glycogen phosphorylase, causing exercise-induced muscle pain and cramping. Myoglobulinuria results from a breakdown of muscle protein in an attempt to liberate amino acids for conversion to glucose. Myoglobin contains heme, binds oxygen, and provides oxygen to muscle for oxidation. BUN and measures the ability of the kidney to excrete the nitrogenous waste products produced by the body.
- Duchenne muscular dystrophy (DMD) is a genetic disease that shows X-linked recessive inheritance. The DMD gene is located on the short (p) arm of chromosome X in band 21 (i.e., Xp21) and encodes for the dystrophin protein. Dystrophin anchors within skeletal muscle fibers to the extracellular matrix, thereby stabilizing the cell membrane. A mutation of the DMD gene alters the normal function of dystrophin, leading to progressive muscle weakness and wasting. The muscle weakness begins as early as 1 year of age.
- Myasthenia gravis is an autoimmune disease characterized by circulating antibodies against the nACh receptor (nicotinic acetylcholine receptor; anti-nAChR) and decreased number of nACh receptors. Clinical findings of myasthenia gravis include muscle weakness that fluctuates daily or even within hours, and extraocular muscle involvement with ptosis and diplopia being the first disability.
- Polymyositis is a connective tissue disease. Clinical findings of polymyositis include progressive, bilateral weakness of the proximal muscles.

Chapter 3

The Cell Membrane: Eicosanoids and Receptors/Signal Transduction

I. The Lipid Component of the Cell Membrane (Figure 3-1)

A. The lipid component consists of four phospholipids: **phosphatidylcholine, sphingomyelin, phosphatidylethanolamine,** and **phosphatidylserine.**

B. The lipid component exhibits **asymmetry** in which phosphatidylcholine and sphingomyelin are located in the **outer leaflet** (extracellular side), and phosphatidylethanolamine and phosphatidylserine are located in the **inner leaflet** (cytoplasmic side).

C. The four phospholipids are **amphiphilic**; that is, they have a **hydrophilic (polar) head** and a **hydrophobic (nonpolar) tail.**

D. The lipid component exhibits **fluidity**, which means that the phospholipids diffuse laterally within the lipid bilayer.

E. **CHOLESTEROL** is a component of the cell membrane and is thought to be distributed in both the outer and inner leaflets.

F. **GLYCOLIPIDS** are sugar-containing sphingolipids and are confined exclusively to the outer leaflet. The types of glycolipids include:
1. **Cerebrosides,** which contain a single sugar moiety (e.g., galactose)
2. **Other Neutral Glycolipids** (e.g., red blood cell group antigens A, B, and O), which contain many sugar moieties (e.g., glucose, galactose, N-acetyl-D-galactosamine, fucose)
3. **Gangliosides** (e.g., ganglioside GM_1), which contain many sugar moieties and negatively charged N-acetylneuraminic acid (or sialic acid)

G. **PRODUCTION OF EICOSANOIDS.** The lipid component produces **arachidonic acid,** which leads to the formation of **eicosanoids** through the following process.
1. In response to physical injury or inflammatory response, **phospholipase A_2 or C** catalyzes the breakdown of membrane lipids to **arachidonic acid.**
2. Arachidonic acid may be converted to straight-chain eicosanoids called **leukotrienes (LTB_4, LTC_4, LTD_4)** by **lipoxygenase.**
3. Arachidonic acid may be converted to cyclical eicosanoids called **prostaglandins** (PGE_1, PGE_2 PGF_{2a}), **prostacyclin (PGI_2),** and **thromboxane (TXA_2)** by **cyclooxygenase (COX I and COX II).** COX I produces eicosanoids used in many normal physiologic processes; hence, it is sometimes referred to as "good COX." COX II produces eicosanoids used in the inflammatory response; hence, it is sometimes referred to as "bad COX."
4. **Pharmacology**
   a. **Aspirin (acetylsalicylic acid, Bayer, Bufferin)** is a nonsteroidal anti-inflammatory drug (NSAID) that irreversibly inhibits cyclooxygenase and is used clinically to ameliorate effects of myocardial infarction, inhibit platelet aggregation, reduce pain, reduce fever, and as a general anti-inflammatory agent.

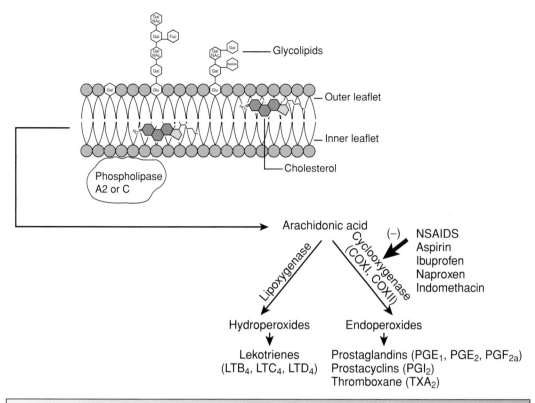

Eicosonoid	Function
LTB$_4$	Stimulates leukocyte chemotaxis.
LTC$_4$	Potent bronchoconstrictor. Component of slow-reacting substance of anaphylaxis (SRS-A)
LTD$_4$	Potent bronchoconstrictor. Component of slow-reacting substance of anaphylaxis (SRS-A)
PGE$_1$	Potent vasodilator (used to maintain patency of ductus arteriosus). Misoprostol (a PGE1 analogue) is used with mifepristone (RU-486; a progesterone receptor blocker) to induce therapeutic abortion. Inhibits gastric HCL secretion. Stimulates gastric secretion of bicarbonate and mucus (misoprostol is used to treat peptic ulcers).
PGE$_2$	Causes contraction of uterine smooth muscle at parturition (induces labor or therapeutic abortion in 2nd trimester). Potent vasodilator. Potent bronchodilator. Inhibits platelet aggregation. Inhibits mast cell secretion. Potentiates the inflammatory response.
PGF$_{2a}$	Causes contraction of uterine smooth muscle at parturition (induces labor or therapeutic abortion in 2nd trimester).
PGI$_2$	Potent vasodilator. Inhibits platelet aggregation. Potentiates the inflammatory response.
TXA$_2$	Potent vasodilator. Stimulates platelet aggregation.

● **Figure 3-1 Diagram of the lipid component of the cell membrane and its biologic actions.** Note that two molecules of cholesterol are shown in the outer and inner leaflets. COX, cyclooxygenase; Gal, galactose; Glu, glucose; GalNAc, N-acetyl-D-galactosamine; Fuc, fucose; NANA, N-acetylneuraminic acid (or sialic acid).

b. **Ibuprofen (Advil, Motrin, Nuprin)** and **Naproxen (Aleve)** are NSAIDs (propionic acid derivatives) that reversibly inhibit cyclooxygenase and are used clinically to reduce pain, to treat rheumatoid arthritis, and to treat osteoarthritis.

c. **Indomethacin** is an NSAID (an acetic acid derivative) that reversibly inhibits cyclooxygenase and is used clinically to treat acute gout, to treat ankylosing spondylitis, and to promote closure of the ductus arteriosus.

Ⅱ The Protein Component of the Cell Membrane (Figure 3-2)

A. The protein component exhibits **patching or capping**, which means that proteins diffuse laterally within the lipid bilayer.

B. The protein component consists of **peripheral** and **integral proteins**.

C. PERIPHERAL PROTEINS can be easily disassociated from the lipid bilayer by changes in ionic strength or pH.

D. INTEGRAL PROTEINS are difficult to disassociate from the lipid bilayer unless detergents (e.g., sodium dodecyl sulfate or Triton X-100) are used.

E. TRANSMEMBRANE PROTEINS are integral proteins that span the lipid bilayer, exposing the protein to both the extracellular space and the cytoplasm.

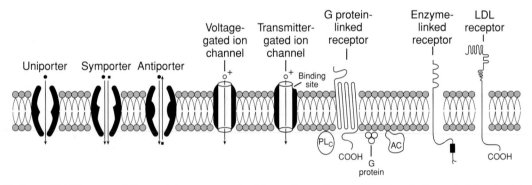

● **Figure 3-2 Diagram of the protein component of the cell membrane.** PL_C, phospholipase C; AC, adenylate cyclase; LDL, low-density lipoprotein.

Ⅲ Membrane Transport Proteins allow for the passage of polar molecules (e.g., ions, sugars, amino acids, nucleotides, and metabolites) across a membrane. There are two main classes of transport proteins: carrier proteins and ion channel proteins.

A. CARRIER PROTEINS (TRANSPORTERS). Carrier proteins or transporters bind a specific molecule and undergo **conformational changes** in order to transport the molecule across the membrane. Carrier proteins that transport a single molecule are called **uniporters**. Other carrier proteins function as **coupled transporters** in which the transport of one molecule depends on the simultaneous transport of another molecule either in the same direction (**symporters**) or in the opposite direction (**antiporters**). Carrier proteins participate predominately in **active transport**, whereby molecules are transported "**uphill**" of the concentration and membrane potential (i.e., electrochemical gradient). Some important carrier proteins are indicated in **Table 3-1**.

TABLE 3-1	FUNCTIONAL ASPECTS OF CARRIER PROTEIN (TRANSPORTERS)
Carrier Protein (Transporter)	**Functional Aspects**
Ca^{2+} adenosine triphosphatase (ATPase)	Is a uniporter carrier protein most commonly found in the sarcoplasmic reticulum (SR) of skeletal muscle that pumps Ca^{2+} from the cytoplasm back into the SR
Na^+-K^+ ATPase	Is an antiporter carrier protein found in almost all cells that pumps Na^+ out of the cell and K^+ into the cell to maintain a low intracellular [Na^+] **Ouabain** is a specific inhibitor that competes for the K^+-binding site. **Cardiac glycosides (digoxin and digitoxin)** are Na^+-K^+ ATPase blockers that elevate intracellular Na^+ levels within cardiac myocytes.
H^+-K^+ ATPase	Is an antiporter carrier protein most commonly found in the parietal cells of the stomach mucosa that pumps H^+ into the lumen of the stomach to form HCl gastric acid
MDR1 MDR2	Are expressed by human cancer cells and unfortunately confer resistance to cancer chemotherapeutic drugs by transporting the hydrophobic drugs out of the cancer cell
Chloroquine transporter	Is expressed by *Plasmodium falciparum* (which causes malaria) and confers resistance to the antimalarial drug chloroquine by transporting the drug out of *P. falciparum*
Cystic fibrosis (CF) transporter	Transports Cl^- out of the cell
Na^+-K^+-$2Cl^-$ cotransporter	Is a symporter carrier protein that transports Na^+ across the luminal membrane into the cytoplasm by cotransport with K^+ and Cl^- into the cytoplasm, which occurs because cytoplasmic [Na^+] is kept low by Na^+-K^+ ATPase **Furosemide (Lasix; last 6 h), bumetanide (Bumex), and torsemide (Demadex)** inhibit the Na^+-K^+-$2Cl^-$ cotransporter by acting primarily on the **distal straight tubule of the loop of Henle ("loop diuretics").** Loop diuretics are the most efficacious diuretics available and are sometimes called **"high ceiling diuretics."**
Na^+-Cl^- cotransporter	Is a symporter carrier protein that transports Na^+ across the luminal membrane into the cytoplasm by cotransport with Cl^- into the cytoplasm, which occurs because cytoplasmic [Na^+] is kept low by Na^+-K^+ ATPase **Hydrochlorothiazide (HydroDIURIL), chlorthalidone (Hygroton), indapamide (Lozol), and metolazone (Mykrox)** inhibit the Na^+-Cl^- cotransporter by acting primarily on the **distal convoluted tubule,** resulting in decreased Na^+ reabsorption **("thiazide diuretics").**

MDR, multidrug resistance protein.

B. **ION CHANNEL PROTEINS.** Ion channel proteins form **hydrophilic pores** in order to transport **inorganic ions** across the membrane and are generally called **ion channels.** Ion channels participate only in passive **transport (facilitated diffusion),** whereby molecules are transported "downhill" of the concentration and membrane potential (i.e., electrochemical gradient). Ion channels are **ion selective** and **gated** (i.e., open briefly and then close). Stimuli that open gates include mechanical stress (**mechanical-gated ion channels**), changes in voltage across the cell membrane (**voltage-gated ion channels**), and ligand binding (**ligand-gated ion channels**). One of the more important types of ligand-gated ion channels is the **transmitter-gated ion channel** that binds neurotransmitters and mediates ion movement. Depending on the type of ion involved, transmitter-gated ion channels may have an excitatory or inhibitory effect. Some important ion channel proteins are indicated in **Tables 3-2** and **3-3.**

TABLE 3-2	FUNCTIONAL ASPECTS OF VOLTAGE-GATED ION CHANNEL PROTEINS
Voltage-gated Ion Channel Protein	**Functional Aspects**
L-type Ca^{2+} channel protein (dihydropyridine receptor)	Is an important determinant of vascular tone and cardiac contractility In vascular smooth muscle cells, contraction is caused by transmembrane Ca^{2+} influx into the cytoplasm through the L-type Ca^{2+} channel protein and Ca^{2+} release from the sarcoplasmic reticulum through the fast Ca^{2+} release channel protein. In the SA and AV nodes, phase 0 of the slow action potential is caused by Ca^{2+} influx through the L-type Ca^{2+} channel protein. In ventricular myocytes, phase 2 of the fast action potential is caused by Ca^{2+} influx through the L-type Ca^{2+} channel protein. This transmembrane Ca^{2+} influx is called **"trigger Ca^{2+}"** and is involved in myocyte contraction. **Nifedipine** and **amlodipine** are Ca^{2+} channel blockers that act on vascular smooth muscle cells and cause arterial vasodilation. **Diltiazem** and **verapamil** are Ca^{2+} channel blockers that act preferentially on the SA and AV nodal cells. They have two major actions: slow the rise of phase 0 of the action potential, which leads to a slowed conduction velocity through the AV node, and prolong the repolarization of the AV node, which increases the effective refractory period of the AV node.
Fast Ca^{2+} release channel protein (ryanodine receptor)	Plays a role in skeletal, smooth, and cardiac muscle contraction.
T-type Ca^{2+} channel protein	In the SA and AV nodes, phase 4 of the action potential is caused by Ca^{2+} influx through the T-type Ca^{2+} channel protein and Na^+ influx through slow (funny) Na^+ channels.
K^+ channel protein	In cardiac myocytes, phase 2 of the action potential is caused by the depolarizing Ca^{2+} influx through the L-type Ca^{2+} channel protein and the hyperpolarizing K^+ efflux through the K^+ ion channel protein. **Ibutilide** is a class III antiarrhythmic K^+ channel protein antagonist (blocker) that also enhances a slow Na^+ influx that further prolongs repolarization. **Sotalol** is a mixed class II (nonselectively antagonizes β-adrenergic receptors) and a class III antiarrhythmic K^+ channel protein antagonist (blocker). **Bretylium** is an antihypertensive agent (performs a "chemical sympathectomy" by inhibiting the release of norepinephrine) and a class III antiarrhythmic K^+ channel protein antagonist (blocker). **Amiodarone** is mainly a class III antiarrhythmic K^+ channel protein antagonist (blocker).
Slow (funny) Na^+ channel protein	In the SA and AV nodes, phase 4 of the slow action potential is caused by Ca^{2+} influx through T-type Ca^{2+} channel proteins and Na^+ influx through slow (funny) Na^+ channel proteins.
Fast Na^+ channel protein	In cardiac myocytes, phase 0 of the fast action potential is caused by Na^+ influx through fast Na^+ channel proteins. **Quinidine, procainamide, and disopyramide** are class IA antiarrhythmic Na^+ channel protein antagonists (blockers) that bind preferentially to **open** Na^+ channel proteins. **Lidocaine, tocainide, and mexiletine** are class IB antiarrhythmic Na^+ channel protein antagonists (blockers) that bind preferentially to **open and inactivated** Na^+ channel proteins. A major distinguishing characteristic of class IB antiarrhythmics is their **fast dissociation** from Na^+ channel proteins. **Flecainide, propafenone, moricizine, and encainide** are class IC antiarrhythmic Na^+ channel protein antagonists (blockers) that are the most potent Na^+ channel protein blockers.

L, long-lasting; SA, sinoatrial; AV, atrioventricular; T, transient.

TABLE 3-3	FUNCTIONAL ASPECTS OF TRANSMITTER-GATED ION CHANNEL PROTEINS

Transmitter-gated Ion Channel Protein	Functional Aspects
Nicotinic acetylcholine (nACh) receptor	When ACh binds to the nACh receptor, the gate is opened and the influx of Na^+ and Ca^{2+} and efflux of K^+ occurs. The N_2 or N_N nACh receptor is found in the central nervous system (CNS), autonomic ganglia, and adrenal medulla. The N_1 or N_M nACh receptor is found at the neuromuscular junction in skeletal muscle. The influx of Na^+ is primarily responsible for the depolarization of the postsynaptic membrane and mediates the excitatory postsynaptic potential (EPSP). **Succinylcholine (Anectine, Quelicin, Sucostrin)** is an nACh receptor agonist that competes with ACh for the nACh receptor. Succinylcholine maintains an open Na^+ channel, eventually causing skeletal muscle relaxation and paralysis. Succinylcholine is used to induce paralysis during surgery by means of a **depolarizing blockade.** **Tubocurarine, pancuronium, vecuronium, and rocuronium** are nACh receptor antagonists (blockers) that block endogenous ACh binding. These blockers are used to induce paralysis during surgery by means of a **nondepolarizing blockade.**
N-methyl-D-aspartate (NMDA) receptor	When **glutamate** and the cofactor **glycine** bind to the NMDA receptor, the gate is opened and the influx of Na^+ and Ca^{2+} and efflux of K^+ occurs. The NMDA receptor is found throughout the CNS (e.g., hippocampus, cerebral cortex, and spinal cord). Glutamate is the **major excitatory neurotransmitter in the CNS.** **Amantadine** is a noncompetitive NMDA receptor antagonist (blocker). **Memantine** is a noncompetitive, use-dependent NMDA receptor antagonist. **Ketamine** (Ketalar; Special K; K) is an NMDA receptor antagonist that acts as a CNS depressant and a dissociative anesthetic. Ketamine has sedative, analgesic, and hallucinogenic effects and is used as a "date rape" drug. **Phencyclidine (PCP; angel dust)** and **dizocilpine (MK-801)** are NMDA receptor antagonists that cause hallucinogenic behavior and require the NMDA receptor to be open in order to gain access to their binding sites (i.e., open channel blockers).
γ-Aminobutyric acid$_A$ (GABA$_A$) receptors	When GABA binds to the GABA$_A$ receptor, the gate is opened and the influx of Cl^- occurs (causes hyperpolarization of the cell). GABA$_A$ receptor is found in most areas of the CNS. GABA$_A$ receptor generates fast inhibitory postsynaptic potentials (IPSPs). GABA is the **major inhibitory neurotransmitter in the CNS.** **Thiopental, methohexital, pentobarbital, secobarbital, amobarbital,** and **phenobarbital** are GABA$_A$ receptor modulators that enhance the **efficacy** of GABA by increasing the **duration** of Cl^- **channel opening,** leading to membrane hyperpolarization and decreased neuronal excitability. **Midazolam, clorazepate, alprazolam, lorazepam, chlordiazepoxide, clonazepam, diazepam, triazolam, estazolam, temazepam, flurazepam, and quazepam** are GABA$_A$ receptor modulators that enhance the **potency** of GABA by increasing the **frequency of Cl^- channel opening,** leading to membrane hyperpolarization and decreased neuronal excitability. **Flunitrazepam (Rohypnol; "roofies"; Forget Me Pill)** is a fast-acting benzodiazepine that causes amnesia and is used as a "date rape" drug.
Glycine receptor	When glycine binds to the glycine receptor, the gate is opened and the influx of Cl^- occurs (causes **hyperpolarization** of the cell). Glycine is the **major inhibitory neurotransmitter in the spinal cord.**

IV **G Protein-linked Receptors (Figure 3-3).** G protein-linked receptors are proteins that span the cell membrane seven times (**seven-pass receptor**) and are linked to **trimeric guanosine triphosphate (GTP)-binding proteins (called G proteins)** composed of an **α-chain**, a **β-chain**, and a **γ-chain**. These receptors activate a chain of cellular events either through the **adenylate cyclase (AC) pathway** (by increasing or decreasing cyclic adenosine monophosphate [cAMP] levels) or the **phospholipase C (PL$_C$) pathway.**

A. **AC PATHWAY ($\uparrow$ cAMP LEVELS).** When norepinephrine (NE) binds to the β_1, β_2, or β_3 receptor, inactive **G$_S$ protein** (which exists as a trimer with guanosine diphosphate [GDP] bound to the α_S chain) exchanges its GDP for GTP to become **active G$_S$ protein**. This allows the α_S chain to disassociate from the β_S chain and γ_S chain and **stimulate adenylate cyclase to increase cAMP levels**. Active G$_S$ protein is short-lived since the α_S chain has **guanosine triphosphatase (GTPase) activity**, which quickly hydrolyzes GTP to GDP to form inactive G$_S$ protein. cAMP activates the enzyme **cAMP-dependent protein kinase (or protein kinase A; PKA)**, which catalyzes the **covalent phosphorylation** of serine and threonine within certain intracellular proteins to increase their activity. The enzyme **serine/threonine protein phosphatase** reverses the effects of protein kinase A by dephosphorylating serine and threonine. **Cholera toxin** (an enzyme that catalyzes **adenosine diphosphate (ADP) ribosylation of the α_S chain**) blocks α_S chain GTPase activity so that the effects of active G$_S$ protein continue indefinitely. Within intestinal epithelium, this causes Na^+ ion and water movement into the gut lumen, resulting in severe **diarrhea**.

B. **AC PATHWAY ($\downarrow$ cAMP LEVELS).** When NE binds to the α_2-adrenergic receptor, inactive **G$_i$ protein** (which exists as a trimer with GDP bound to the α_i chain) exchanges its GDP for GTP to become **active G$_i$ protein**. This allows the α_i chain to disassociate from the β_i chain and γ_i chain and **inhibit adenylate cyclase to decrease cAMP levels**. The β_i and γ_i complex stimulates a K^+ channel protein (probably K_{IR}; inward rectifier) so that the channel opens and K^+ flows out of the cell, causing a hyperpolarization of the cell (probably the main effect). **Pertussis toxin** (an enzyme that catalyzes **ADP ribosylation of the α_i chain**) blocks the dissociation of the α_i chain from the β_i chain and γ_i chain so that adenylate cyclase is not inhibited.

C. **PL$_C$ PATHWAY.** When acetylcholine (ACh) binds to the M_3 muscarinic acetylcholine receptor, **inactive G$_q$ protein** (which exists as a trimer with GDP bound to the α-chain) exchanges its GDP for GTP to become **active G$_q$ protein**. Active G$_q$ protein activates **phospholipase C**, which cleaves **phosphatidylinositol biphosphate (PIP$_2$)** into **inositol triphosphate (IP$_3$)** and **diacylglycerol (DAG)**. IP$_3$ causes the **release of Ca^{2+} from the endoplasmic reticulum**, which activates the enzyme **Ca^{2+}/calmodulin-dependent protein kinase (or CaM-kinase)**, which catalyzes the **covalent phosphorylation** of serine and threonine within certain intracellular proteins to increase their activity. DAG activates the enzyme **protein kinase C (PKC)**, which catalyzes the **covalent phosphorylation** of serine and threonine within certain intracellular proteins to increase their activity.

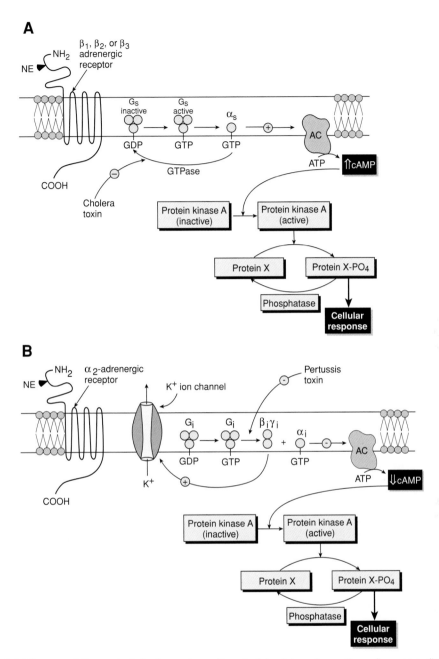

● **Figure 3-3 Diagram of G protein-linked receptor action. A:** Adenylate cyclase pathway (increase cyclic adenosine monophosphate [cAMP] levels). **B:** Adenylate cyclase pathway (decrease cAMP levels). (*continued*)

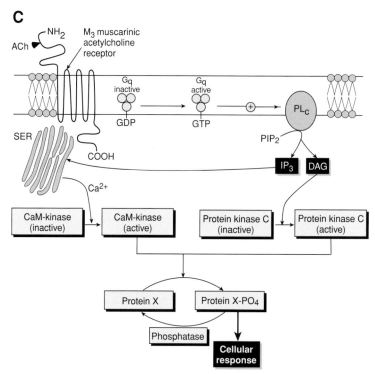

● **Figure 3-3** *Continued* **C:** Phospholipase C pathway. NE, norepinephrine; ACh, acetylcholine; AC, adenylate cyclase; SER, smooth endoplasmic reticulum; PL_C, phospholipase C; CaM, Ca^{2+}/calmodulin-dependent protein kinase; IP_3, inositol triphosphate; DAG, diacylglycerol; PIP_2, phosphatidylinositol biphosphate.

 Types of G Protein-linked Receptors. Some important G protein-linked receptors are indicated in **Table 3-4**.

TABLE 3-4	FUNCTIONAL ASPECTS OF G PROTEIN-LINKED RECEPTORS
G Protein-linked Receptor	**Functional Aspects**
Muscarinic acetylcholine (mACh) receptors (M_1, M_2, M_3, M_4, M_5)	The mACh receptors bind **acetylcholine.** The **M_1 receptor** is found in the central nervous system (CNS) and autonomic ganglia (mediates the slow excitatory postsynaptic potential) where it elicits its action through the PL_C pathway ($\uparrow IP_3$ + DAG). The **M_2 receptor** is found in the heart (SA and AV nodes, atrial and ventricular cardiac myocytes) where it elicits its action through the AC pathway ($\downarrow$ cAMP levels + opens a K^+ channel protein so that K^+ flows out of the cell, causing hyperpolarization). The **M_3 receptor** is found in smooth muscle and secretory glands where it elicits its action through the PL_C pathway ($\uparrow IP_3$ + DAG). The **M_4 receptor** is found in the CNS where it elicits its action through the AC pathway ($\downarrow$ cAMP levels + opens a K^+ channel protein so that K^+ flows out of the cell, causing hyperpolarization). The **M_5 receptor** is found in the CNS where it elicits its action through the PL_C pathway ($\uparrow IP_3$ + DAG). **Methacholine, carbachol, bethanechol,** and **pilocarpine** (an alkaloid) are mACh receptor agonists. **Atropine, scopolamine, pirenzepine,** and **ipratropium** are mACh receptor antagonists.

TABLE 3-4	FUNCTIONAL ASPECTS OF G PROTEIN-LINKED RECEPTORS (*Continued*)
G Protein-linked Receptor	**Functional Aspects**
Adrenergic receptors (α_1, α_2, β_1, β_2, β_3)	The adrenergic receptors bind **epinephrine** and **norepinephrine.** The **α_1 receptor** is found in the dilator pupillae muscle, arteriolar smooth muscle, GI and GU sphincters, arrector pili muscle, GU smooth muscle, and liver where it elicits its action through the PL$_C$ pathway ($\uparrow$ IP$_3$ + DAG). The **α_2 receptor** is found in pancreatic β cells, platelets, and autonomic ganglia (mediates the slow inhibitory postsynaptic potential) where it elicits its action through the AC pathway ($\downarrow$ cAMP + opens a K$^+$ channel protein so that K$^+$ flows out of the cell, causing hyperpolarization). The **β_1 receptor** is found in the heart and juxtaglomerular cells where it elicits its action through the AC pathway ($\uparrow$ cAMP). The **β_2 receptor** is found in vascular smooth muscle (within skeletal muscle), bronchiolar smooth muscle, GI and urinary bladder smooth muscle, uterine smooth muscle, skeletal muscle, and liver where it elicits its action through the AC pathway ($\uparrow$ cAMP). The **β_3 receptor** is found in adipose tissue where it elicits its action through the AC pathway ($\uparrow$ cAMP). **Phenylephrine, oxymetazoline, and tetrahydrozoline** are α_1 agonists. **Clonidine** and **methyldopa** (a prodrug metabolized to methyl-epinephrine) are α_2 agonists. **Phenoxybenzamine** and **phentolamine** are nonselective α_1 and α_2 antagonists. **Prazosin, terazosin**, and **doxazosin** are α_1 antagonists. **Tamsulosin** is an α_{1A} antagonist. **Yohimbine** is an α_2 antagonist. **Isoproterenol** is a nonselective β_1 and β_2 agonist. **Dobutamine** is a β_1 agonist. **Metaproterenol, terbutaline, albuterol**, and **salmeterol** are β_2 agonists. **Propranolol, nadolol,** and **timolol** are β_1 and β_2 antagonists. **Labetalol** and **carvedilol** are α_1, β_1, and β_2 antagonists. **Pindolol** is a partial β_1 and β_2 agonist. **Acebutolol** is a partial β_1 agonist. **Esmolol, metoprolol**, and **atenolol** are β_1 antagonists.
Opiate receptors (μ, δ, κ, σ)	The **μ receptor** elicits its action through the PL$_C$ pathway ($\uparrow$ IP$_3$ + DAG and closes voltage-gated Ca^{2+} channels when acting presynaptically) and the AC pathway ($\downarrow$ cAMP levels and opens a K$^+$ channel protein so that K$^+$ flows out of the cell, causing hyperpolarization when acting postsynaptically). The μ, δ, κ, σ receptors bind the naturally occurring opioids **β-endorphin, enkephalins,** and **dynorphins.** The **μ, δ, κ, σ receptors** are found throughout the CNS and spinal cord. **Morphine (Roxanol, MS Contin), meperidine (Demerol), methadone (Dolophine), fentanyl (Sublimaze, Duragesic), alfentanil, sufentanil, remifentanil, hydromorphone (Dilaudid),** and **heroin** are μ-receptor agonists and are used to treat severe pain. **Hydrocodone (Hycodan), oxycodone (Roxicodone, Supeudol), codeine, and propoxyphene (Darvon)** are μ-receptor agonists and are used to treat moderate to mild pain. **Butorphanol** and **buprenorphine** are partial μ-receptor agonists. **Nalbuphine** is a mixed agonist with κ-agonist activity and μ-antagonist activity. **Naloxone (Narcan) and naltrexone (Trexan) are** μ-receptor antagonists and are used to treat opioid toxicity, respiratory depression, and opioid addiction.

PL$_C$, phospholipase C; IP$_3$, inositol triphosphate; DAG, diacylglycerol; SA, sinoatrial; AV, atrioventricular; AC, adenylate cyclase; cAMP, cyclic adenosine monophosphate; GI, gastrointestinal; GU, genitourinary.

VI **Enzyme-linked Receptors (Figure 3-4).** All enzyme-linked receptors are composed structurally of single or multiple polypeptides that span the cell membrane once (**one-pass transmembrane receptors**). These receptors are unique in that their cytoplasmic domain has **intrinsic enzyme activity** or **associates directly with an enzyme.** Some important enzyme-linked receptors are indicated in **Table 3-5.**

TABLE 3-5	FUNCTIONAL ASPECTS OF ENZYME-LINKED RECEPTORS
Enzyme-linked Receptor	**Functional Aspects**
Receptor guanylate cyclase (e.g., ANP receptor)	When the appropriate signal binds to receptor guanylate cyclase, its intrinsic enzyme guanylate cyclase activity produces cGMP. cGMP activates **cGMP-dependent protein kinase (protein kinase G; PKG),** which catalyzes the **covalent phosphorylation** of serine and threonine within certain intracellular proteins to increase their activity.
Receptor tyrosine phosphatase (e.g., CD45)	When the appropriate signal binds to a receptor tyrosine phosphatase, its intrinsic tyrosine phosphatase will catalyze the **dephosphorylation** of tyrosine within certain intracellular proteins to increase their activity.
Receptor serine/threonine kinase (e.g., TGF-β receptor)	When the appropriate signal binds to a receptor serine/threonine kinase, its intrinsic serine/threonine kinase activity will catalyze the **covalent phosphorylation** of serine and threonine within certain intracellular proteins to increase their activity.
Tyrosine kinase–associated receptor (e.g., cytokine receptors, growth hormone receptor, prolactin hormone receptor, antigen-specific receptors on B and T lymphocytes, IL-2 receptor, and erythropoietin receptor)	When the appropriate signal binds to a tyrosin kinase–associated receptor, the tyrosine kinase that is associated with the receptor will catalyze the **covalent phosphorylation** of tyrosine within certain intracellular proteins to increase their activity. One important tyrosine kinase that is associated with the receptor is the Src protein. Src protein is a tyrosine kinase that is the gene product of the *src* **proto-oncogene.**
Receptor tyrosine kinase (e.g., EGF receptor, PDGF receptor, FGF receptor, NGF receptor, VEGF receptor, and insulin receptor)	See legend for Figure 3-4.

cGMP, cyclic guanosine monophosphate; TGF, transforming growth factor; IL-2, interleukin-2; EGF, epidermal growth factor; PDGF, platelet-derived growth factor; FGF, fibroblast growth factor; NGF, nerve growth factor; VEGF, vascular endothelial growth factor.

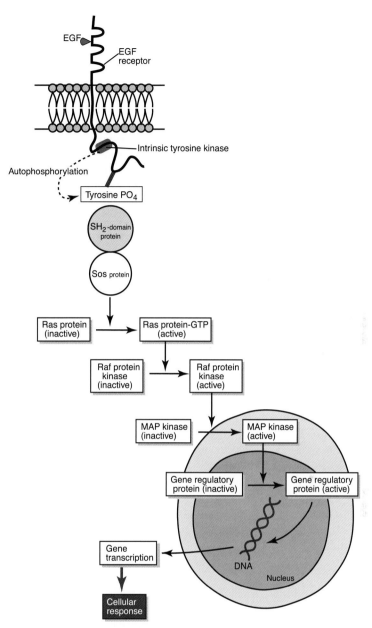

● **Figure 3-4 Signal transduction of a receptor tyrosine kinase.** When the appropriate signal binds to a receptor tyrosine kinase, its intrinsic tyrosine kinase activity will catalyze the **autophosphorylation** of tyrosine (producing **phosphotyrosine**) within the receptor. There is a vast array of intracellular proteins that bind to the phosphotyrosine residues, all of which share a sequence homology (called SH_2 domain) and are called **SH_2-domain proteins.** The SH_2-domain protein interacts with **Sos protein.** The Sos protein activates **Ras protein** by causing Ras protein to bind guanosine triphosphate (GTP). Ras protein is a monomeric G protein that is the gene product of the **ras proto-oncogene.** The activated Ras protein activates **Raf protein kinase.** The activated Raf protein kinase activates **mitogen-activated protein kinase (MAP kinase)** by covalent phosphorylation of tyrosine and threonine. The activated MAP kinase leaves the cytoplasm and enters the nucleus where it phosphorylates gene regulatory proteins that then cause **gene transcription.** EGF, epidermal growth factor; Sos, son-of-sevenless; Ras, rat sarcoma; MAP, mitogen-activated protein; SH_2, sequence homology.

Low-density Lipoprotein (LDL) Receptor. The LDL receptor has an extracellular portion that consists of one domain with seven cysteine-rich areas called the **LDL-binding region**; a second domain with EGF homology; and a third domain with serine and threonine-rich areas linked to oligosaccharides. When LDL (the principal carrier of serum cholesterol) binds to the LDL receptor, **receptor-mediated endocytosis** occurs in the following steps.

A. Receptor-mediated endocytosis forms **clathrin-coated vesicles** that fuse with an **endosome** or **compartment for uncoupling of receptor and ligand (called the CURL)**, where the LDL and LDL receptor are disassociated from each other due to the low pH. The LDL receptor is recycled back to the cell membrane.

B. **ENDOLYSOSOMES** fuse with the endosome and LDL is lysosomally degraded to **cholesterol**, which is released into the cytoplasm.

C. The cholesterol inhibits the enzyme **3-hydroxy-3-methylglutaryl coenzyme A (HMG-CoA) reductase**, which catalyzes the committed step in cholesterol biosynthesis and thereby suppresses de novo cholesterol biosynthesis. This process contributes to keeping serum cholesterol levels in the normal range.

D. **CLINICAL CONSIDERATION: FAMILIAL HYPERCHOLESTEROLEMIA (FH)**

    1. FH is an autosomal dominant genetic disorder caused by more than 400 different mutations in the *LDLR* gene on **chromosome 19p13.1-13.3** for the low-density lipoprotein receptor, which binds LDL and delivers LDL into the cell cytoplasm.

    2. Mutations in the *LDLR* gene are grouped into six classes:
        a. **Class 1** mutations prevent LDLR synthesis.
        b. **Class 2** mutations prevent LDLR transport to the cell membrane.
        c. **Class 3** mutations prevent LDL binding to LDLR.
        d. **Class 4** mutations prevent LDL internalization into the cell cytoplasm by coated pits.
        e. **Class 5** mutations prevent LDLR recycling back to the cell membrane after LDL + LDLR dissociation.
        f. **Class 6** mutations prevent LDLR targeting to the apical membrane adjacent to the blood capillaries.

    3. **Clinical features include:** premature heart disease as a result of atheromas (deposits of LDL-derived cholesterol in the coronary arteries), xanthomas (cholesterol deposits in the skin and tendons), and arcus lipoides (deposits of cholesterol around the cornea of the eye). Homozygote and heterozygote phenotypes are known; homozygotes develop severe symptoms early in life and rarely live past 30 years of age, and heterozygotes have plasma cholesterol levels twice that of normal.

Chapter 4

Epithelium

I **Introduction.** Epithelium is a tissue that **covers the body surface, lines body cavities** (e.g., peritoneal, pleural), **lines tubules** (e.g., gastrointestinal tract, blood vessels, kidney tubules), and **forms glands** (e.g., exocrine, endocrine). Epithelium is **avascular** and has a **high regeneration capacity** ranging from a **few days** (e.g., epithelium lining small intestine) to **1 month** (e.g., epidermis of the skin).

II **Classification of Epithelium (Table 4-1)**

TABLE 4-1	CLASSIFICATION AND LOCATION OF VARIOUS EPITHELIA
Type of Epithelium	**Location in the Body**
Simple squamous	Type I pneumocytes of alveoli, parietal layer of Bowman capsule, endothelium of blood and lymph vessels, mesothelium of body cavities, corneal endothelium
Simple cuboidal	Lining of respiratory bronchioles, thyroid follicular cells, germinal epithelium of ovary, lens of eye, pigment epithelium of retina, ependymal cells of choroid plexus
Simple columnar	Lining of pulmonary bronchioles, lining of gastrointestinal tract, lining of anal canal above anal valves, lining of uterus and uterine tubes, lining of large excretory ducts of glands, lining of efferent ductules
Stratified squamous	Epidermis of skin, lining of oral cavity and esophagus, lining of anal canal below anal valves, lining of vagina, corneal epithelium, lining of female urethra, lining of fossa navicularis of the penile urethra
Stratified columnar	Lining of membranous and penile urethra up to fossa navicularis
Pseudostratified	Lining of trachea and primary bronchi; lining of epididymis, ductus deferens, and ejaculatory duct
Transitional	Lining of renal calyces, renal pelvis, ureters, urinary bladder, and prostatic urethra

Apical Region (Figure 4-1). The apical region of an epithelial cell is characterized by the following specializations.

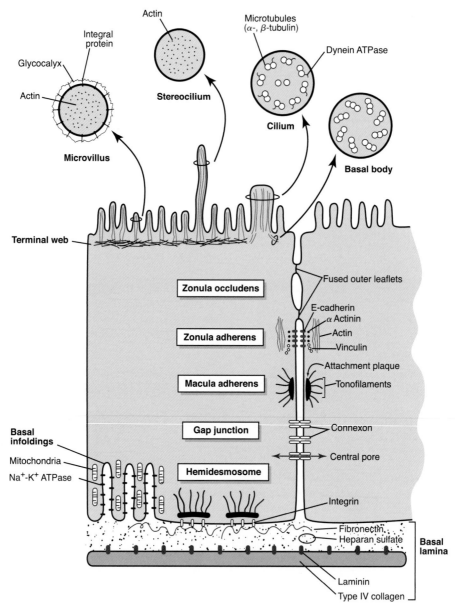

● **Figure 4-1** Diagram of a hypothetical epithelial cell demonstrating the specializations in the apical, lateral, and basal regions.

A. **MICROVILLI** contain a core of **actin** filaments that are anchored to the **terminal web**. The actin filaments are cross-linked by villin. Microvilli of intestinal epithelium are coated with a **glycocalyx** that consists of **terminal oligosaccharides of integral membrane proteins**. The glycocalyx has enzymatic activity involved in carbohydrate digestion.

B. **STEREOCILIA** are long microvilli found on epididymal epithelium and hair cells of the inner ear.

C. **CILIA** are motile cell processes that contain a core of microtubules (α- and β-tubulin) called the **axoneme**. The axoneme consists of nine doublet microtubules uniformly spaced around two central microtubules (**9 + 2 arrangement**). **Nexin** connects the nine doublet microtubules. Each doublet has **short arms** that consist of **dynein adenosine triphosphatase (ATPase)**, which splits adenosine triphosphate (ATP) to provide energy for cilia movement. At the base of each cilium is a **basal body** that consists of nine triplet microtubules and no central microtubules (**9 + 0 arrangement**).

 Lateral Region (Figure 4-1). The lateral region of an epithelial cell is characterized by the following specializations.

A. **ZONULA OCCLUDENS (TIGHT JUNCTION)**
1. The zonula occludens (or tight junction) extends around the **entire perimeter** of the cell. The outer leaflets of the cell membrane of the two adjoining cells **fuse** at various points.
2. The zonula occludens is the gatekeeper of the **paracellular pathway,** thereby regulating the passage of fluid, electrolytes, macromolecules, and immune cells through the intercellular space between epithelial cells. Various epithelia have been classified either as "tight" or "leaky" based on the permeability of the zonula occludens.
3. The zonula occludens can be rapidly formed and disassembled (e.g., during leukocyte migration across endothelium).
4. The proteins **occludin** and **claudin** play a role in regulating the paracellular pathway.

B. **ZONULA ADHERENS**
1. The zonula adherens extends around the **entire perimeter** of the cell.
2. The cell membranes of the two adjoining cells are separated by an intercellular space filled with an amorphous material.
3. There is a dense area on the cytoplasmic side of each cell that consists of **actin** filaments, which are linked by α-**actinin** and **vinculin** to a transmembrane protein called **E-cadherin** (or adherens cell adhesion molecule [A-CAM]).

C. **MACULA ADHERENS (DESMOSOME)**
1. The macula adherens (desmosome) occurs at **small discrete sites.**
2. The cell membranes of the two adjoining cells are separated by an intercellular space filled with a **thin dense line** of material. An **attachment plaque** on the cytoplasmic side of each cell anchors **tonofilaments.**
3. Several protein components of the desmosome have been identified:
   a. **Desmoglein I** and **desmocollin I and II** are calcium-binding proteins that mediate calcium-dependent cell adhesion.
   b. **Desmoplakin I and II** are located in the attachment plaque.

D. **GAP JUNCTION (NEXUS)**
1. The gap junction (nexus) occurs at **small discrete sites** for the **metabolic and electrical coupling** of cells.
2. The cell membranes of the two adjoining cells are separated by an intercellular space that is bridged by **connexons.**
3. Connexons consist of complexes of the transmembrane protein called **connexin.**

4. Connexons contain central pores that allow passage of ions, cyclic adenosine monophosphate (cAMP), amino acids, steroids, and small molecules (<1200 d) between cells. The opening and closing of the pores is regulated by intracellular levels of calcium.

5. Gap junctions are also found between osteocytes, astrocytes, cardiac muscle cells, smooth muscle cells, and endocrine cells.

 Basal Region (Figure 4-1). The basal region of an epithelial cell is characterized by the following specializations.

A. BASAL INFOLDINGS

1. Basal infoldings are invaginations of the cell membrane that contain **ion pumps** (e.g., Na^+-K^+ ATPase) found in close association with **mitochondria**, which provide the substrate ATP.

2. Basal infoldings are found in the proximal and distal convoluted tubules of the kidney and in ducts of salivary glands.

B. HEMIDESMOSOMES

1. Hemidesmosomes are junctions that anchor epithelial cells to the underlying basal lamina via a transmembrane protein called **integrin** and hemidesmosomal proteins called **BP230** and **BP180**. As a result, hemidesmosomes provide a connection between the **cytoskeleton** of the epithelial cell and the **extracellular matrix**.

C. BASAL LAMINA (OR BASEMENT MEMBRANE)

1. The principal constituents are **fibronectin** (binds to integrin of the hemidesmosome), **heparan sulfate, laminin,** and **type IV collagen**.

2. The basal lamina **forms a barrier** between epithelium and connective tissue. **In normal conditions**, lymphocytes may pass through the basal lamina (e.g., during immune surveillance). **In cancerous conditions**, neoplastic cells may pass through the basal lamina (e.g., during malignant invasion).

3. The basal lamina **serves as a filter** (e.g., in the renal glomerulus).

4. The basal lamina **plays a role in regeneration** (e.g., epithelial, nerve, or muscle cells use the basal lamina as scaffolding during regeneration or wound healing).

 Clinical Considerations

A. PRIMARY CILIARY DYSKINESIA (PCD; IMMOTILE CILIA SYNDROME)/ KARTAGENER SYNDROME

1. PCD is an autosomal recessive genetic disorder caused by mutations in the *DNAH5* gene on **chromosome 5p15-p14** for **ci**liary **dy**nein **a**xonemal **h**eavy chain **5** (28% of the cases) or the *DNAI1* gene on **chromosome 9p21-p13** for **dy**nein **a**xonemal **i**ntermediate chain **1** (10% of the cases).

2. Approximately 60% of PCD-affected individuals do not have mutations in the *DNAH5* gene or *DNAI1* gene. It is speculated that mutations in other genes for dynein light chains, spoke head proteins, and other axonemal proteins may be causative.

3. These mutations result in defective outer dynein arms, which results in cilia that are immotile (**ciliary immotility**), beat abnormally (**ciliary dyskinesia**), or are absent (**ciliary aplasia**).

4. **Clinical features include:** chronic cough, chronic rhinitis, chronic sinusitis, chronic/ recurrent ear infections, recurrent sinus/pulmonary infections due to a defect of cilia in the respiratory pathways, neonatal respiratory distress, digital clubbing, sterility in males (retarded sperm movement), sterility in females (immotility of oviduct cilia), situs inversus totalis (mirror-image reversal of all visceral organs with no apparent consequences; PCD with situs inversus totalis is called **Kartagener syndrome**), and heterotaxy (discordance of right and left patterns of ordinarily asymmetric structures with significant malformations, e.g., asplenia or polysplenia). The gold standard diagnostic test is the appearance of ciliary ultrastructural defects obtained by electron microscopy of a respiratory epithelium biopsy.

B. PEMPHIGUS (BUBBLE) VULGARIS

1. Pemphigus vulgaris is an autoimmune blistering disease in which autoantibodies are formed against a **desmosomal protein** called **desmoglein.** The autoantibodies interfere with the attachment of epidermal cells to each other (acantholysis). The cause for the formation of the autoantibodies is unknown.
2. **Clinical features include:** flaccid blisters that begin in the oropharynx and then spread to the skin of the face, scalp, chest, axillae, and groin; the blisters rupture easily so the patient may present only with skin erosions. All patients will develop oropharyngeal disease at some point.

C. BULLOUS PEMPHIGOID

1. Bullous pemphigoid is an autoimmune blistering disease in which autoantibodies are formed against **hemidesmosomal glycoproteins** called **BP230** and **BP180.** The autoantibodies interfere with the attachment of the epidermis to the basal lamina. The cause for the formation of the autoantibodies is unknown.
2. **Clinical features include:** widespread blistering eruption in middle-aged or elderly patients (>60 years of age) who are taking multiple medications (e.g., penicillamine, furosemide); blisters commonly occur in the flexural areas, groin, and axillae. Deposits of autoantibodies and complement are found in a linear pattern at the junction of the epidermis and dermis (i.e., basal lamina zone), and pruritus (itching) is a common feature.

D. CARCINOMA is a malignant neoplasm derived from epithelium.

E. ADENOCARCINOMA is a malignant neoplasm derived from glandular epithelium.

F. SQUAMOUS CARCINOMA is a malignant neoplasm derived from squamous epithelium.

G. TRANSITIONAL CARCINOMA is a malignant neoplasm derived from transitional epithelium (e.g., urinary tract).

VII Selected Photomicrographs (Figure 4-2)

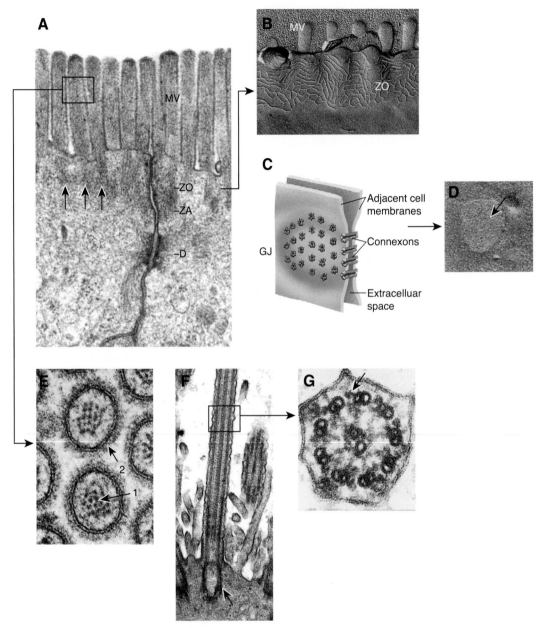

● **Figure 4-2 Epithelial components. A:** Electron micrograph (EM) of a junctional complex that exists between adjoining epithelial cells. Note the zonula occludens (ZO), zonula adherens (ZA), and macula adherens of desmosome (D). Note the actin core of the microvilli (MV) extending into the terminal web (*arrows*) within the cytoplasm. **B:** A freeze-fracture replica of a zonula occludens or tight junction. A beltlike band of anastomosing strands (ZO) can be observed. The strands are seen as ridges of intramembranous particles on the P-face or complementary grooves on the E-face. Microvilli (MV) are apparent. **C:** Diagram of a gap junction (GJ) or nexus between adjoining cells. **D:** A freeze-fracture replica of a gap junction or nexus shows a cluster of intramembranous particles (*arrow*) on the P-face. Each intramembranous particle corresponds to a connexon. Gap junctions are constructed from transmembrane proteins (called connexins) that form structures called connexons. Two connexons bridge across the intercellular space to form a channel (or pore) connecting two cells. **E:** EM of microvilli in cross section demonstrating the actin core (*arrow 1*) and the fuzzy glycocalyx (*arrow 2*). **F:** EM of a cilium in longitundinal section. Note the microtubule core extending into the basal body within the cytoplasm. **G:** EM of a cilium in cross section. Note the arrangement of microtubules in a 9 + 2 arrangement and the dynein arm (*arrow*).

Chapter 5

Connective Tissue

I. **Introduction.** Types of connective tissue include loose connective tissue (e.g., fascia, lamina propria), dense connective tissue (e.g., tendons), adipose tissue, cartilage, and bone. The common features of all connective tissues are the **ground substance, fibers, and cells,** as described below.

II. **Ground Substance** contains the following components.

A. Proteoglycans consist of a **core protein,** which binds many side chains of glycosaminoglycans (GAGs), and a **link protein,** which binds hyaluronic acid. GAGs are highly sulfated (SO_4^{2-}) and consist of **repeating disaccharide units** of a **hexosamine** (e.g., N-acetylglucosamine, N-acetylgalactosamine) and a **uronic acid** (e.g., glucuronic acid). Specific GAGs include the following.

1. **Hyaluronic acid** is found in most connective tissues and binds to the link protein of a large number of proteoglycans to form a proteoglycan aggregate.
2. **Chondroitin sulfate** is found in cartilage and bone.
3. **Keratan sulfate** is found in cartilage and bone, cornea, and intervertebral disc.
4. **Dermatan sulfate** is found in dermis of skin, blood vessels, and heart valves.
5. **Heparan sulfate** is found in the basal lamina (e.g., glomerular kidney basement membrane).

B. **GLYCOPROTEINS**
1. **Fibronectin** is a component of the basal lamina.
2. **Laminin** is a component of the basal lamina.
3. **Chondronectin** is found in cartilage.
4. **Osteocalcin, osteopontin, and bone sialoprotein** are found in bone.

C. **THE MINERAL (INORGANIC) COMPONENT** varies depending on the type of connective tissue.

D. **WATER (TISSUE FLUID).** The high concentration of negative charges due to sulfation (SO_4^{2-}) and carboxylation (COO–) of GAGs attracts water into the ground substance.

III. **Fibers**

A. **COLLAGEN** contains two characteristic amino acids, **hydroxyproline** and **hydroxylysine.**
1. **Synthesis of collagen** involves intracellular and extracellular events.
   a. **Intracellular events** include:
      i. **Synthesis of preprocollagen** within rough endoplasmic reticulum (rER)
      ii. **Hydroxylation of proline and lysine** within rER catalyzed by **peptidyl proline hydroxylase** and **peptidyl lysine hydroxylase** (Vitamin C is essential in this step. When vitamin C deficiency [i.e., scurvy] occurs, wounds fail to heal, bone formation is impaired, and teeth become loose.)

          iii. **Glycosylation of hydroxylysine** within rER
          iv. **Formation of triple helix procollagen** within rER (involves registration peptides)
          v. **Addition of carbohydrates** within Golgi complex
          vi. **Secretion of procollagen**
      b. **Extracellular events** include:
          i. **Cleavage of procollagen** to form **tropocollagen** by extracellular peptidases
          ii. **Self-assembly of tropocollagen** into fibrils (**67-nm periodicity**)
          iii. **Cross-linking of adjacent** tropocollagen molecules catalyzed by lysyl oxidase
  2. **Types of collagen (Table 5-1)**

TABLE 5-1	DISTRIBUTION OF COLLAGEN TYPES IN THE BODY
Type	**Location in Body**
I	Fibrocartilage, bone, dermis of skin, tendons, cornea, fascia In **wound healing,** type I replaces the initial type III collagen **Most ubiquitous type of collagen** Involved in Ehlers-Danlos syndrome and osteogenesis imperfecta
II	Hyaline cartilage, elastic cartilage, nucleus pulposus, vitreous body
III	Liver, spleen, tunica media of blood vessels, muscularis externa of gastrointestinal tract In **wound healing,** type III is laid down first In **keloid formation,** increased amounts of type III are laid down Traditionally called **reticular fibers** Involved in Ehlers-Danlos syndrome
IV	Basal lamina Involved in Alport syndrome (hereditary nephritis)

  B. **ELASTIC FIBERS** consist of an amorphous core of the **elastin** protein surrounded by microfibrils of the **fibrillin** protein. Elastic fibers contain two unique amino acids called **desmosine** and **isodesmosine**, which are involved in cross-linking.

Cells

  A. **RESIDENT OR FIXED CELLS** are a stable population of cells that remain in the connective tissue. These include the following types of cells.
    1. **Fibroblasts/fibrocytes** are fixed cells that are involved in the secretion of collagen and ground substance.
    2. **Macrophages (histiocytes)**
      a. Macrophages arise from **monocytes** within the circulating blood and bone marrow.
      b. Macrophages have a **phagocytic function.**
          i. F_C **antibody receptors** on the macrophage cell membrane bind antibody-coated foreign material and subsequently phagocytose the material for lysosomal digestion.
          ii. **C3 (a component of complement) receptors** on the macrophage cell membrane bind bacteria and subsequently phagocytose the bacteria (called opsonization) for lysosomal digestion.
          iii. Certain phagocytosed material (e.g., bacilli of tuberculosis and leprosy, *Trypanosoma cruzi*, *Toxoplasma*, *Leishmania*, asbestos) cannot undergo lysosomal digestion, so macrophages will fuse to form **foreign body giant cells.**

iv. In sites of chronic inflammation, macrophages may assemble into epithelial-like sheets called **epithelioid cells of granulomas.**

c. Macrophages have an **antigen-presenting function.**

   i. **Exogenous antigens** circulating in the bloodstream are phagocytosed by macrophages and undergo degradation in endosomal acid vesicles.

   ii. Antigen proteins are degraded into **antigen peptide fragments,** which are presented on the macrophage cell surface in conjunction with class II major histocompatibility complex (MHC).

   iii. **CD4+ helper T cells** with antigen-specific T-cell receptors (TcR) on their cell surface recognize the antigen peptide fragment.

d. Macrophages are activated by **lipopolysaccharides** (a surface component of gram-negative bacteria) and **interferon-γ.**

e. Macrophages secrete **interleukin-1** (IL-1; stimulates mitosis of T lymphocytes), **interleukin-6** (IL-6; stimulates differentiation of B lymphocytes into plasma cells), **pyrogens** (mediate fever), **tumor necrosis factor-α (TNF-α),** and **granulocyte–macrophage colony-stimulating factor (GM-CSF).**

f. Macrophages have granules that are endolysosomes that contain **acid hydrolases, aryl sulfatase, acid phosphatases,** and **peroxidase.**

g. Macrophages impart natural (innate) immunity along with neutrophils and natural killer (NK) cells.

3. **Mast cells**

a. Mast cells arise from stem cells in the bone marrow.

b. Mast cells have a function in **type I anaphylactic reactions, inflammation, and allergic reactions.**

c. Mast cells have **immunoglobulin E (IgE) antibody receptors** on their cell membranes that **bind IgE** produced by plasma cells upon **first exposure** to an allergen (e.g., plant pollen, snake venom, foreign serum), which sensitizes the mast cells.

d. Mast cells secrete the following substances upon **second exposure** to the same allergen, causing the classic **wheal-and-flare reaction** in the skin:

   i. **Heparin,** an anticoagulant and cofactor for lipoprotein lipase (LPL)

   ii. **Histamine** (produced by decarboxylation of histidine), which increases vascular permeability, causes vasodilation, causes smooth muscle contraction of bronchi, and stimulates HCl secretion from parietal cells in the stomach.

   iii. **Leukotrienes C_4 and D_4** (are eicosanoids and components of slow-reacting substance of anaphylaxis [SRS-A]), which increase vascular permeability, cause vasodilation, and cause smooth muscle contraction of bronchi

   iv. **Eosinophil chemotactic factor (ECF-A),** which attracts eosinophils to the inflammation site

4. **Adipocytes**

a. Adipocytes in **multilocular (brown) adipose tissue** contain numerous fat droplets and **numerous mitochondria that lack elementary particles** on the inner membrane. The energy produced by these mitochondria is dissipated as heat instead of being stored as adenosine triphosphate (ATP). Brown adipose tissue is present in **human infants after birth** to assist in **regulation of body temperature** but disappears within a few years. Multilocular adipose tissue has a brown color due to the numerous mitochondria that contain **cytochromes,** which have a color similar to hemoglobin.

b. Adipocytes in **unilocular (white) adipose tissue** contain a large, single fat droplet surrounded by a thin rim of cytoplasm. This tissue accounts for all of the stored fat in humans and has a yellow color due to the presence of carotene.

5. **Chondroblasts and chondrocytes** are discussed in Chapter 6.

6. **Osteoblasts and osteocytes** are discussed in Chapter 7.

B. **TRANSIENT OR FREE CELLS** enter connective tissue from blood, usually during inflammation. These cells include neutrophils, eosinophils, basophils, monocytes, B lymphocytes, plasma cells, and T lymphocytes, which are discussed in Chapter 9.

Ⅴ Clinical Considerations

A. **OSTEOGENESIS IMPERFECTA (OI).** OI is a group of disorders (types I through VII) with a continuum ranging from perinatal lethality → severe skeletal deformities → nearly asymptomatic individuals.
  1. OI (types I through IV) are autosomal dominant genetic disorders caused by mutations where at least two different genes have been implicated thus far:
     a. *COL1A1* gene on chromosome 17q21.3-q22 for collagen pro-**α**-1 (I) chain of type I procollagen
     b. *COL1A2* gene on chromosome 7q22.1 for collagen pro-**α**-2 (I) chain of type I procollagen
  2. **Clinical features include:** extreme bone fragility with spontaneous fractures, short stature with bone deformities, gray or brown teeth, **blue sclera of the eye**, and progressive postpubertal hearing loss. Milder forms of OI may be confused with child abuse. Severe forms of OI are fatal in utero or during the early neonatal period.

B. **ALPORT SYNDROME (HEREDITARY NEPHRITIS)**
  1. Alport syndrome is an X-linked genetic disorder (80% of cases) caused by a mutation in the *COL4A5* gene on Xq22 chromosome for collagen pro-**α**-5 (IV) chain of type IV procollagen.
  2. **Clinical features include:** an initial manifestation as asymptomatic persistent microscopic hematuria; glomerular disease that leads to end-stage renal disease; ocular abnormalities (e.g., anterior lenticonus, which is a conical protrusion on the anterior aspect of the lens due to thinning of the lens capsule); sensorineural hearing loss due to impaired adhesion of the organ of Corti to the basilar membrane; and an **irregularly thickened glomerular basement membrane** with interlacing lamellae.

C. **CLASSIC-TYPE EHLERS-DANLOS SYNDROME (EDS)**
  1. EDS is an autosomal dominant genetic disorder caused by mutations where at least two different genes have been implicated thus far:
     a. *COL5A1* gene on chromosome 9q34.2-q34.3 for collagen pro-**α**-1 (V) chain of type V procollagen
     b. *COL5A2* gene on chromosome 2q31 for collagen pro-**α**-2 (V) chain of type V procollagen
  2. **Clinical features include:** extremely stretchable and fragile skin, hypermobile joints, aneurysms of blood vessels, rupture of the bowel, abnormal wound healing, and widened atrophic scars.

D. **MARFAN SYNDROME (MFS)**
  1. MFS is an autosomal dominant genetic disorder caused by a mutation in the *FBN1* gene on chromosome 15q21.1 for the fibrillin-1 protein, which is an essential component of **microfibrils** found in both elastic and nonelastic tissue. Microfibrils play a role in the formation of the elastic matrix (i.e., **elastic fibers**), elastic matrix–cell attachments, and regulation of growth factors.
  2. **Clinical features include:** unusually tall individuals; exceptionally long, thin limbs; pectus excavatum ("hollow chest"); scoliosis; **ectopia lentis (dislocation of the lens)**; severe near-sightedness (myopia); and **dilatation or dissection of the aorta** at the level of the sinuses of Valsalva, which may lead to cardiomyopathy or even a rupture of the aorta, dural ectasia, and mitral valve prolapse.

E. HOMOCYSTINURIA is a genetic defect involving the enzyme cystathionine synthetase, resulting in abnormal cross-linking of collagen.

F. KELOID FORMATION is a deviation in normal wound healing whereby an excessive accumulation of collagen occurs, resulting in a raised, tumorous scar.

G. AMYLOIDOSIS is a group of diseases that have in common the **deposition of amyloid** (a proteinaceous substance) in the intercellular space of various organs.

    1. By light microscopy, amyloid is an eosinophilic, amorphous substance. By electron microscopy, amyloid is composed of **nonbranching fibrillar proteins** (95%) and a glycoprotein called **P component**, which is pentagonal in shape (5%).

    2. A number of different nonbranching fibrillar proteins have been identified, which include:

        a. **Amyloid light chain**, an immunoglobulin protein secreted by plasma cells

        b. **Amyloid-associated protein**, synthesized by the liver

        c. β_2**-Microglobulin**, a component of the MHC class I proteins

        d. β_2**-Amyloid**, a 4000-d peptide

        e. **Islet amyloid polypeptide (amylin)**, which is increased within pancreatic islets of Langerhans in patients with type 2 diabetes

    3. Types of amyloidosis include the following.

        a. **Immunocyte dyscrasias with amyloidosis (primary amyloidosis)** is the most common form of amyloidosis and is associated with the amyloid light chain protein. Some patients with **multiple myeloma** (a plasma cell neoplasia) demonstrate amyloidosis along with the presence of light chains (**Bence Jones proteins**) in the serum and urine.

        b. **Reactive systemic amyloidosis (secondary amyloidosis)** occurs as a secondary complication to chronic inflammation (e.g., rheumatoid arthritis, regional enteritis, ulcerative colitis) and is associated with the amyloid-associated protein.

        c. **Hemodialysis-associated amyloidosis** occurs in patients on **long-term hemodialysis** and is associated with the β_2-microglobulin protein.

        d. **Senile cerebral amyloidosis** occurs in patients with **Alzheimer disease** and is associated with β_2-amyloid protein deposition in cerebral plaques.

        e. **Endocrine amyloid** occurs in patients with **type 2 diabetes** and is associated with islet amyloid polypeptide deposition in the pancreatic islets.

VI Selected Photomicrographs (Figure 5-1)

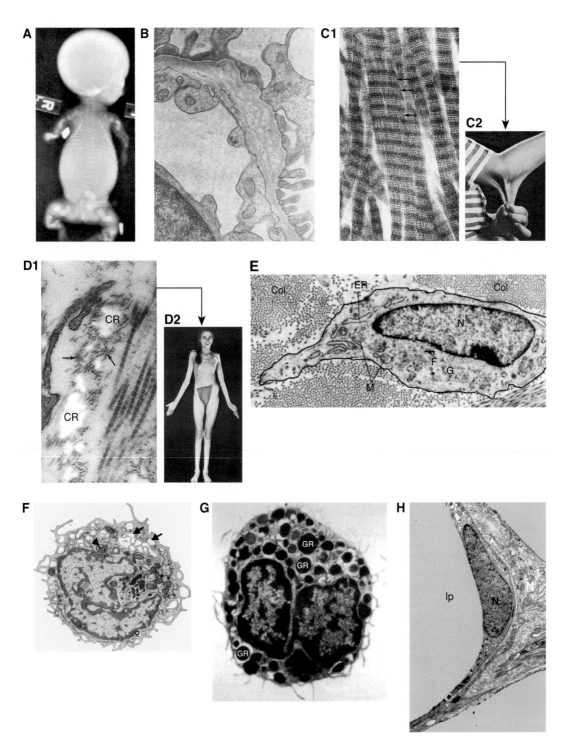

● **Figure 5-1 Connective tissue. A:** Osteogenesis imperfecta. Radiograph shows multiple bone fractures of the upper and lower limbs resulting in an accordionlike shortening of the limbs. **B:** Alport syndrome (hereditary nephritis). Electron micrograph (EM) shows an irregularly thickened glomerular basement membrane with interlacing lamellae instead of forming a normal single dense band. **C1:** EM of collagen fibers. Note the 67-nm periodicity (*arrows*). **C2:** Ehlers-Danlos syndrome. Note the extremely stretchable skin at the elbow. **D1:** EM of elastic fibers. Note the amorphous core (CR) of elastin protein and the microfibrils (*arrows*) of the fibrillin protein. **D2:** Marfan syndrome. Note the tall stature, exceptionally long limbs, and arachnodactyly (elongated hands and feet with very slender digits). **E:** EM of a fibroblast. Fibroblasts (F) have a centrally located, cigar-shaped nucleus (N). The cytoplasm is characterized by a well-developed rough endoplasmic reticulum (rER), mitochondria (M), Golgi (G), and secretory vesicles reflecting active collagen (Col) synthesis. **F:** EM of a macrophage. Macrophages have an ovoid nucleus that is frequently indented on one side to become bean shaped. The cell surface is uneven, varying from short projections to long, thin, fingerlike projections. The cytoplasm is characterized by phagolysosomes (*arrowhead*) and phagocytic vacuoles (*arrows*) reflecting their phagocytic activity. **G:** EM of a mast cell. Mast cells have a centrally located, ovoid-shaped nucleus (but irregular borders may be apparent as in this EM). The cytoplasm is characterized by numerous secretory granules (Gr) that display variations in morphology. **H:** EM of an adipocyte. Adipocytes have an eccentrically located nucleus (N) and a thin rim of cytoplasm giving the "signet ring" appearance. The cytoplasm is characterized by a small Golgi, few mitochondria, sparse rER, abundant free ribosomes, and a large lipid droplet (lp) that is not membrane bound.

Chapter 6

Cartilage

I   **Introduction.** Cartilage is a type of connective tissue that includes **hyaline cartilage** (e.g., articular ends of long bones), **elastic cartilage** (e.g., pinna of ear), and **fibrocartilage** (e.g., annulus fibrosus of the intervertebral disc). Cartilage has all the common features of connective tissue, which include ground substance, fibers, and cells, as indicated in the following sections.

II   **Ground Substance** consists of:

A.   **PROTEOGLYCANS,** containing side chains of **glycosaminoglycans (GAGs),** specifically **chondroitin sulfate** and **keratan sulfate**

B.   **GLYCOPROTEINS,** including **chondronectin** and **chondrocalcin** (a calcium-binding protein)

C.   **NO MINERAL (INORGANIC) COMPONENT,** because cartilage is not mineralized

D.   **WATER (TISSUE FLUID)**—high degree of hydration (75%)

III   **Fibers**

A.   **TYPE I COLLAGEN** is found in fibrocartilage.

B.   **TYPE II COLLAGEN** is found in hyaline and elastic cartilage.

IV   **Cells**

A.   **CHONDROGENIC CELLS** are found in the **perichondrium,** where they undergo mitosis and differentiate into chondroblasts.

B.   **CHONDROBLASTS** arise from chondrogenic cells and may undergo mitosis.

C.   **CHONDROCYTES** reside in lacunae. They form **isogenous groups** that are surrounded by a **territorial matrix** that stains basophilic due to the higher local concentration of chondroitin sulfate. Chondrocytes may undergo mitosis.

V   **Blood Vessels and Nerves** are absent. Like epithelium, cartilage is **avascular.** It receives its nutrients by **diffusion** through the ground substance.

Chondrogenesis occurs in the embryo when mesodermal cells withdraw their processes and condense into aggregations called **centers of chondrification**. Cartilage may then grow in the following ways.

A. **INTERSTITIAL GROWTH** occurs by mitosis of preexisting chondrocytes.

B. **APPOSITIONAL GROWTH** occurs by differentiation of chondrogenic cells in the perichondrium into chondroblasts.

Hormonal Influence

A. **PROTEIN HORMONES**
   1. **Growth hormone (GH)** stimulates hepatocytes in the liver to produce **somatomedin C (or insulin-like growth factor 1; IGF-1)**, which stimulates cartilage growth.

B. **STEROID HORMONES**
   1. **Triiodothyronine (T$_3$), thyroxine (T$_4$),** and **testosterone** stimulate cartilage growth.
   2. **Estradiol, cortisone,** and **hydrocortisone** inhibit cartilage growth.

 Repair. In the adult, damaged cartilage shows limited repair (regeneration) and may form scar tissue instead of cartilage. In young children, damaged cartilage shows a greater capacity for repair.

Chapter 7

Bone

I **Introduction.** Bone is a type of connective tissue that has a **supportive and protective function** and also serves as a **reservoir for Ca^{2+} and $PO_4{}^{3-}$**. Bone has all the common features of connective tissue, which include ground substance, fibers, and cells, as indicated in the following sections.

II **Ground Substance** consists of:

A. **PROTEOGLYCANS** containing a side chain of glycosaminoglycans (GAGs), specifically **chondroitin sulfate** and **keratan sulfate**

B. **GLYCOPROTEINS,** such as **osteonectin** and **osteocalcin** (a calcium-binding protein)

C. **A MINERAL (INORGANIC) COMPONENT** that includes $Ca_{10}(PO_4)_6OH_2$ (**hydroxyapatite crystals**), $C_6H_5O_7{}^{3-}$ (**citrate ions**), and $CO_3{}^{2-}$ (**carbonate ions**). The mineral component makes up approximately 75% of the bone mass and contributes to the **hardness/rigidity** of bone.

D. **WATER (TISSUE FLUID),** which contributes to a low degree of hydration (7%)

III **Fibers** consist of **type I collagen** that provides **tensile strength** to bone.

IV **Cells**

A. **OSTEOPROGENITOR CELLS** differentiate into osteoblasts during osteogenesis and bone repair and undergo mitosis.

B. **OSTEOBLASTS**
   1. Osteoblasts are derived from osteoprogenitor cells.
   2. Osteoblasts secrete **osteoid,** which is unmineralized bone matrix consisting of proteoglycans, glycoproteins, and type I collagen.
      a. For mineralization to occur, osteoblasts secrete **osteocalcin** and **alkaline phosphatase,** which hydrolyzes phosphate-containing substrates as well as Ca^{2+} β-glycerophosphate to release Ca^{2+} and $PO_4{}^{3-}$.
      b. In addition, osteoblasts release **matrix vesicles** (membrane-bound vesicles), which concentrate Ca^{2+} and $PO_4{}^{3-}$ and are the most important factor for mineralization to occur.
      c. Clinical markers for osteogenesis or bone repair: **serum alkaline phosphatase** and **serum osteocalcin**
   3. Osteoblasts secrete **interleukin-1 (IL-1),** which is a potent stimulator of osteoclast activity.

   4. Osteoblasts possess the **parathyroid hormone (PTH) receptor** and the **1,25-(OH)$_2$ vitamin D receptor.**
   5. Osteoblasts do *not* undergo mitosis.

C. OSTEOCYTES
   1. Osteocytes and their cytoplasmic processes are surrounded by bone matrix as they reside in spaces called **lacunae** and **canaliculi**, respectively. Cytoplasmic processes of neighboring osteocytes communicate via **gap junctions.**
   2. Osteocytes do *not* undergo mitosis.

D. OSTEOCLASTS
   1. Osteoclasts are derived from **granulocyte–monocyte progenitor cells** within the bone marrow.
   2. Osteoclasts are multinucleated cells that reside in shallow depressions of the bone called **Howship lacunae.**
   3. Osteoclasts function in **bone resorption** in the following ways:
      a. Secrete **lysosomal enzymes** (e.g., β-glucuronidase, aryl sulfatase) to digest the proteoglycans of the bone matrix
      b. Secrete **collagenase** to digest type I collagen of the bone matrix
   4. Osteoclasts have a **ruffled border** (infoldings of the cell membrane) closest to the bone that contains **H$^+$ adenosine triphosphatase (ATPase)** and **carbonic anhydrase**, which produces H$^+$ ions that create an acidic environment to digest the mineral component of the bone matrix.
   5. Clinical markers for bone resorption: **urine hydroxyproline** (amino acid unique to collagen) and **urine pyridinoline cross-links**
   6. Osteoclasts possess the **calcitonin receptor.**
   7. Osteoclasts do *not* undergo mitosis.

V. Blood Vessels and Nerves are present in Haversian canals and Volkmann canals. However, they are absent in lacunae and canaliculi.

VI. Osteogenesis always occurs by replacing preexisting connective tissue. In the embryo, two types of osteogenesis occur.

A. INTRAMEMBRANOUS OSSIFICATION occurs in the embryo when mesoderm condenses into sheets of highly vascular connective tissue, which then forms a primary ossification center. Bones that form via intramembranous ossification include **flat bones of the skull.**

B. ENDOCHONDRAL OSSIFICATION occurs in the embryo when mesoderm initially forms a hyaline cartilage model, which then develops a primary ossification center at the diaphysis. Later, secondary ossification centers form at the epiphysis at each end of the bone. Bones that form via endochondral ossification include the **humerus, femur, tibia, and other long bones.**
   1. **Growth in length of long bones** occurs at the **epiphyseal plate**, which includes a number of zones, as indicated to follow.
      a. **Zone of reserve** contains resting chondrocytes.
      b. **Zone of proliferation** contains chondrocytes undergoing mitosis and forming isogenous groups.
      c. **Zone of hypertrophy** contains hypertrophied chondrocytes, which secrete alkaline phosphatase to increase calcium and phosphate levels.
      d. **Zone of calcification** contains dead chondrocytes and calcified cartilage matrix called spicules.

e. **Zone of ossification** contains osteoprogenitor cells that congregate on spicules and differentiate into osteoblasts. Osteoblasts deposit bone on the surface of a spicule to form a **mixed spicule**, which consists of calcified cartilage matrix and bone.

2. **Growth in diameter of long bones** occurs at the **diaphysis** by deposition of bone at the periphery (**appositional growth**) as osteoprogenitor cells within the **periosteum** differentiate into osteoblasts.

 Bone Repair. In the adult, bone shows a high capacity for repair through the proliferation of osteoprogenitor cells. After a bone fracture, the following actions take place.

A. Ruptured blood vessels form a **hematoma**, which bridges the fracture gap and provides a meshwork for the influx of inflammatory cells that secrete products to activate osteoprogenitor cells to form osteoblasts.

B. After 1 week, the hematoma is organized into a **soft tissue callus (procallus)** that anchors the ends of the fracture but provides no rigidity for weight bearing.

C. Osteoblasts begin to deposit **immature woven bone**. Woven bone is formed whenever osteoblasts produce osteoid rapidly and is characterized by an irregular arrangement of collagen.

D. Mesenchymal cells in the procallus form **hyaline cartilage** at the periphery that envelops the fracture site. The hyaline cartilage undergoes endochondral ossification.

E. The collection of bone at the fracture is now called a **bony callus**. As the bony callus mineralizes, controlled weight bearing can be tolerated.

F. Eventually all the woven bone of the bony callus is remodeled into **mature lamellar bone**. Lamellar bone is characterized by a regular layered arrangement of collagen.

 Hormonal Influence

A. PROTEIN HORMONES

1. **Growth hormone (GH)** stimulates hepatocytes in the liver to produce **somatomedin C (or insulin-like growth factor 1; IGF-1)**, which promotes skeletal growth and bone remodeling.

2. **PTH** acts directly on osteoblasts to secrete **macrophage colony-stimulating factor (M-CSF)** and cause the expression of a cell surface protein called RANKL. M-CSF stimulates monocytes to differentiate into macrophages and express a cell surface receptor called **RANK**. RANKL (on the osteoblasts) and RANK (on the macrophage) interact and cause the differentiation of macrophages into osteoblasts. Osteoblasts **increase bone resorption**, thereby **elevating blood Ca^{2+} levels.**

3. **Calcitonin** acts directly on osteoclasts to **decrease bone resorption**, thereby lowering blood Ca^{2+} levels.

B. STEROID HORMONES

1. **T_3 and T_4** stimulate endochondral ossification and linear growth of bone.

a. **Androgens** and **Estrogens.** The closure of the epiphyseal plate is closely related to the development of the ovaries and testes. In **precocious sexual development**, skeletal growth is stunted due to premature closure of the epiphyseal plate. In **gonadal hypoplasia**, closure of the epiphyseal plate is delayed, and arms or legs become disproportionately long.

2. **Cortisol** inhibits bone formation.

3. **1,25-(OH)$_2$ vitamin D** acts directly on osteoblasts to secrete IL-1, which stimulates osteoclasts to increase bone resorption, thereby **elevating blood Ca^{2+} levels.**

IX Cartilage and Bone Comparison (Table 7-1)

TABLE 7-1	CARTILAGE AND BONE COMPARISON	
Characteristic	**Cartilage**	**Bone**
Ground substance	Chondroitin sulfate, keratan sulfate Chondronectin, chondrocalcin No mineralization High degree of hydration (75%)	Chondroitin sulfate, keratan sulfate Osteonectin, osteocalcin Hydroxyapatite, citrate, bicarbonate Low degree of hydration (7%)
Fibers	Type I collagen (fibrocartilage) Type II collagen (hyaline and elastic)	Type I collagen (provides tensile strength)
Vascularity	Avascular; nutrients received via diffusion	Highly vascular
Nerves	Absent	Present
Growth	Interstitial Appositional	Appositional only
Repair	Low	High
Mitosis	Chondrogenic—yes Chondroblasts—yes Chondrocytes—yes	Osteoprogenitor—yes Osteoblasts—no Osteocytes—no Osteoclasts—no
Communication	No junctions between chondrocytes	Gap junctions between osteocytes
Hormonal influence	GH, T_3, T_4, testosterone, estradiol, cortisone, hydrocortisone	GH, PTH, calcitonin, T_3, T_4, androgens, estrogens, cortisol, 1,25-(OH_2) vitamin D
Vitamin influence	N/A	Vitamin D Vitamin C Vitamin A

GH, growth hormone; T_3, triiodothyronine; T_4, thyroxine; PTH, parathyroid hormone.

X Clinical Considerations of Bone

A. PRIMARY OSTEOPOROSIS (SENILE OR POSTMENOPAUSAL) is a critical loss of bone mass associated with a deficiency of either **GH (senile)** or **estrogen (postmenopausal)**. **Decreased estrogen levels** result in **increased secretion of IL-1** (a potent stimulator of osteoclasts) from monocytes and **increased osteoclast activity**. Osteoporosis is widely recognized as a serious consequence of **chronic glucocorticoid** use to manage diseases including rheumatoid arthritis, inflammatory bowel diseases (e.g., Crohn disease), asthma, emphysema, and rejection of organ transplant. Clinical findings include being asymptomatic in early stages; presentation of vertebral compression fractures, femoral head fractures, or wrist fractures; or slow healing of fractured bones. Severity is assessed by bone densitometry.

B. OSTEOSARCOMA is a malignant tumor in which the tumor cells characteristically **produce bone**. This tumor is usually found in patients between **10 and 20 years old** and most often around the **knee**. **Retinoblastoma** and mutations in the *TP53* gene **(Li-Fraumeni syndrome)** have been implicated in increased risk for osteosarcomas.

C. PAGET DISEASE is characterized by **uncontrolled osteoclast activity**, causing widespread bone resorption followed by intense osteoblast activity, producing woven bone that fills in the erosion. The net effect is paradoxically an increase in bone mass that is architecturally unsound because the woven bone persists.

D. OSTEOMALACIA (in adults) and rickets (in children) are characterized by **lack of minerals within osteoid**, which occurs as a result of **vitamin D deficiency**.

1. To understand osteomalacia and rickets, normal **vitamin D metabolism** must be explained as indicated to follow.
   a. Vitamin D sources include dietary intake and production by skin keratinocytes stimulated by ultraviolet light.
   b. Vitamin D is hydroxylated by liver hepatocytes to **25-(OH) vitamin D**.
   c. 25-(OH) vitamin D is hydroxylated in the kidney to **1,25-(OH)$_2$ vitamin D**, the active metabolite that functions similar to a steroid hormone.
   d. **1,25-(OH)$_2$D stimulates absorption of Ca^{2+} and PO$_4^{3-}$ ions** from the intestinal lumen into the blood, thereby **elevating blood Ca^{2+} and PO$_4^{3-}$ levels.** Ca^{2+} and PO$_4^{3-}$ are used in the normal mineralization of osteoid.
2. **Physical signs of osteomalacia** in adults include bowed legs, increased tendency to fracture, and scoliotic deformity of the vertebral column. **Physical signs of rickets** in nonambulatory children include: craniotabes (elastic recoil of the skull upon compression), "rachitic rosary" (excess osteoid at the costochondral junction), and "pigeon-breast deformity" (anterior protrusion of sternum).

E. ACROMEGALY is characterized by thick bones as a result of excess GH.

F. SCURVY is characterized by **lack of collagen** within osteoid, which occurs as a result of **vitamin C deficiency**. Vitamin C is necessary for the hydroxylation of proline and lysine amino acids during collagen synthesis. Physical signs of scurvy include: poor bone growth and poor fracture repair due to lack of collagen within osteoid, as well as hemorrhages in the skin (purpura), gingival mucosa, and joints due to a weakened tunica media of blood vessels.

G. VITAMIN A. An excess of vitamin A causes a premature closure of the epiphyseal plate, resulting in a person of small stature.

H. OSTEOGENESIS IMPERFECTA (OI). OI is a group of disorders (types I through VII) with a continuum ranging from perinatal lethality → severe skeletal deformities → nearly asymptomatic individuals.
   1. OI types I through IV are autosomal dominant genetic disorders caused by mutations where at least two different genes have been implicated thus far:
      a. *COL1A1* gene on **chromosome 17q21.3-q22** for <u>col</u>lagen pro-**α**-**1** (**I**) chain of type I procollagen
      b. *COL1A2* gene on **chromosome 7q22.1** for <u>col</u>lagen pro-**α**-**2** (**I**) chain of type I procollagen
   2. **Clinical features include:** extreme bone fragility with spontaneous fractures, short stature with bone deformities, gray or brown teeth, **blue sclera of the eye**, and progressive postpubertal hearing loss. Milder forms of OI may be confused with child abuse. Severe forms of OI are fatal in utero or during the early neonatal period.

XI Clinical Considerations of Joints

A. DEGENERATIVE JOINT DISEASE (OSTEOARTHRITIS; OA) is characterized by progressive erosion ("wear and tear" of articular cartilage without a prominent inflammatory reaction (which seems to be a secondary event). Chondrocytes produce IL-1, which initiates matrix breakdown, and **tumor necrosis factor-α (TNF-α)/TNF-β**, which stimulates release of lytic enzymes from chondrocytes and inhibits matrix synthesis. OA is considered a disease of the cartilage.

B. RHEUMATOID ARTHRITIS (RA) is characterized by erosion of articular cartilage and ankylosis (fusion) of the joint due to a chronic proliferative synovitis (i.e., inflammatory reaction of the synovium). RA is an autoimmune disease that may affect many different tissues but typically begins in the proximal interphalangeal (PIP) and metacarpophalangeal (MP) joints of the hand and then spreads to other joints. Women are affected three to five times more often than men.

XII Selected Photomicrographs

A. Spongy bone, compact bone, and osteoclast (Figure 7-1)

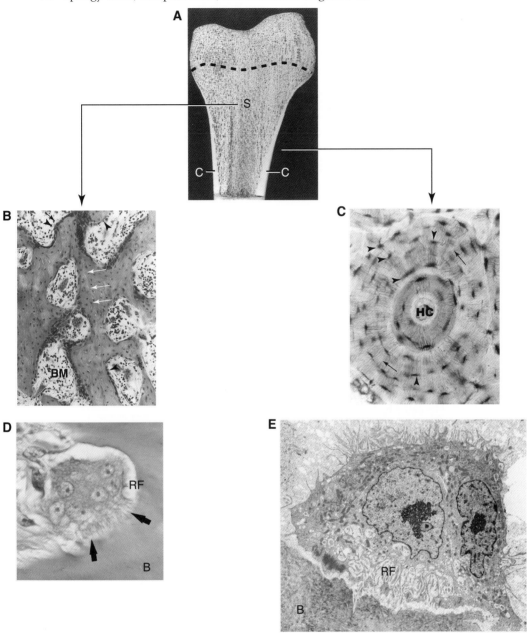

● **Figure 7-1 A:** Coronal section through the epiphysis of an adult tibia. Gross anatomically, two different types of bone can be described: spongy bone (S) arranged as trabeculae that are adapted to mechanical forces, and compact bone (C) forming a rigid outer shell. The *dotted line* is the site of the former epiphyseal plate. **B:** Light micrograph of spongy bone (hematoxylin & eosin [H&E]-stained section). Trabeculae of spongy bone are shown with a lamellar (layered linearly) arrangement of osteocytes (*arrows*) and bone matrix. Osteoblasts (*arrowheads*) can be observed on the surface of the trabeculae. The interstices between the trabeculae are filled with bone marrow (BM). **C:** Light micrograph of compact bone (ground bone section). An osteon or Haversian system of compact bone is shown with a lamellar (layered concentrically) arrangement of osteocytes within lacunae (*arrowheads*) and bone matrix. Osteocytes have many cytoplasmic processes within canaliculi (*arrows*) that extend throughout the bone matrix and communicate with other osteocytes. Within the center of an osteon is a Haversian canal (HC) that contains blood vessels and nerves. **D:** Light micrograph of an osteoclast. Note the multinucleated osteoclast attached to the resorbing bone (B). The ruffled border (RF) is clearly shown at the resorbing surface (*arrows*). **E:** Electron micrograph of an osteoclast. The ruffled border (RF) adjacent to the resorbing bone (B) is shown.

B. Epiphyseal growth plate (Figure 7-2)

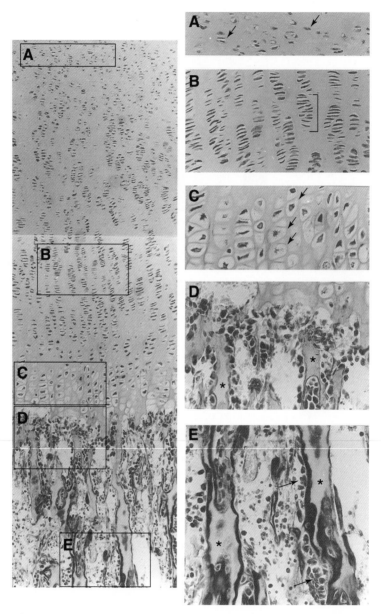

● **Figure 7-2 Light micrograph of endochondral ossification at the epiphyseal plate. A:** Zone of reserve consists of hyaline cartilage and chondrocytes (*arrows*). **B:** Zone of proliferation consists of hyaline cartilage and chondrocytes undergoing mitosis, forming stacks of chondrocytes (*bracket*). **C:** Zone of hypertrophy consists of hyaline cartilage and hypertrophied chondrocytes (*arrows*) that are secreting alkaline phosphatase to increase Ca^{2+} and PO_4^{3-} levels in the ground substance. **D:** Zone of calcification consists of dead chondrocytes and calcified cartilage matrix called spicules (*asterisk*). **E:** Zone of ossification consists of osteoprogenitor cells in the marrow cavity that differentiate into osteoblasts (*arrows*). Osteoblasts deposit bone (*black areas*) on the surface of a spicule to form a mixed spicule (*asterisk*).

C. Osteoporosis, osteosarcoma, Paget disease (Figure 7-3)

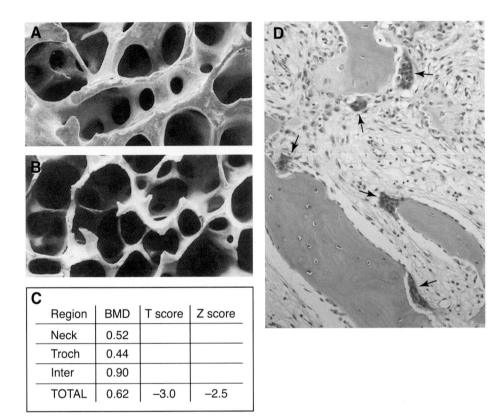

Region	BMD	T score	Z score
Neck	0.52		
Troch	0.44		
Inter	0.90		
TOTAL	0.62	–3.0	–2.5

● **Figure 7-3 Osteoporosis and Paget disease. A:** Scanning electron micrograph (SEM) of normal bone biopsy from a normal individual. **B:** SEM of bone biopsy from female with osteoporosis. Compare A and B. **C:** Table of the results after measurement of bone mass using dual energy x-ray absorptiometry (DEXA) scan of the hip. All bone densitometry techniques measure the amount of calcium present in the bone. BMD is the bone mass density expressed as g/cm^2. The T score compares the patient's bone density to a young, normal reference population. A T score > –1.0 is defined as normal bone. A T score < –2.5 is defined as osteoporosis. The Z score compares the patient's bone density to an age-matched reference population. A Z score > –2.0 is defined as bone density appropriate for the patient's age. A Z score < –2.0 is defined as bone density inappropriate for the patient's age, indicating a medical or lifestyle condition that has hastened bone loss. **D:** Light micrograph of Paget disease. Note the bone spicules surrounded by an increased number of osteoclasts (*arrows*) causing widespread bone resorption.

D. Degenerative joint disease (osteoarthritis), rheumatoid arthritis (Figure 7-4)

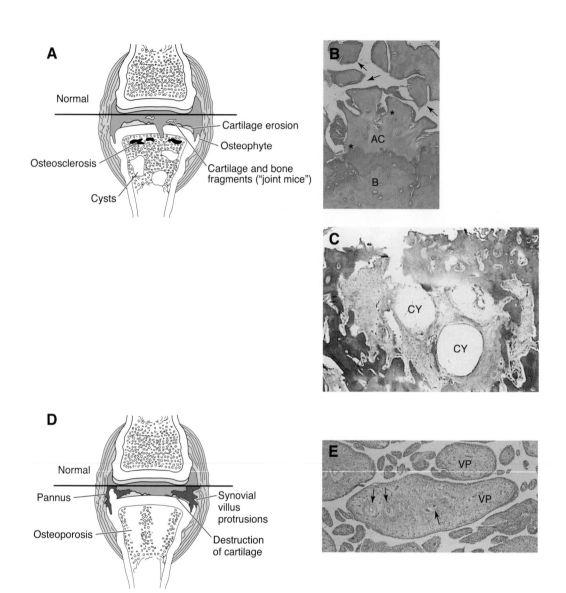

● **Figure 7-4 Osteoarthritis and rheumatoid arthritis. A–C:** Degenerative joint disease (osteoarthritis; OA). **A:** Diagram shows the hallmarks of OA, which include articular cartilage erosion, osteophyte formation, cartilage and bone fragments ("joint mice"), and osteosclerosis. **B:** Articular cartilage (AC) erosion produces cartilage fragments (*arrows*) that float within the joint space ("joint mice"). Fibrillations (microscopic vertical splits) of the articular cartilage (*asterisks*) are also seen. B, bone. **C:** As the fibrillations become progressively more deep, synovial fluid may accumulate in the subchondral bone and form cysts (CY). **D, E:** Rheumatoid arthritis (RA). **D:** Diagram shows the hallmarks of RA, which include synovial villus protrusion with inflammation, pannus, destruction of articular cartilage, and osteoporosis. **E:** Synovial villous protrusions (VP) are shown that are hyperemic (i.e., increased vascularity; *arrows*) and filled with an inflammatory infiltrate. These protrusions creep over the articular cartilage forming a pannus, which eventually erodes all the articular cartilage. In time, the pannus bridges the opposing bones (fibrous ankylosis) that eventually ossify, resulting in bony ankylosis (fusion of the joint).

Chapter 8

Muscle

I. Skeletal Muscle. The terms muscle fiber and muscle cell are synonymous.

A. MUSCLE FIBER TYPES (FIGURE 8-1). Skeletal muscle fibers can be classified mainly into **red fibers (type I)** and **white (type II) fibers** that have quite different characteristics based on their function.

1. **Red fibers (type I)** are **slow-twitch fibers** and are largely present, for example, in the long muscles of the back (antigravity muscles).
2. **White fibers (type II)** are **fast-twitch fibers** and are largely present, for example, in the extraocular muscles of the eye.
3. **Intermediate fibers** have characteristics intermediate between red and white fibers.

B. CROSS-STRIATIONS (FIGURE 8-1)

1. The **A band** contains both thin and thick myofilaments and is the **dark band** seen when using an electron microscope.
2. The **I band** contains only thin myofilaments and is the **light band** seen when using an electron microscope.
3. The **H band** bisects the A band and contains only thick myofilaments.
4. The **Z disc** bisects the I band. The distance between two Z discs delimits a sarcomere, which is the basic unit of contraction for the myofibril.

C. THIN MYOFILAMENTS

1. **F-actin** has an active site that interacts with the cross-bridges of myosin.
2. **Tropomyosin** blocks the active site on F-actin during relaxation.
3. **Troponin C** is a calcium-binding protein.

D. THICK MYOFILAMENTS

1. **Myosin** contains **cross-bridges** that have **actin-binding sites** and **adenosine triphosphatase (ATPase) activity**.

E. CHANGES IN CONTRACTED AND STRETCHED MUSCLE (FIGURE 8-1). The cross-striational pattern of skeletal muscle changes when it is contracted or stretched. These changes are caused by the degree of interdigitation of the thin and thick myofilaments

A

Characteristic	Red Fiber Type I	White Fiber Type II
Speed of contraction	Slow twitch	Fast twitch
Myoglobin content*	High	Low
Generation of ATP	Aerobic glycolysis† Oxidative phosphorylation	Anaerobic glycolysis‡
Number of mitochondria	Many	Few
Glycogen content	Low	High
Succinate dehydrogenase NADH dehydrogenase	High	Low
Glycolytic enzymes	Low	High

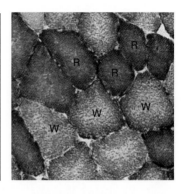

B

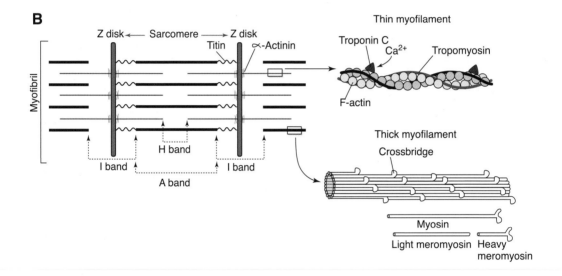

C

Band	Contracted	Relaxed	Stretched
A band	No change		No change
I band	Shortens		Lengthens
H band	Shortens		Lengthens
Z disks	Move closer together		Move farther apart

● **Figure 8-1 Skeletal muscle. A:** Characteristics of muscle fiber types. Light micrograph (LM) of skeletal muscle stained for reduced nicotinamide adenine dinucleotide (NADH) dehydrogenase, which specifically identifies red (type I) slow-twitch fibers (R) and white (type II) fast-twitch fibers (W). *Myoglobin is an oxygen-binding protein similar to hemoglobin and accounts for the reddish appearance of red (type I) fibers. †Aerobic glycolysis (conversion of glucose to carbon dioxide and water) is a relatively slow process so that it can meet the demands of red fibers, but it yields 36 to 38 moles of adenosine triphosphate (ATP) per mole of glucose. ‡Anaerobic glycolysis (conversion of glucose to lactate) is a relatively fast process so that it can meet the demands of white fibers, but it yields only 2 moles of ATP per mole of glucose. **B:** Organization of thin and thick myofilaments in skeletal muscle. **C:** Changes in contracted and stretched muscle compared to relaxed muscle.

F.   THE TRIAD. A triad consists of one **transverse tubule (T tubule)** located at the A–I junction flanked on either side by two **terminal cisternae (TC)**.

   1. T tubules are invaginations of the cell membrane and transmit an action potential to the depths of a muscle fiber. T tubules contain a voltage-sensitive protein called the **L-type Ca^{2+} channel protein** (also called the **dihydropyridine receptor**).

   2. TC are dilated sacs of sarcoplasmic reticulum (SR) that store, release, and reaccumulate Ca^{2+} critical for muscle contraction. TC and SR contain a **fast Ca^{2+} release channel protein** (also called the **ryanodine receptor-1; RyR-1**) that releases Ca^{2+} from the TC and SR into the cytoplasm and a **Ca^{2+} ATPase that** pumps Ca^{2+} from the cytoplasm into the TC and SR.

G.   NEUROMUSCULAR JUNCTION (also called **myoneural junction** or **motor endplate**)

   1. Synaptic terminals of **α-motoneurons** contain synaptic vesicles, which store **acetylcholine (ACh)**. ACh is synthesized by the condensation of **acetyl coenzyme A (CoA)** and **choline**, which is catalyzed by **choline-O-acetyltransferase**. Choline is obtained by active uptake from the extracellular fluid.

   2. The cell membrane of the synaptic terminal is called the **presynaptic membrane** and is where exocytotic release of ACh occurs. The cell membrane of the muscle fiber is called the **postsynaptic membrane**, and it contains the **nicotinic acetylcholine receptor (nAChR)**.

   3. The space between the presynaptic and postsynaptic membrane is called the **synaptic cleft**, and it contains the basal lamina associated with the enzyme **acetylcholinesterase (AChE)**, which hydrolyzes ACh (ACh $\rightarrow$ acetate + choline).

   4. nAChR is a **transmitter-gated ion channel** such that when nAChR binds ACh, the "gate" is opened and allows Na^+ influx. Na^+ influx causes depolarization of the postsynaptic membrane called the **endplate potential**.

   5. Endplate potentials spread to areas of the cell membrane and T tubule by **electrotonic conduction** until a threshold is reached and an action potential is generated. (Note: An action potential is not generated per se at the neuromuscular junction.)

H.   PHARMACOLOGY

   1. **Tubocurarine, pancuronium, vecuronium,** and **atracurium** are nondepolarizing drugs that competitively block nACh receptors (i.e., an **nACh receptor antagonist**). The effect of these drugs can be reversed by anticholinesterase drugs that increase the amount of acetylcholine within the synaptic cleft.

   2. **Succinylcholine (Anectine, Quelicin, Sucostrin)** is a depolarizing drug that competes with acetylcholine for the nACh receptor (i.e., an **nACh receptor agonist**). Succinylcholine maintains an open Na^+ channel, eventually causing skeletal muscle relaxation and paralysis. The effect of succinylcholine cannot be reversed by anticholinesterase drugs. Succinylcholine may cause **malignant hyperthermia**, which is a major cause of anesthesia-related deaths.

   3. **Botulinus Toxin** is a potent toxin produced by *Clostridium botulinus* bacteria that inhibits the release of acetylcholine.

I.   INNERVATION. A single axon of an α-motoneuron may innervate one to five muscle fibers (forming a small motor unit), or the axon may branch and innervate more than 150 muscle fibers (forming a large motor unit). **A motor unit is the functional contractile unit of a muscle** (not a muscle fiber).

J.   DENERVATION. If a nerve to a muscle is severed, **fasciculations** (small irregular contractions) occur, caused by release of ACh from the degenerating axon. Several days after denervation, **fibrillations** (spontaneous repetitive contractions) occur, caused by a supersensitivity of the muscle to ACh as nACh receptors spread out over the entire cell membrane of the muscle fiber.

K. SKELETAL MUSCLE REPAIR (regeneration) is limited. Skeletal muscle fibers develop embryologically from **rhabdomyoblasts**. After injury or extensive exercise, **satellite cells** present in the adult proliferate and fuse to form new skeletal muscle fibers. Adult skeletal muscle fibers do not undergo mitosis.

L. STRETCH (SENSORY) RECEPTORS

1. **Muscle spindles** activate the **myotatic (stretch) reflex** and consist of **nuclear bag fibers** or **nuclear chain fibers**.

    a. **Nuclear bag fibers** contain nuclei that are bunched together centrally and that transmit sensory information to group **Ia afferent neurons**.

    b. **Nuclear chain fibers** contain nuclei that are linearly arranged and that transmit sensory information (muscle length and rate of change in muscle length) to group **Ia and group II afferent neurons**.

    c. Nuclear bag fibers and nuclear chain fibers are innervated by **γ-motoneurons** that set the sensitivity of the muscle spindle. The activity of γ-motoneurons is controlled by descending pathways of higher brain centers (upper motoneurons) such that after spinal cord transection, hyperactivity of γ-motoneurons plays a role in **spasticity** and **hypertonia**.

2. **Golgi tendon organs** activate the **inverse myotatic (stretch) reflex** and consist of a bundle of collagen fibers within the tendon that transmit sensory information (force on the muscle) to group **Ib afferent neurons**.

M. CLINICAL CONSIDERATIONS

1. **Duchenne Muscular Dystrophy (DMD)**

    a. DMD is an X-linked recessive genetic disorder caused by various mutations in the *DMD* gene on **chromosome Xp21.2** for **dystrophin**, which anchors the cytoskeleton (actin) of skeletal muscle cells to the extracellular matrix via a transmembrane protein (**α-dystrophin and β-dystrophin**), thereby stabilizing the cell membrane. The *DMD* gene is the largest known human gene.

    b. **Serum Creatine Phosphokinase (CK) Measurement.** The measurement of serum CK is one of the diagnostic tests for DMD. [Serum CK] greater than or equal to 10 times normal is diagnostic.

    c. **Skeletal Muscle Biopsy.** A skeletal muscle biopsy shows histologic signs of fiber size variation, foci of necrosis and regeneration, hyalinization, and deposition of fat and connective tissue. Immunohistochemistry shows almost complete absence of the dystrophin protein.

    d. **Clinical features include:** symptoms appearing in early childhood with delays in sitting and standing independently; progressive muscle weakness (proximal weakness > distal weakness) often with calf hypertrophy; progressive muscle wasting; waddling gait; difficulty in climbing; wheelchair bound by 12 years of age; cardiomyopathy by 18 years of age; death by ≈ 30 years of age due to cardiac or respiratory failure.

2. **Myasthenia Gravis (MG)**

    a. MG is a relatively uncommon autoimmune disorder characterized by circulating autoantibodies against the **nicotinic acetylcholine receptor (anti-nAChR)**. The linkage between nAChR autoantibodies and myasthenia gravis is not absolute. In this regard, ~10% to 20% of MG patients have no detectable nAChR autoantibodies. Some of these patients have circulating autoantibodies against the **muscle-specific receptor tyrosine kinase (anti-MuSK)**, although their role in the pathogenesis of MG is not clear.

    b. MG also involves **T lymphocytes**, whose main role is the stimulation of B-lymphocyte antibody production. A majority of anti-nAChR–positive MG patients have thymus abnormalities (e.g., thymic hyperplasia or thymoma).

  c. **Clinical features include:** fluctuating skeletal muscle weakness, often with true fatigue. Fatigue is manifest by worsening contractile force of the muscle, not a sensation of tiredness. Weakness may fluctuate throughout the day, but is commonly worse later in the day or evening. In ocular MG, the muscle weakness is limited to the eyelids and extraocular muscle (e.g., ptosis, diplopia); in generalized MG, the muscle weakness affects not only ocular muscles but also bulbar, limb, and respiratory muscles. Age of onset is 20 to 30 years in females and 60 to 80 years in males.

 3. **Malignant Hyperthermia (MH)**

  a. MH is a rare autosomal dominant (50% of all cases) genetic disorder caused by **single nucleotide polymorphic** mutations in the *RYR1* gene on **chromosome 19q13.1** for the ryanodine receptor-1 (or **fast Ca^{2+} release channel protein**), which releases Ca^{2+} from the TC and SR into the cytoplasm to activate skeletal muscle contraction.

  b. MH manifests following treatment with **anesthetic agents** (e.g., succinylcholine, halothane, sevoflurane, desflurane, isoflurane). In the presence of these anesthetic agents, single nucleotide polymorphic mutations result in the **uncontrolled release of Ca^{2+}** from the TC and SR causing **tetany, increased skeletal muscle metabolism**, and **heat production**.

  c. **Clinical features include:** onset occurring within 1 hour of administration of general anesthesia; early signs including muscle rigidity (especially masseter stiffness), sinus tachycardia, increased CO_2 production, and skin cyanosis with mottling; hyperthermia increasing up to 113°F; and hypotension, disseminated intravascular coagulation, mixed acidosis, complex dysrhythmias, electrolyte abnormalities, and rhabdomyolysis (dissolution of muscle).

⚫ Cardiac Muscle will be discussed in Chapter 10.

⚫ Smooth Muscle (Figure 8-2)

A. **SINGLE-UNIT SMOOTH MUSCLE (SU)**

 1. SU is found in the **uterus, gastrointestinal (GI) tract, ureter,** and **urinary bladder.** SU demonstrates spontaneous oscillating membrane potentials called **slow waves** that determine the pattern of action potentials. Action potentials that produce contraction are superimposed on a background of slow waves. SU has **gap junctions** that permit coordinated contraction. SU activity is modulated by:

  a. **Postganglionic parasympathetic neurons** that release ACh, which binds to M_3 muscarinic ACh receptors (mAChR)

  b. **Postganglionic sympathetic neurons** that release norepinephrine (NE), which binds to α_1- and β_2-adrenergic receptors

  c. **Hormones (Oxytocin, Epinephrine, Cholecystokinin [CCK]).** For example, oxytocin binds to the oxytocin receptor, which is a G protein–linked receptor that generates inositol triphosphate (IP_3). IP_3 opens IP_3-gated Ca^{2+} channels in the terminal cisternae and sarcoplasmic reticulum.

B. **MULTIUNIT SMOOTH MUSCLE (MU)**

 1. MU is found in the **dilator and sphincter pupillae muscles of the iris, ciliary muscle of the lens,** and **ductus deferens.** MU behaves as individual motor units and is highly innervated. MU has no gap junctions. MU activity is generated by:

  a. **Postganglionic parasympathetic neurons** that release ACh, which binds to M_3 muscarinic ACh receptors (mAChR)

  b. **Postganglionic sympathetic neurons** that release NE, which binds to α_1-and β_2-adrenergic receptors

C. **SU/MU SMOOTH MUSCLE** has properties of both SU and MU smooth muscle and is found in the **tunica media of blood vessels**.

A

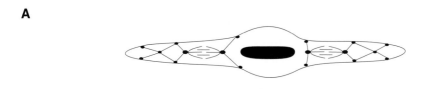

B

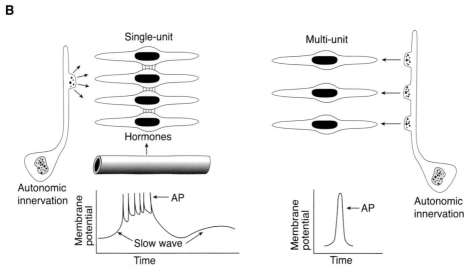

● **Figure 8-2 Smooth muscle. A:** Organization of the cytoskeleton and actin/myosin filaments. Intermediate filaments connect dense bodies in the cytoplasm and dense plaques beneath the cell membrane. Movement of actin and myosin filaments during contraction transmits the force throughout the smooth muscle cell. **B:** Characteristics of single-unit and multiunit types of smooth muscle. Single-unit smooth muscle has characteristics that include gap junctions, autonomic nerves that synapse en passant and diffuse neurotransmitters to numerous cells, hormonal control, and action potentials (AP) superimposed on slow waves. Multiunit smooth muscle has characteristics that include no gap junctions, autonomic nerves that synapse en passant and diffuse neurotransmitters to an individual cell, and spiked action potentials (AP).

Comparisons and Contrasts of Skeletal, Cardiac, and Smooth Muscle (Table 8-1)

TABLE 8-1	COMPARISON OF SKELETAL, CARDIAC, AND SMOOTH MUSCLE	
Skeletal Muscle	**Cardiac Muscle**	**Smooth Muscle**
Types: Red fibers (type I) White fibers (type II) Intermediate fibers	Types: Cardiac myocytes Purkinje myocytes Myocardial endocrine cells	Types: Single unit Multiunit Single unit/multiunit
Long parallel cylinders with multiple peripheral nuclei	Short branching cylinders with single central nucleus	Spindle-shaped, tapering ends with single central nucleus
A band, I band, H band, and Z discs are present	A band, I band, H band, and Z discs are present	Dense bodies and dense plaques connected by intermediate filaments; actin and myosin filaments
T tubules present at A–I junction and form triads with terminal cisternae	T tubules present at Z discs and form diads with a terminal cisterna	Caveolae present
Extensive sarcoplasmic reticulum	Intermediate sarcoplasmic reticulum	Limited sarcoplasmic reticulum
Cell junctions absent	Intercalated discs present (fascia adherens, desmosomes, gap junctions)	Gap junctions present in single unit Gap junctions absent in multiunit
Muscle spindles present	Muscle spindles absent	Muscle spindles absent
Neuromuscular junction	Synapse en passant	Synapse en passant
Voluntary regulation of "all-or-none" contraction by α-motoneurons	Involuntary regulation of pacemaker-generated heart beat by autonomic nervous system	Involuntary regulation of contraction by autonomic nervous system and hormonal control
α-Motoneuron releases acetylcholine (ACh) at neuromuscular junction, which binds to nicotinic ACh receptor (nAChR)	Postganglionic parasympathetic neuron releases ACh, which binds to M_2 muscarinic ACh receptor (mAChR) Postganglionic sympathetic neuron releases norepinephrine (NE), which binds to β_1-adrenergic receptor	Postganglionic parasympathetic neuron releases ACh, which binds to M_3 mAChR Postganglionic sympathetic neuron releases NE, which binds to α_1- and β_2-adrenergic receptors Hormonal control: Oxytocin, epinephrine, cholecystokinin (CCK)
Troponin C is the Ca^{2+}-binding protein	Troponin C is the Ca^{2+}-binding protein	Calmodulin is the Ca^{2+}-binding protein
Intracellular Ca^{2+} stored in the terminal cisternae (TC)/sarcoplasmic reticulum (SR) is released for contraction	Extracellular Ca^{2+} enters ("trigger Ca^{2+}") and induces more Ca^{2+} release from TC/SR	Extracellular Ca^{2+} enters ("trigger Ca^{2+}") and induces more Ca^{2+} release from SR (neural control) or Intracellular Ca^{2+} stored in the SR is released (hormone control)
Upstroke of action potential due to inward Na^+ current	Upstroke of action potential due to inward Ca^{2+} current	Upstroke of action potential due to inward Ca^{2+} current in the sinoatrial (SA) node Upstroke of action potential due to inward Na^+ current in the atria, ventricles, and Purkinje fibers
No action potential plateau	No action potential plateau	No action potential plateau in SA node Action potential plateau due to inward Ca^{2+} current in atria, ventricles, and Purkinje fibers
Action potential lasts ~1 msec	Action potential lasts ~10 msec	N/A
Growth by hypertrophy	Growth by hypertrophy	Growth by hypertrophy and hyperplasia
Regeneration limited Satellite cells give rise to myoblasts	No regeneration	Regeneration high Pericytes give rise to new cells
No mitosis	No mitosis	Mitosis

V **Selected Photomicrographs**

A. Skeletal muscle (Figure 8-3)

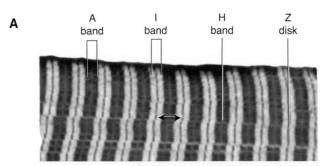

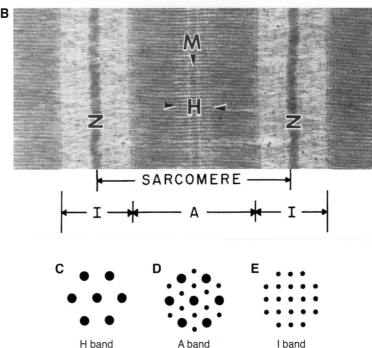

● **Figure 8-3 Skeletal muscle. A:** Light micrograph (LM) of skeletal muscle cut longitudinally. Note the A band (dark) and I band (light). The I band is bisected by the Z disc. A sarcomere (Z disc to Z disc) is indicated by the *double-headed arrow*. **B:** Electron micrograph (EM) of skeletal muscle cut longitudinally. Note the A band (dark), I band (light), and H band. The M line is also indicated. The I band is bisected by the Z disc (Z). A sarcomere is indicated. **C–E:** EM of skeletal muscle cut in cross section showing the characteristic arrangement of myofilaments in the H band, A band, and I band, respectively. The H band shows only thick myofilaments (*large black dots*). The A band shows both thick myofilaments (*large black dots*) surrounded by six thin myofilaments (*small black dots*). The I band shows only thin myofilaments (*small black dots*). **F:** EM of the sarcoplasmic reticulum (SR), which is an extensive network of smooth endoplasmic reticulum (sER) that ends as dilated sacs called terminal cisternae (TC). A T tubule (T), which is an invagination of the cell membrane, is indicated. Two terminal cisternae are always found in close association with T tubule (T) forming a triad. The drug dantrolene blocks release of Ca^{2+} from the SR.

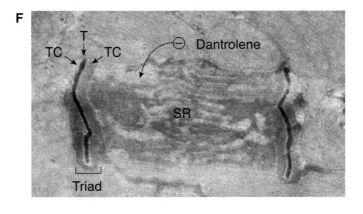

B. Neuromuscular junction and muscle spindle (Figure 8-4)

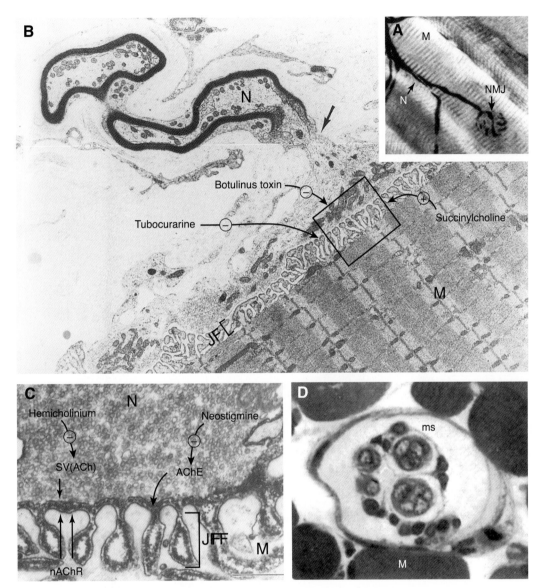

● **Figure 8-4 Neuromuscular junction and muscle spindle. A:** Light micrograph (LM) of a neuromuscular junction (NMJ) in whole mount. M, muscle; N, nerve. **B:** Electron micrograph of a neuromuscular junction. A myelinated axon (N) loses its myelin sheath (at the *arrow*) and ends in a synaptic terminal on the surface of a skeletal muscle fiber (M). At the junction of the nerve and muscle fiber, the cell membrane of the muscle fiber is thrown into junctional folds (JF; *brackets*). The *boxed area* is shown at high magnification in C. **C:** High magnification of the neuromuscular junction (*boxed area* in B). A collection of synaptic vesicles (SV) that contain acetylcholine (ACh) is indicated along with the presynaptic membrane (*single arrow*) where ACh is released. The postsynaptic membrane (*double arrows*) that contain nACh receptors (nAChR) is shown. The *bracket* indicates the postsynaptic membrane of the skeletal muscle fiber thrown into junctional folds (JF). The synaptic cleft (*large arrow*) containing the electron-dense basal lamina and acetylcholinesterase (AChE) is shown. **D:** LM of a muscle spindle (ms) showing both the nuclear bag fibers and nuclear chain fibers. Note the surrounding muscle fibers (M).

C.   Cardiac muscle and smooth muscle (Figure 8-5)

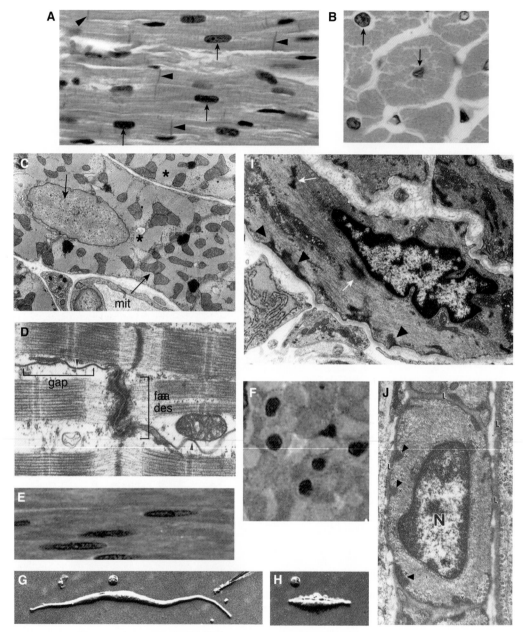

● **Figure 8-5 Cardiac muscle and smooth muscle. A:** Light micrograph (LM) of cardiac muscle in longitudinal section. Note the intercalated discs (*arrowheads*) and centrally located nuclei (*arrows*). The cytoplasm demonstrates a striated appearance although less prominent than in skeletal muscle. **B:** LM of cardiac muscle in cross section. Note the centrally located nuclei (*arrows*). **C:** Electron micrograph (EM) of cardiac muscle in longitudinal section. Note the centrally located nucleus (*arrow*), numerous mitochondria (mit), and striations (*). **D:** EM of an intercalated disc in cardiac muscle. An intercalated disc is found at the junction of two cardiac myocytes and is typically arranged in a stair-step pattern. The intercalated disc consists of a fascia adherens (fa), desmosomes (des), and gap junction (gap). The gap junction is always oriented parallel to the myofilaments. **E:** LM of smooth muscle in longitudinal section. Note the centrally located nuclei and lack of cytoplasmic striations. **F:** LM of smooth muscle in cross section. Note the centrally located nucleus. **G, H:** Viable smooth muscle cell in relaxed state (G) and contracted state (H). **I:** EM of smooth muscle in longitudinal section. Note the centrally located nucleus and lack of cytoplasmic striations. Note the cytoplasmic dense bodies (*arrows*) and the dense plaques (*arrowheads*) located at the cell membrane. The dense bodies and dense plaques are connected by an array of intermediate filaments that participate in contraction generated by actin and myosin interaction. **J:** EM of smooth muscle in cross section. Note the dense plaques (*arrowheads*) located at the cell membrane. N, nucleus.

Chapter 9

Nervous Tissue

I   **The Neuron** is the structural and functional unit of the nervous system. The neuron consists of a **perikaryon (cell body)**, **dendrite**, and **axon**, each of which contains certain ultrastructural components (Table 9-1). The axon arises from an extension of the perikaryon called the **axon hillock**. The part of the axon between the axon hillock and the start of the myelin sheath is called the **initial segment** and is where the action potential is initiated.

TABLE 9-1	ULTRASTRUCTURAL COMPONENTS OF NEURON
Neuron Part	**Components**
Perikaryon	Nucleus with prominent nucleolus, rER and polyribosomes (Nissl substance), Golgi, some sER, mitochondria, lysosomes, microfilaments (actin), neurofilaments (intermediate), microtubules, and: Pigments: **Lipofuscin granules** are pigmented residual bodies derived from lysosomal degradation that accumulate with age. **Melanin** is a black cytoplasmic pigment found in the substantia nigra and locus coeruleus. Melanin disappears from nigral neurons in Parkinson disease. Inclusion bodies: **Lewy bodies** are round, eosinophilic inclusions composed of α-synuclein that are characteristic of Parkinson disease. **Negri bodies** are inclusions that are pathognomonic of rabies. **Hirano bodies** are rodlike, eosinophilic inclusions that are found in Alzheimer disease. **Neurofibrillary tangles** are degenerated neurofilaments that are found in Alzheimer disease. **Cowdry type A** is an intranuclear inclusion that is found in herpes simplex encephalitis.
Dendrite	Similar to the perikaryon
Axon	Some sER, mitochondria, neurofilaments (intermediate), microtubules, and neurosecretory vesicles *Absent: rER and polyribosomes (Nissl substance), Golgi, and lysosomes*

rER, rough endoplasmic reticulum; sER, smooth endoplasmic reticulum.

A. AXONAL TRANSPORT

1. **Fast anterograde transport** is responsible for transporting **vesicles** (containing enzymes, proteins, phospholipids, and neurotransmitters) necessary for neurotransmission. This transport occurs at the rate of 200 to 400 mm/day, is mediated by **microtubules**, and uses **kinesin**, which is a motor protein with **adenosine triphosphatase (ATPase) activity**.

2. **Slow anterograde transport** is responsible for transporting **cytosolic and cytoskeletal components (enzymes, actin, myosin, etc.)** from the perikaryon to the synaptic terminal. This transport occurs at the rate of 1 to 5 mm/day.

3. **Fast retrograde transport** is responsible for transporting **nerve growth factor, tetanus toxin, polio virus, rabies virus, and herpes simplex virus** from the synaptic terminal to the perikaryon. This transport occurs at the rate of 100 to 200 mm/day, is mediated by **microtubules**, and uses **dynein**, which is a motor protein with ATPase activity.

B. **CONDUCTION VELOCITY (TABLE 9-2)** of action potentials down an axon is influenced by **axon diameter** and **degree of myelination.** Large diameter and highly myelinated axons have a high conduction velocity (fast). Small diameter and unmyelinated axons have a low conduction velocity (slow).

TABLE 9-2			CLASSIFICATION OF NERVE FIBERS
Fiber	Diameter (μm)[a]	Conduction Velocity (m/sec)	Function
Sensory axons			
Ia (A-α)	12–20	70–120	Proprioception, muscle spindles
Ib (A-α)	12–20	70–120	Proprioception, Golgi tendon organs
II (A-β)	5–12	30–70	Touch, pressure, vibration, muscle spindles
III (A-δ)	2–5	12–30	Touch, pressure, fast pain, temperature
IV (C)	0.5–1	0.5–2	Slow pain and temperature, unmyelinated fibers
Motor axons			
Alpha (A-α)	12–20	15–120	α-Motor neurons of ventral horn (innervate extrafusal muscle fibers)
Gamma (A-δ)	2–10	10–45	γ-Motor neurons of ventral horn innervate intrafusal muscle fibers)
Preganglionic autonomic fibers (B)	<3	3–15	Myelinated preganglionic autonomic fibers
Postganglionic autonomic fibers (C)	1	2	Unmyelinated postganglionic autonomic fibers

Type A = high myelination.
Type B = myelination.
Type C = no myelination.
[a]Myelin sheath included if present.

C. **NODE OF RANVIER** is a segment of the axon exposed to the extracellular milieu due to gaps in the myelin sheath. It is the site where action potentials are regenerated due to the **presence of Na$^+$ channels (i.e., saltatory conduction).**

D. **FUEL SOURCES.** Although **glucose** is a major fuel source for neurons, glucose is not the only fuel source. If the diet includes little or no carbohydrates (e.g., fasting, low-carbohydrate dieting, or starvation), then **ketone bodies** (acetoacetate, 3-hydroxybutyrate) are synthesized by **liver mitochondria** when fatty acids are in high concentration in the blood. These ketone bodies will supply **75% of the energy** to the brain. **Glucose synthesized from dietary protein or muscle breakdown and glycerol** released by metabolism of triglycerides will supply the remaining **25% of energy** to the brain.

Ⅱ Neurotransmitters (Table 9-3)

TABLE 9-3	TABLE OF NEUROTRANSMITTERS AND FUNCTIONS
Neurotransmitter	**Characteristics**
Acetylcholine (ACh)	Binds to nicotinic ACh receptor (nAChR), which is a **transmitter-gated ion channel** permeable to Na^+, K^+, and Ca^{2+} ions Binds to M_1, M_2, and M_3 muscarinic ACh receptors (mAChR), which are **G protein–linked receptors** Is the neurotransmitter of: Neuromuscular junction, preganglionic parasympathetic neurons, preganglionic sympathetic neurons (ACh + nAChR) Postganglionic parasympathetic neurons (ACh + M_2 or M_3 mAChR) Somatic and visceral motor nuclei in the brainstem; basal nucleus of Meynert, which degenerates in Alzheimer disease; and striatum (caudatoputamen), which degenerates in Huntington disease (ACh + M_1 mAChR) Postganglionic sympathetic neurons that innervate eccrine sweat glands for thermoregulation and blood vessels in skeletal muscle for dilation (ACh + mAChR)
Catecholamines Norepinephrine	Binds to α_1-, α_2-, β_1-, β_2-, or β_3-adrenergic receptors, which are **G protein–linked receptors** Is the neurotransmitter of postganglionic sympathetic neurons and locus ceruleus in pons and midbrain Is metabolized by MAO and COMT to form metabolites NMN, MOPEG, and VMA Plays a role in anxiety states, panic attacks, depression, and mania
Epinephrine	Binds to α_1-, α_2-, β_1-, β_2-, or β_3-adrenergic receptors, which are **G protein–linked receptors** Plays an insignificant role in the CNS Is secreted by chromaffin cells of the adrenal medulla
Dopamine	Binds to D_1 and D_2 dopamine receptors, which are **G protein–linked receptors** Is the neurotransmitter of the arcuate nucleus in hypothalamus, ventral tegmental area, and substantia nigra Plays a role in Parkinson disease (dopamine decreased) and schizophrenia (dopamine increased)
Serotonin (5-hydroxytryptamine; 5-HT)	Binds to $5\text{-HT}_{1A,B,C,D,E,F}$ receptors, which are **G protein–linked receptors** ($\downarrow$ cAMP) found in the CNS (raphe nuclei of the brainstem and hippocampus) Binds to $5\text{-HT}_{2A,B,C}$ serotonin receptors, which are **G protein–linked receptors** ($\uparrow IP_3$ + DAG) found in the CNS Binds to the 5-HT_3 serotonin receptor, which is a **transmitter-gated ion channel** permeable to Na^+ and K^+ ions Binds to $5\text{-HT}_{4,6,7}$ serotonin receptors, which are **G protein–linked receptors** ($\uparrow$cAMP) found in the CNS
γ-Aminobutyric acid (GABA)	Binds to $GABA_A$ receptor, which is a **transmitter-gated ion channel** permeable to Cl^- ions Binds to $GABA_B$ receptor, which is a **G protein–linked receptor** Is the **major inhibitory neurotransmitter of the CNS**

(Continued)

86   CHAPTER 9

Neurotransmitter	Characteristics

Actual

TABLE 9-3   TABLE OF NEUROTRANSMITTERS AND FUNCTIONS (Continued)

Neurotransmitter	Characteristics
Glycine	Binds to glycine receptor which is a **transmitter-gated ion channel** permeable to Cl^- ions Is the **major inhibitory neurotransmitter of the spinal cord**
Glutamate	Binds to N-methyl-D-aspartate (NMDA), kainate, or quisqualate A receptors, which are **transmitter-gated ion channels** permeable to Na^+, K^+, and Ca^{2+} ions Is the **major excitatory neurotransmitter of the CNS**
Opioid peptides (**B-endorphin,** leu-enkephalin, met-enkephalin)	Bind to μ, δ, κ, and σ receptors, which are **G protein–linked receptors** Play a role in pain suppression
Neuropeptides	Use **G protein–linked receptors**

MAO, monoamine oxidase; COMT, catechol O-methyltransferase; NMN, normetanephrine; MOPEG, 3-methoxy-4-hydroxyphenylglycol; VMA, vanillylmandelic acid; CNS, central nervous system; cAMP, cyclic adenosine monophosphate; IP₃, inositol triphosphate; DAG, diacylglycerol.

III Parasympathetic Pharmacology

A. CHOLINERGIC AGONISTS
1. **Carbachol, Methacholine, Bethanechol, Pilocarpine,** and **Nicotine** are cholinergic agonists that bind directly to muscarinic acetylcholine receptors (mAChRs).
2. **Edrophonium, Neostigmine,** and **Physostigmine** are indirect cholinergic agonists that inhibit acetylcholinesterase.

B. CHOLINERGIC ANTAGONISTS ("BLOCKERS")
1. **Atropine** is the classic cholinergic antagonist ("mAChR blocker," muscarinic blocker, or antimuscarinic) that blocks mAChR. Atropine overdose is associated with dry mouth, dry skin, and inhibition of sweating ("dry as a bone"); red, flushed, hot skin ("red as a beet"); blurred vision ("blind as a bat"); and delirium and hallucinations ("mad as a hatter").
2. **Scopolamine, Propantheline, Methantheline, Benztropine, Cyclopentolate,** and **Pirenzepine** are other cholinergic antagonists that block mAChR.

IV Sympathetic Pharmacology

A. ADRENERGIC AGONISTS
1. **Phenylephrine, Tetrahydrozoline, Oxymetazoline, Naphazoline, Methoxamine,** and **Clonidine** are α-adrenergic agonists that bind directly to α_1- and α_2-adrenergic receptors.
2. **Methyldopa** is a prodrug to the α_2-adrenergic agonist methylnorepinephrine.
3. **Isoproterenol, Dobutamine, Metaproterenol, Albuterol, Terbutaline, Salmeterol,** and **Ritodrine** are β-adrenergic agonists that bind directly to β_1-, β_2-, and β_3-adrenergic receptors.

4. **Tyramine, Amphetamine,** and **Methamphetamine** are indirect adrenergic agonists that act by either increasing norepinephrine release or inhibiting norepinephrine reuptake.
5. **Ephedrine** and **Phenylpropanolamine** are mixed adrenergic agonists that act either directly or indirectly.

B. **ADRENERGIC ANTAGONISTS ("BLOCKERS")**
  1. **Prazosin (Minipress), Terazosin, Doxazosin, Phenoxybenzamine, Phentolamine, Tamsulosin,** and **Yohimbine** are α-adrenergic antagonists ("α-blockers") that block α_1- and α_2-adrenergic receptors.
  2. **Metoprolol (Lopressor), Propranolol (Inderal), Atenolol, Esmolol, Acebutolol, Pindolol, Timolol, Celiprolol,** and **Nadolol** are β-adrenergic antagonists ("β-blockers") that block β_1-, β_2-, and β_3-adrenergic receptors.
  3. **Labetalol** and **Carvedilol** are α- and β-adrenergic antagonists ("α- and β-blockers") that block α_1-, α_2-, β_1-, β_2-, and β_3-adrenergic receptors.

V **Neuroglial Cells** are the nonneural cells of the nervous system.

A. **OLIGODENDROCYTES** produce myelin in the central nervous system (CNS). One oligodendrocyte can myelinate several (up to 30) axons.

B. **ASTROCYTES** have the following characteristics and functions: project foot processes to capillaries that contribute to the blood-brain barrier, play a role in the metabolism of neurotransmitters (e.g., glutamate, γ-aminobutyric acid [GABA], serotonin), buffer the $[K^+]$ of the CNS extracellular space, form the external and internal glial-limiting membrane in the CNS, form glial scars in a damaged area of the CNS (i.e., astrogliosis), undergo hypertrophy and hyperplasia in reaction to CNS injury, and contain the **glial fibrillary acidic protein (GFAP)** and **glutamine synthetase**, which are good markers for astrocytes.

C. **MICROGLIA** are derived from **monocytes** and have phagocytic function.

D. **EPENDYMAL CELLS** line the central canal and ventricles of the brain. These cells are not joined by tight junctions so that exchange between the cerebrospinal fluid (CSF) and CNS extracellular fluid occurs freely.

E. **CHOROID EPITHELIAL CELLS**
  1. These cells are a continuation of the ependymal layer that is reflected over the choroid plexus villi and **secrete CSF** by selective transport of molecules from blood.
  2. These cells are joined by tight junctions, which is the basis of the **blood-CSF barrier.**
  3. CSF is normally **clear.** A **yellow color (xanthochromia)** indicates previous bleeding (subarachnoid hemorrhage) or increased [protein]. A **pinkish color** is usually due to a bloody tap. **Turbidity** is due to the presence of leukocytes.
  4. CSF normal values include:
     a. **CSF pressure = 70 to 80 mm H_2O**
     b. **CSF cell count = <6 lymphocytes/mm^3**; 0 neutrophils (presence of neutrophils is always pathologic)
     c. **CSF [protein] = 20 to 45 mg/dL** (serum proteins are generally too large to cross the blood-CSF barrier)
     d. **CSF [glucose] = 40 to 70 mg/dL**
  5. **In acute bacterial meningitis,** the CSF has the following characteristics: cloudy, ↑↑ pressure, ↑↑ neutrophils, ↑↑ [protein], and ↓↓ [glucose].

F.   SCHWANN CELLS produce myelin in the peripheral nervous system (PNS) and are derived from neural crest cells. One Schwann cell myelinates only one axon. Schwann cells invest all myelinated and unmyelinated axons of the PNS and are separated from each other by nodes of Ranvier.

VI   The Blood-Brain Barrier (BB)

A.   The BB represents an anatomic and physiologic separation of blood from the CNS extracellular fluid. The BB consists of **zonula occludens (tight junctions)** between non-fenestrated intracerebral capillary endothelial cells with few pinocytic vesicles, the surrounding **basal lamina**, and **astrocytic foot processes**, which promote the formation of tight junctions.

B.   Water, gases, and small lipid-soluble molecules freely diffuse across the BB. Glucose and amino acids cross via carrier-mediated transport mechanisms.

C.   The BB excludes many drugs from the CNS. Note: Dopamine does not cross the BB, but L-DOPA (used to treat Parkinson disease) does cross the BB.

D.   The BB does not exist in some areas of the CNS, such as the median eminence, neurohypophysis, lamina terminalis, pineal gland, area postrema, and choroid plexus.

E.   Infarction of brain tissue destroys the BB and results in vasogenic edema.

VII   Nerve Degeneration and Regeneration

A.   PNS
   1.   **Degeneration. Anterograde (Wallerian) degeneration** of the axon and myelin sheath occurs distal to the site of injury. Macrophages infiltrate to remove cellular debris.
      a.   **Chromatolysis** (loss of rough endoplasmic reticulum [rER], movement of nucleus to the periphery, and hypertrophy of the perikaryon) occurs.
      b.   During this time, **muscle fasciculations** (small irregular contractions) occur, caused by release of ACh from the degenerating synaptic terminal.
   2.   **Regeneration.** Schwann cells proliferate and form a cord that is penetrated by the growing axon. The axon grows at 3 mm/day until it reaches the skeletal muscle.
      a.   If the axon does not penetrate the cord of Schwann cells, the axon will not reach the skeletal muscle.
      b.   During this time, **muscle fibrillations** (spontaneous repetitive contractions) occur caused by a supersensitivity of the muscle to ACh.

B.   CNS
   1.   **Degeneration.** Microglia phagocytose myelin and injured axons. Glial scars (astrogliosis) form.
   2.   **Regeneration.** Effective regeneration does not occur in the CNS.

VIII   Clinical Considerations

A.   ASTROCYTIC TUMORS
   1.   There are three levels of astrocytic tumors based on histopathology: **astrocytomas** (grades I and II; benign), **anaplastic astrocytomas** (grade III; malignant), and **glioblastomas** (grade IV; malignant).
   2.   The formation of a grade II astrocytoma is associated with both the **inactivation of the *TP53* gene** (a tumor suppressor gene) on chromosome 17p, which encodes for the p53 protein and the **loss of chromosome 22q.**

3. The progression to a grade III anaplastic astrocytoma is associated with both the **loss of chromosome 13q**, which contains the *RB1* gene (a tumor suppressor gene), which encodes for the p110^{RB} protein, and **deletions in chromosome 9p**, which contains the *CDKN2A* gene (a tumor suppressor gene; cyclin dependent kinase 2A), which encodes for the **p16** protein, and the *CDKN2B* gene (a tumor suppressor gene), which encodes for the **p15** protein.

4. The progression to a grade IV glioblastoma is associated with both the **inactivation of the *PTEN* gene** (a tumor suppressor gene) on chromosome 10q23, which encodes for the **phosphatase and tensin homolog** protein, and the **amplification of the *EGFR* gene** on chromosome 7p12, which encodes for the **epidermal growth factor receptor protein**.

5. **Grade IV Glioblastomas**
   a. Grade IV glioblastomas are the most common primary brain tumor in adults and pursue a rapidly fatal course.
   b. Age of onset is 40 to 70 years of age, and they are more in men than women.
   c. They are generally found in the frontal lobes of the cerebral cortex and commonly cross the corpus callosum, producing a butterfly appearance on magnetic resonance imaging (MRI).
   d. Grade IV glioblastomas are hemorrhagic tumors with multifocal areas of necrosis and cystic degeneration.
   e. Histologic features include hemorrhagic necrosis with a proliferation of blood vessels, pseudopalisading of neoplastic cells around foci of necrosis and blood vessels, highly pleomorphic malignant cells (bizarre giant tumor cells), and atypical mitotic figures.
   f. Clinical features include: seizures, headaches, and focal neurologic deficits depending on the area of the CNS involved.

B. MULTIPLE SCLEROSIS (MS)

1. MS is the most common autoimmune inflammatory demyelinating disease of the central nervous system.
2. The cause of MS remains unknown. However, it is theorized that the start of MS is mediated by autoreactive lymphocytes and later MS is dominated by microglial activation and chronic neurodegeneration.
3. The pathologic hallmarks of MS are **demyelinated plaques**, which are most commonly found in the white matter of the optic chiasm, cerebellar peduncles, angles of the ventricles, and floor of the fourth ventricle. The demyelinated plaques are characterized histologically by a selective loss of myelin, decreased number of oligodendrocytes, axonal injury, microglial cells with phagocytosed lipid, and edema.
4. **Clinical features include:** age of onset between 20 and 40 years of age; classic triad of scanning speech (patient sounds drunk), intention tremor, and nystagmus; sensory (e.g., paresthesias) and motor (e.g., muscle weakness) abnormalities; optic neuritis with unilateral loss of vision; cerebellar incoordination; and **Lhermitte sign** (electric shock-like sensation that runs down the back and/or limbs upon flexion of the neck).

C. FRIEDREICH ATAXIA (FRDA)

1. FRDA is an autosomal recessive genetic disorder caused by a 600 to 1200 unstable repeat sequence of $(GAA)_n$ in intron 1 of the *FXN* gene on **chromosome 9q13-a21.1** for the **frataxin** protein, which is located on the inner mitochondrial membrane and plays a role in the synthesis of respiratory chain complexes I through III, mitochondrial iron content, and antioxidation defense.
2. A long-standing hypothesis is that FRDA is a result of mitochondrial accumulation of iron, which may promote oxidative stress injury.

3. **Clinical features include:** degeneration of the posterior columns and spinocerebellar tracts; loss of sensory neurons in the dorsal root ganglion; slowly progressive ataxia of all four limbs with onset at 10 to 15 years of age; optic nerve atrophy; scoliosis; bladder dysfunction; swallowing dysfunction; pyramidal tract disease; cardiomyopathy (arrhythmias); and diabetes.

D. ALZHEIMER DISEASE (AZ)

1. AZ is a neurodegenerative disease of the central nervous system.
2. The cause of AZ remains unknown.
3. The pathologic hallmarks of AZ are the **senile plaques** and **neurofibrillary tangles**.
4. The formation of senile plaques involves a family of amyloid precursor proteins (APPs), which can be cleaved by specific **secretases**. When APP is cleaved at the amino end by β-secretase and the carboxy end by γ-secretase, a highly amyloidogenic protein is released called **amyloid β-protein 42 (Aβ-42)**. Aβ-42 then aggregates into diffuse plaques, which probably mature into senile plaques.
5. The formation of neurofibrillary tangles involves the **hyperphosphorylated tau protein**. The normal tau protein is a **microtubule-associated protein (MAP)**. However, the hyperphosphorylated tau protein does not associate with microtubules but instead aggregates into helical filaments. Microtubule function is also compromised so that axonal transport is diminished.
6. **Clinical features include:** age of onset at older than 60 years of age; loss of recent memory being one of the first signs; cerebral atrophy due to neuronal loss within the temporal, frontal, and parietal lobes; depression; psychosis; difficulty with language; and agitation.

E. HUNTINGTON DISEASE (HD)

1. HD is an autosomal dominant genetic disorder caused by a $36 \rightarrow 100+$ unstable repeat sequence of $(CAG)_n$ in the coding sequence of the *HD* gene on **chromosome 4p16.3** for the **huntingtin** protein, which is a widely expressed cytoplasmic protein present in neurons within the striatum, cerebral cortex, and cerebellum, although its precise function is unknown.
2. Since CAG codes for the amino acid glutamine, a long tract of glutamines (a polyglutamine tract) will be inserted into the huntingtin protein and cause protein aggregates to form within certain cells (such as is implicated in other neurodegenerative disorders).
3. Normal *HD* alleles have 26 or fewer repeats. They are stably transmitted without any decrease or increase in repeat number.
4. Premutation *HD* alleles have 27 to 35 repeats. They are not stably transmitted. Individuals with permutation *HD* alleles are at risk for having children with HD. A child with HD inherits the expanded repeat from the father.
5. An inverse correlation exists between the number of CAG repeats and the age of HD onset: 60 to 100 CAG repeats = juvenile onset of HD and 36 to 55 CAG repeats = adult onset of HD.
6. **Clinical features include:** age of onset between 35 and 44 years of age; mean survival time 15 to 18 years after onset; a movement jerkiness most apparent at movement termination; chorea (dancelike movements); memory deficits; affective disturbances; personality changes; dementia; diffuse and marked atrophy of the **neostriatum** due to cell death of **cholinergic neurons** and **GABAergic neurons** within the striatum (caudate nucleus and putamen) and a relative increase in dopaminergic neuron activity; and neuronal intranuclear aggregates. The disorder is protracted and invariably fatal. In HD, homozygotes are not more severely affected by the disorder than heterozygotes, which is an exception in autosomal dominant disorders.

F. IDIOPATHIC PARKINSONISM (IP)

1. IP is a movement disorder characterized by **deficiency of dopamine** and **loss of melanin-containing dopaminergic neurons** within the **substantia nigra** and **locus ceruleus**.

2. The **striatal system** consists of the substantia nigra, caudate nucleus and putamen (neostriatum), globus pallidus, subthalamic nucleus, and thalamus. The striatal system is involved in the voluntary movement of skeletal muscles.

3. The substantia nigra connects to the neostriatum via the **nigrostriatal tract**, which uses dopamine as its principal neurotransmitter.

4. A pathologic hallmark of IP are **Lewy bodies**, which are round, eosinophilic intracytoplasmic inclusions with a dense granular core and loosely arranged fibrillary elements toward a peripheral "halo." A Lewy body consists mainly of **α-synuclein** along with ubiquitin, calbindin, complement proteins, microfilament subunits, tubulin, and microtubule-associated proteins 1 and 2.

5. **Clinical features include:** age of onset ~45 years of age; extrapyramidal signs; rest tremor ("pill rolling"); bradykinesia (generalized slowness of movement); cogwheel rigidity (increased resistance to passive movement about a joint); postural instability; expressionless face; and festinating or shuffling gait (progressively shortened accelerated steps).

6. Drug treatment includes:

    a. **Levodopa (L-DOPA, Dopar, Larodopa)** is converted to dopamine by DOPA decarboxylase in many peripheral body tissues and the brain. L-DOPA crosses the blood-brain barrier.

    b. **Levodopa plus Carbidopa (Sinemet).** Carbidopa inhibits DOPA decarboxylase only in peripheral body tissues. Carbidopa does not cross the blood-brain barrier.

    c. **Selegiline (Eldepryl, Deprenyl)** inhibits type B monoamine oxidase (MAO), which selectively metabolizes dopamine in preference to other catecholamines.

    d. **Bromocriptine** is an ergot alkaloid, which is a D_2 dopamine receptor agonist.

    e. **Pergolide (Permax)** is a D_1 and D_2 dopamine receptor agonist.

    f. **Amantadine (Symmetrel)** increases the synthesis and secretion of dopamine and delays the reuptake of dopamine.

Ⅸ Selected Photomicrographs

A. Neurons (Figure 9-1)

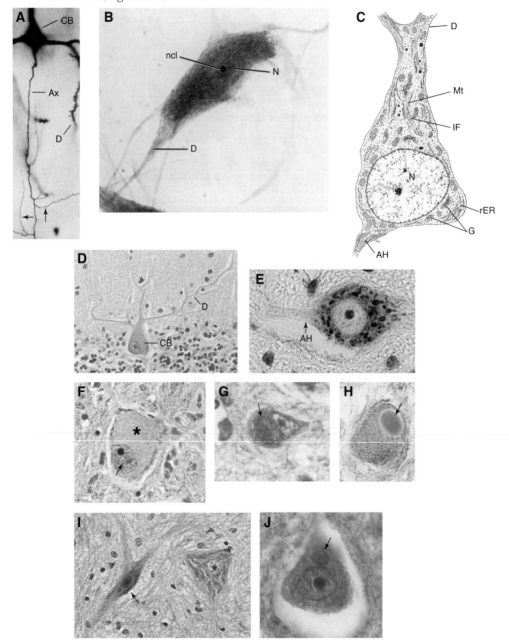

● **Figure 9-1 A:** A multipolar neuron showing the perikaryon (cell body; CB), axon (Ax), axon collaterals (*arrows*), and dendrites with dendritic spines (D). **B:** Light micrograph (LM) of a multipolar neuron showing the nucleus (N), nucleolus (ncl), and dendrite (D). **C:** Diagram of a multipolar neuron showing nucleus (N), dendrites (D), microtubules (Mt), intermediate filaments (IF), rough endoplasmic reticulum (rER), Golgi (G), and axon hillock (AH). **D:** LM of a Purkinje neuron from the cerebellum. CB, cell body; D, dendrites. **E:** LM of a multipolar neuron showing the nucleus with prominent nucleolus and axon hillock (AH). Note that most of the cytoplasmic staining is due to rER and polyribosomes (Nissl substance). **F:** LM of a neuron undergoing chromatolysis. Note the loss of rER and polyribosomes (*), movement of nucleus to the periphery (*arrow*), and hypertrophy of the cell body. **G:** Hurler disease is a lysosomal storage disease that involves the L-iduronidase enzyme where abnormal amounts of heparan sulfate and dermatan sulfate accumulate within the cytoplasm of neurons (*arrow*). **H:** Parkinson disease involves the depigmentation of neurons in the substantia nigra and the appearance of round cytoplasmic inclusions called Lewy bodies (*arrow*). **I:** LM of an atrophic neuron (*arrow*), which has a reduced amount of cytoplasm and an indistinct nucleus. A normal neuron is shown for comparison. **J:** LM of a neuron infected with the rabies virus showing the presence of a cytoplasmic inclusion called the Negri body (*arrow*).

B.   Peripheral nerve (Figure 9-2)

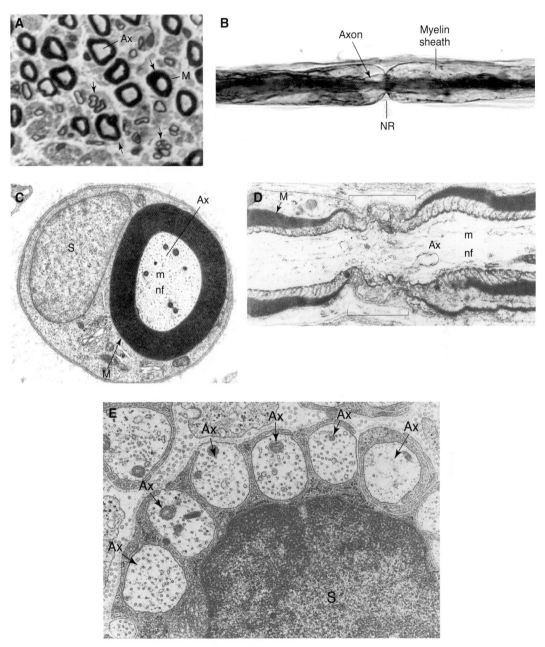

● **Figure 9-2 Peripheral nerve.** A peripheral nerve contains both myelinated and unmyelinated axons. **A:** Light micrograph (LM) of a cross section of a peripheral nerve stained with osmic acid. This area shows only myelinated axons of various diameters (*arrows*). Note the myelin sheath (M; *black*) and axon (Ax; *white*). **B:** LM shows a single myelinated nerve fiber with its axon surrounded by a myelin sheath. Note the node of Ranvier (NR) where two Schwann cells meet, forming a gap in the myelin sheath that exposes the axon to the extracellular milieu. **C:** Electron micrograph (EM) of a cross section of a peripheral nerve. This area shows only a myelinated axon. Note the Schwann cell (S) nucleus and cytoplasm, myelin sheath (M), and axon (Ax) containing microtubules (m) and neurofilaments (nf). **D:** EM of a longitudinal section of a peripheral nerve. Note the myelin sheath (M), axon (Ax) containing microtubules (m) and neurofilaments (nf), and node of Ranvier (*brackets*) where the myelin sheath is absent. The node of Ranvier is where action potentials are regenerated due to the presence of Na^+ ion channels that allow an influx of Na^+ to occur. **E:** EM of a cross section of a peripheral nerve. This area shows only unmyelinated axons (Ax; *arrows*). Unmyelinated axons are embedded in the cytoplasm of a Schwann cell (S) but no myelin sheath is formed.

C. Neuroglia (Figure 9-3)

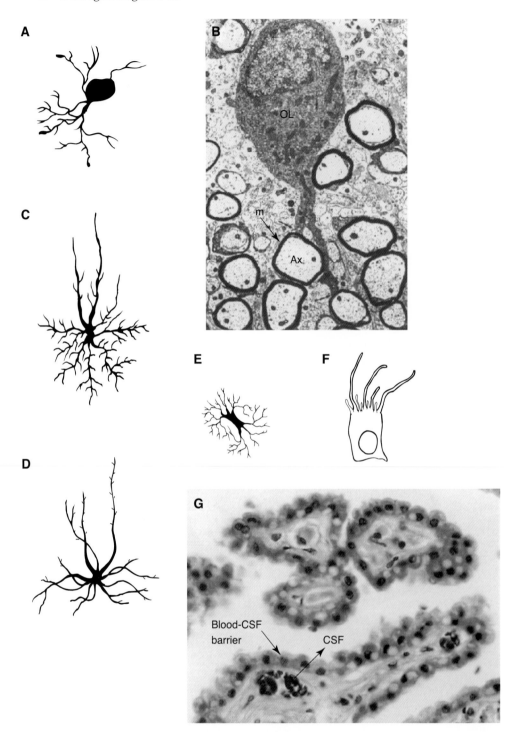

● **Figure 9-3 Neuroglial cells. A:** Drawing of an oligodendrocyte. **B:** Electron micrograph (EM) of an oligodendrocyte (OL). Note the cell processes of the oligodendrocyte extending to two axons (Ax) within the central nervous system and forming a myelin sheath (M). Note that one oligodendrocyte can myelinate several axons. **C:** Drawing of a protoplasmic astrocyte. **D:** Drawing of a fibrous astrocyte. **E:** Drawing of a microglial cell. **F:** Drawing of an ependymal cell. **G:** Drawing of the choroid plexus showing numerous villi with blood vessels in the connective tissue core. The choroidal epithelial cells secrete cerebrospinal fluid (CSF; *arrow*). Tight junctions at the apical portion of the choroidal epithelial cells form the blood-CSF barrier.

D. Blood-brain barrier and synapse (Figure 9-4)

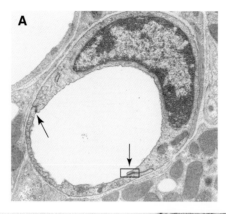

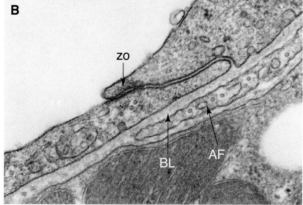

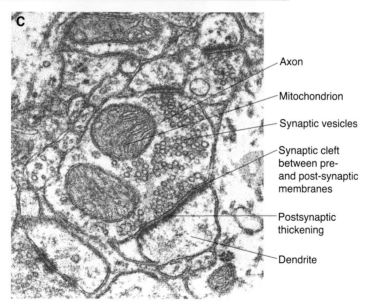

● **Figure 9-4 A:** Electron micrograph (EM) of a capillary within the central the central nervous system. A zonula occlu-dens (*arrows*) between two endothelial cells prevents the escape of macromolecules into the brain. This is the basis of the blood-brain barrier. A paucity of pinocytotic vesicles and astrocytic foot processes also may play a role in the barrier. **B:** High-magnification EM of the boxed area in A showing the zonula occludens (zo; *arrow*) between two endothelial cells. Note the basal lamina (BL) and the astrocytic foot process (AF). **C:** EM of an axodendritic synapse.

E. CNS pathology (Figure 9-5)

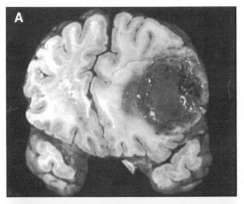

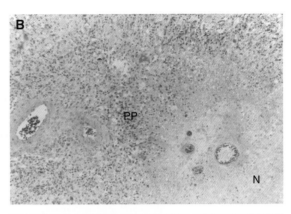

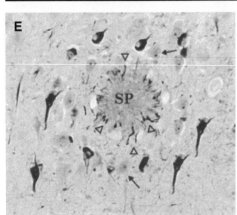

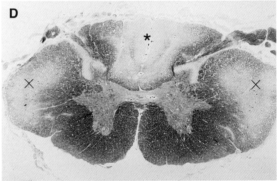

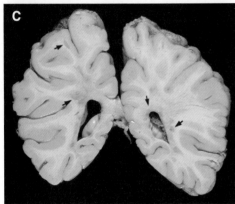

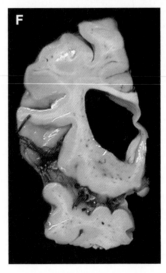

● **Figure 9-5 Central nervous system pathology.** **A, B:** Glioblastoma (grade IV; glioblastoma multiforme). **A:** Coronal brain section shows a glioma in the left frontal cortex containing pigmentation due to hemorrhage. This 65-year-old woman demonstrated personality/behavioral changes during a period of several months. Her condition became increasingly more serious and eventually led to institutionalization for the last 2 weeks of her life. **B:** Light micrograph indicating areas of necrosis (N) that are surrounded by areas of hypercellularity with highly anaplastic tumor cells crowded along the edges of the necrotic regions producing so-called pseudopalisading (PP). **C:** Multiple sclerosis. Coronal section of the brain of a patient with multiple sclerosis showing multiple plaques of demyelination. The most prominent plaques of demyelination (*arrows*) are in the periventricular white matter, left internal capsule, and isthmus of the left temporal lobe. **D:** Friedreich ataxia. A cross section of the spinal cord shows demyelination of the posterior columns (*) and lateral columns (X). **E:** Alzheimer disease. A senile plaque (SP) is shown, which consists of a core of extracellular amyloid surrounded by a halo of dystrophic neurites (*arrowheads*). In addition, a number of dark-staining pyramidal neurons are present due to the neurofibrillary tangles within the cytoplasm. A major component of neurofibrillary tangles is the tau protein, which enhances microtubule assembly. Normal pyramidal neurons are also present (*arrows*). **F:** Huntington disease. Brain from Huntington disease patient with marked atrophy of the head of the caudate nucleus and putamen (Vonsattel grade 3). **G:** Idiopathic parkinsonism. Gross coronal sections through the midbrain of a patient with idiopathic Parkinson disease (*left*) and a control (*right*). Note the marked loss of pigment in the Parkinson disease case.

Chapter 10

Heart and Blood Vessels

I **Heart Layers.** The heart consists of three layers.

A. ENDOCARDIUM. The endocardium is lined by endothelium and is underlain by the **subendocardial space**, which contains blood vessels, nerves, and Purkinje myocytes. The endocardium is continuous with the tunica intima of blood vessels.

B. MYOCARDIUM. The myocardium consists of cardiac myocytes, Purkinje myocytes, and myocardial endocrine cells, which will be discussed later. The myocardium is continuous with the tunica media of blood vessels.

C. EPICARDIUM. The epicardium consists of connective tissue and a layer of mesothelium. In gross anatomy, the epicardium is called the **visceral layer of the pericardial sac (or visceral pericardium)**. The visceral pericardium is reflected to form the **parietal layer of the pericardial sac** (or **parietal pericardium**).

II **Cardiac Myocytes (Figure 10-1; also see Chapter 8).** Cardiac myocytes contract through intrinsically generated action potentials, which are then passed on to neighboring myocytes by gap junctions; that is, the heartbeat is **myogenic**. There are two types of action potentials.

A. SLOW ACTION POTENTIALS. Slow action potentials are observed in the sinoatrial node (SA node) and atrioventricular node (AV node). Slow action potentials are due to the presence of **slow (funny) Na^+ channels** and are divided into three phases.

 1. Phases
   a. Phase 0 is due to the Ca^{2+} influx into nodal cells through **L-type Ca^{2+} channels**.
   b. Phase 3 is due to the K^+ efflux through K^+ channels out of nodal cells.
   c. Phase 4 is due to the Ca^{2+} influx into nodal cells through **T-type Ca^{2+} channels** (transient type) and Na^+ influx into nodal cells through **slow (funny) Na^+ channels**. Note that phase 4 is a gradual depolarization.

 2. Pharmacology
   a. **Class IV Ca^{2+} channel blockers** (diltiazem and verapamil) block L-type Ca^{2+} channels and thus decrease SA node activity and AV nodal conduction.
   b. **Adenosine** binds to the P_1 purinergic receptors and acts by ↓ cyclic adenosine monophosphate (cAMP) levels and stimulates a K^+ channel protein so that the channel opens and K^+ flows out of the cell, causing a hyperpolarization of the cell and thus a decrease in SA node and AV node activity.

B. FAST ACTION POTENTIALS. Fast action potentials are observed in the atrial myocytes, bundle of His, Purkinje myocytes, and ventricular myocytes. Fast action potentials are due to the presence of **fast Na^+ channels** and are divided into five phases.

 1. Phases
   a. Phase 0 is due to Na^+ influx into cardiac myocytes through **fast Na^+ channels**.

    b. **Phase 1** is due to **inactivation of fast Na$^+$ channels** and **K$^+$ efflux** out of cardiac myocytes through K$^+$ **channels.**

    c. **Phase 2** is due to **Ca^{2+} influx** into cardiac myocytes through **L-type Ca^{2+} channels (long-lasting type).** This Ca^{2+} influx ("trigger Ca^{2+}") is involved in the contraction of cardiac myocytes.

    d. **Phase 3** is due to **inactivation of Ca^{2+} channels** and **K$^+$ efflux** out of cardiac myocytes through K$^+$ channels.

    e. **Phase 4** is due to **high K$^+$ efflux, removal of the excess Na$^+$** that entered in phase 0 by **Na$^+$-K$^+$ adenosine triphosphatase (ATPase),** and **removal of the excess Ca^{2+}** that entered in phase 2 by the **Na$^+$-Ca^{2+}exchanger.**

2. **Pharmacology**

    a. **Class I Na$^+$ channel blockers** include class IA, IB, and IC. **Class IA** (quinidine, procainamide, disopyramide) blocks open Na$^+$ channels and thus decreases phase 0 and phase 4 (increases QRS complex). **Class IB** (lidocaine, tocainide, mexiletine, phenytoin) blocks activated and inactivated Na$^+$ channels and thus decreases phase 0. **Class IC** (flecainide, propafenone, moricizine) blocks Na$^+$ channels and thus decreases phase 0.

    b. **Class III K$^+$ channel blockers** (amiodarone and bretylium) block K$^+$ channels, thus prolonging the action potential.

    c. **Cardiac glycosides** (digoxin and digitoxin) are Na$^+$-K$^+$ ATPase blockers that elevate intracellular Na$^+$ ions. The elevated Na$^+$ overwhelms the Na$^+$-Ca^{2+} exchanger so that more Ca^{2+} can be reaccumulated by terminal cisternae (TC). During the next contraction, more Ca^{2+} is released from TC, increasing the force of contraction. Cardiac glycosides are used in congestive heart failure (CHF) to increase the strength of contraction. The antiarrhythmic effect of cardiac glycosides is due to their indirect effect on the autonomic nervous system (increase parasympathetic activity and decrease sympathetic activity).

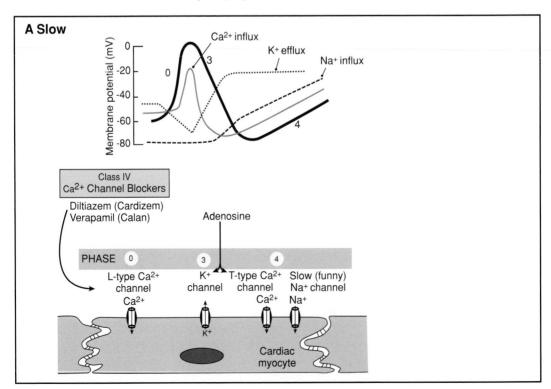

● **Figure 10-1 A:** Slow action potential. A slow action potential (*thick black line*) and its associated ion fluxes observed in the sinoatrial (SA) node are shown. Note the action of **class IV Ca^{2+}** channel blockers (diltiazem and verapamil) and **adenosine** on the cardiac myocyte. (*continued*)

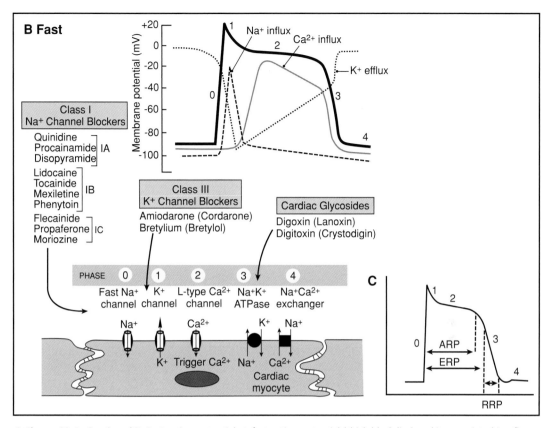

● **Figure 10-1** *Continued* **B:** Fast action potential. A fast action potential (*thick black line*) and its associated ion fluxes observed in ventricular myocytes are shown. Note the action of **class I Na⁺ channel blockers, class III K⁺ channel blockers, and cardiac glycosides** on the cardiac myocyte.

Ⅲ **Purkinje Myocytes (Figure 10-2A)** are modified cardiac myocytes that are specialized for conduction. Purkinje myocytes are *not* neurons. They are joined by gap junctions.

Ⅳ **Myocardial Endocrine Cells** are found in the right and left atria and have secretory granules containing **atrial natriuretic peptide (ANP)**.

A. ANP is secreted in response to increased blood volume or increased venous pressure within the atria (e.g., atrial distention due to left atrial failure). ANP functions include the following.

    1. ANP increases glomerular filtration pressure and glomerular filtration rate (via vasoconstriction of the efferent arteriole) and decreases Na^+ resorption by the proximal convoluted tubule (PCT). These actions produce **natriuresis** (increased Na^+ excretion) in a large volume of dilute urine.

    2. ANP inhibits secretion of **antidiuretic hormone (ADH)** from the neurohypophysis.

    3. ANP inhibits secretion of **aldosterone** from the adrenal cortex (zona glomerulosa).

    4. ANP inhibits secretion of **renin** from juxtaglomerular cells.

    5. ANP causes vasodilation of peripheral and renal blood vessels.

Conduction System (Figure 10-2B)

A. **THE SA NODE** is the pacemaker of the heart and is located at the junction of the superior vena cava and right atrium just beneath the epicardium. From the SA node, the impulse spreads throughout the right atrium and to the AV node via the **anterior, middle, and posterior internodal tracts** and to the left atrium via the **Bachmann bundle**. If all SA node activity is destroyed, the AV node will assume the pacemaker role.

B. **THE AV NODE** is located on the right side of the interatrial septum near the ostium of the coronary sinus in the subendocardial layer.

C. **BUNDLE OF HIS, BUNDLE BRANCHES, PURKINJE MYOCYTES.** The bundle of His travels in the subendocardial space on the right side of the interventricular septum and divides into the **right and left bundle branches**. The left bundle branch is thicker than the right bundle branch. The left bundle branch further divides into an **anterior segment** and a **posterior segment**. The right and left bundle branches both terminate in a complex network of the **Purkinje myocytes**.

D. **CLINICAL CONSIDERATIONS**
   1. **Ectopic pacemakers** are present in the normal heart, and their added activity may induce continuous rhythm disturbances, such as **paroxysmal tachycardias**. When the ectopic pacemaker stops functioning, the SA node may remain quiescent for a period of time (called SA node recovery time). In patients with **sick sinus syndrome**, the SA node recovery time is prolonged with a period of asystole (absence of heartbeat) and loss of consciousness.
   2. **Wolff-Parkinson-White syndrome** is a congenital disorder in which an **accessory conduction pathway** between the atria and ventricles exists. This syndrome is ordinarily asymptomatic. However, a re-entry loop may develop in which impulses travel to the ventricles via the normal conduction pathway but return to the atria via the accessory pathway, causing **supraventricular tachycardia**.
   3. A **first-degree heart block** (Figure 10-2C) occurs when there is an abnormally long delay at the AV node. The delay between the start of the P wave (atrial depolarization) and the QRS complex (ventricle depolarization) occurs at the AV node. This normal delay allows for optimal ventricular filling during atrial contraction.
   4. A **second-degree heart block** (Figure 10-2C) occurs when only a portion of atrial impulses is conducted to the ventricles.
   5. A **third-degree heart block** (Figure 10-2C) occurs when no atrial impulses are conducted to the ventricles.

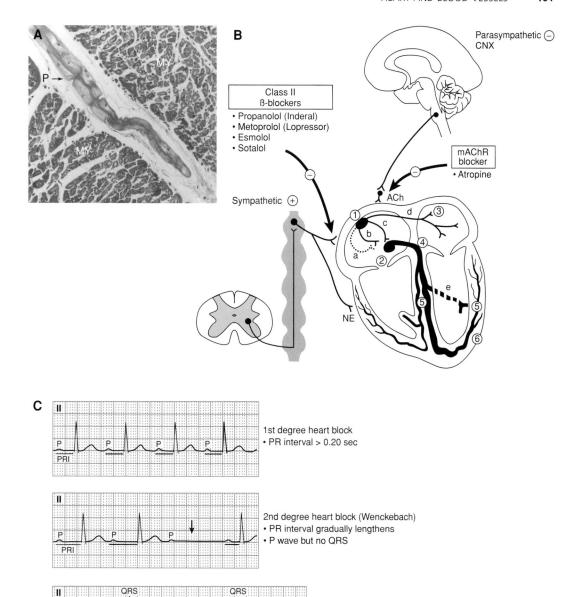

● **Figure 10-2 A:** Purkinje cell. Light micrograph of Purkinje cells (P) traveling within the myocardium (MY). By light microscopy, Purkinje cells appear pale because the large amount of glycogen that is normally contained in the cytoplasm is lost during histologic processing. **B:** Diagram of the conduction system and innervation of the heart. Parasympathetic regulation of heart rate is solely a negative effect. **Atropine** is the classic cholinergic antagonist ("muscarinic acetylcholine receptor [mAChR] blocker," muscarinic blocker, antimuscarinic). Sympathetic regulation of heart rate is solely a positive effect. **Class II β-blockers** block β-adrenergic receptors. 1, sinoatrial node; 2, atrioventricular node; 3, atrial myocytes; 4, bundle of His; 5, Purkinje fibers; 6, ventricular myocytes; a, posterior internodal tract; b, middle internodal tract; c, anterior internodal tract; d, Bachmann bundle; e, posterior segment of left bundle branch. **C:** Electrocardiograms of first-, second-, and third-degree heart blocks. NE, norepinephrine; ACh, acetylcholine.

Parasympathetic Regulation of Heart Rate (Figure 10-2B)

A. EFFECTS

1. **Decreases heart rate** ("vagal arrest") by decreasing Na^+ influx associated with phase 4 depolarization in nodal tissue. This is also called a **negative chronotropism**.
2. **Decreases conduction velocity through the AV node (i.e., increases PR interval)** by decreasing Ca^{2+} influx associated with phase 0 depolarization in nodal tissue. This is also called a **negative dromotropism**.
3. **Decreases contractility of atrial myocytes** by decreasing Ca^{2+} influx associated with phase 2 in atrial myocytes. This is also called a **negative inotropism**.

B. ORGANIZATION.
Preganglionic neuronal cell bodies are located in the **dorsal nucleus of the vagus** and **nucleus ambiguus** of the medulla. Preganglionic axons run in the **vagus nerve (cranial nerve [CN] X)**. Postganglionic neuronal cell bodies are located in the cardiac plexus and atrial wall. Postganglionic axons predominately terminate on the **SA node, AV node, and atrial myocytes** (not ventricular myocytes). Postganglionic axons release **acetylcholine (ACh)** as a neurotransmitter. ACh binds to the M_2 muscarinic ACh receptor (mAChR), which is a G protein–linked receptor that inhibits adenylate cyclase and decreases cAMP levels. The SA node and AV node contain high levels of **acetylcholinesterase** (degrades ACh rapidly) such that any given vagal stimulation is **short-lived. Vasovagal syncope** is a brief period of lightheadedness or loss of consciousness due to an intense burst of CN X activity.

C. PHARMACOLOGY

1. **Atropine** is the classic cholinergic antagonist (mAChR blocker) that blocks the mAChR.

Sympathetic Regulation of Heart Rate (Figure 10-2B)

A. EFFECTS

1. **Increases heat rate** by increasing Na^+ influx associated with phase 4 depolarization in nodal tissue. This is also called **positive chronotropism**.
2. **Increases conduction velocity through the AV node (i.e., decreases PR interval)** by increasing Ca^{2+} influx associated with phase 0 in nodal tissue. This is also called a **positive dromotropism**.
3. **Increases contractility of atrial and ventricular myocytes** by increasing the Ca^{2+} influx associated with phase 2 of the action potential in atrial and ventricular myocytes and increases the activity of the Ca^{2+}-ATPase pump by **phosphorylation of phospholamban** so that more Ca^{2+} reaccumulates during relaxation and therefore is available for release during later heartbeats. This is also called **positive inotropism**.

B. ORGANIZATION.
Preganglionic neuronal cell bodies are located in the intermediolateral columns of the spinal cord. Preganglionic axons enter the paravertebral ganglion and travel to the stellate/middle cervical ganglia. Postganglionic neuronal cell bodies are located in the **stellate and middle cervical ganglia**. Postganglionic axons are distributed to the SA node, AV node, and atrial and ventricular myocytes. **Postganglionic axons release norepinephrine (NE)** as a neurotransmitter. NE binds to the β_1-adrenergic receptor, which is a G protein–linked receptor that stimulates adenylate cyclase and increases cAMP levels. Released NE is either carried away by the bloodstream or taken up by the nerve terminals so that sympathetic stimulation is relatively **long-lived**.

C. PHARMACOLOGY: CLASS II β-BLOCKERS

1. **Propranolol (Inderal)** is a nonselective β_1- and β_2-adrenergic receptor antagonist that blocks the effects of the sympathetic nervous system on the heart. Remember that postganglionic sympathetic axons innervating the heart release NE. NE binds

to the β_1-adrenergic receptor, which is a G_S protein–linked receptor that stimulates the adenylate cyclase and increases cAMP levels. A β-adrenergic receptor antagonist decreases cAMP levels. This results in the following antiarrhythmic effects: **decreased automaticity of the SA node (and ectopic pacemakers)** and **decreased conduction velocity of the AV node** due to reducing the slope of the phase 4 depolarization most likely caused by deactivation of the **T-type Ca^{2+} ion channel** and the **slow (funny) Na^+ ion channel**. Clinical uses include supraventricular arrhythmias, ventricular tachycardia, and digitalis-induced arrhythmia. Propranolol is also used to treat angina and hypertension, which will be discussed later.

2. **Metoprolol (Lopressor)** is a cardioselective β_1-adrenergic receptor antagonist and has similar antiarrhythmic effects as propranolol.

3. **Esmolol (Brevibloc)** is a cardioselective β_1-adrenergic receptor antagonist and has similar antiarrhythmic effects as propranolol.

4. **Sotalol (Betapace)** is a nonselective β_1- and β_2-adrenergic receptor antagonist and has similar antiarrhythmic effects as propranolol. Sotalol is also a K^+ ion channel antagonist.

Ⅷ Clinical Consideration: Myocardial Infarction (MI) (Figure 10-3)

A. Transmural MIs are caused by thrombotic occlusion of a coronary artery.

B. Infarction is localized to the anatomic area supplied by the occluded artery. Coronary artery occlusion occurs most commonly in the **anterior interventricular artery** (also called the **left anterior descending**), followed by the **right coronary artery**, and then the **circumflex artery**.

C. SERUM MARKERS OF MI
1. **Troponin I** is a highly specific cardiac marker that can be detected within 4 hours to 7 to 10 days after MI pain.
2. **Creatine kinase (CK)** consists of M and B subunits. CK-MM is found in skeletal muscle and cardiac muscle. CK-MB is found mainly in cardiac muscle. **CK-MB is the test of choice in the first 24 hours after MI pain.** CK-MB begins to rise 4 to 8 hours after MI pain, peaks at 24 hours, and returns to normal within 48 to 72 hours. This sequence is important because skeletal muscle injury or non-MI conditions may raise serum CK-MB but do not show this pattern. It is common to calculate the ratio **CK-MB/total CK**. A CK-MB/total CK greater than 2.5% indicates MI.
3. **Lactate dehydrogenase (LDH)** consists of H and M subunits. LDH-HHHH (or LDH_1) and LDH-HHHM (or LDH_2) are found in cardiac muscle. **LDH_1 is the test of choice 2 to 3 days after MI pain since CK-MB levels have already returned to normal at this time.** It is common to calculate the ratio LDH_1/LDH_2. A LDH_1/LDH_2 greater than 1.0 indicates MI.

D. ELECTROCARDIOGRAMS (ECGs)
1. **Acute MI.** An acute MI is associated with ST elevation.
2. **Recent MI.** A recent MI (within 1 to 2 days) is associated with deep Q waves and inverted T waves.
3. **Old MI.** An old MI (weeks later) is associated with persistence of deep Q waves but no T-wave inversion.

E. EVOLUTION OF A MI. The histologic changes of an MI are as follows.
1. **Day 1:** coagulation necrosis, wavy myocytes, pyknotic nuclei, eosinophilic cytoplasm, contraction bands
2. **Days 2 to 4:** total coagulation necrosis, loss of nuclei, loss of striations, dilated vessels (hyperemia), and neutrophil infiltration
3. **Days 5 to 10:** macrophage infiltration and phagocytosis of necrotic myocytes
4. **Week 7:** collagenous scar

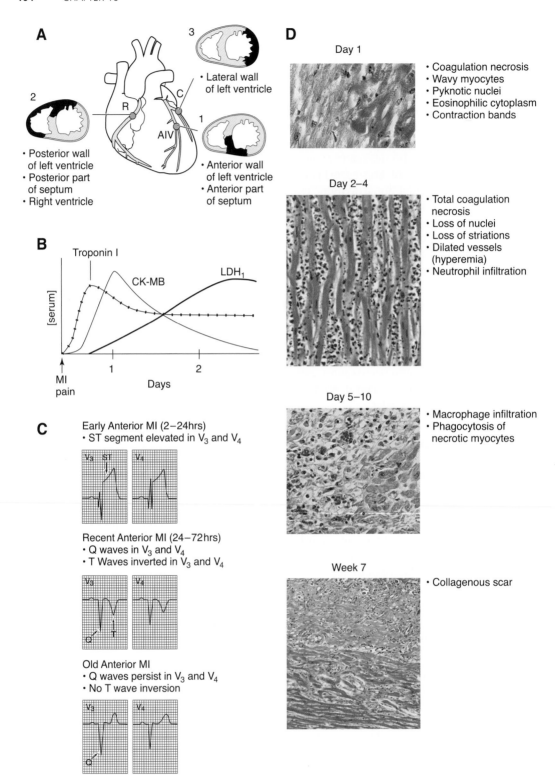

● **Figure 10-3 Myocardial infarction (MI). A:** Coronary artery occlusion occurs most commonly in the anterior inter-ventricular artery (AIV; also called the left anterior descending [LAD]), followed by the right coronary artery (R), and then the circumflex artery (C). This is indicated by the numbers 1, 2, and 3. R, right coronary artery; L, left coronary artery; SA, sinoatrial artery; RM, right marginal artery; S, septal branches; C, circumflex artery; OM, obtuse marginal artery; AM, anterior marginal; AD, anterior diagonal artery. **B:** Serum markers of MI. CK-MB, creatine kinase M and B subunits; LDH, lactate dehydrogenase **C:** Electrocardiograms. An acute MI, a recent MI, and an old MI (weeks later) are shown. **D:** Evolution of an MI from day 1 to week 7. The histologic changes of an MI are indicated.

IX **Tunics of Blood Vessels (Figure 10-4)**

A. TUNICA INTIMA consists of endothelium, a basal lamina, loose connective tissue, and an internal elastic lamina.

B. TUNICA MEDIA consists of smooth muscle cells, type III collagen, elastic fibers, and an external elastic lamina. Many factors affect smooth muscle cells of the tunica media, including:

1. **Sympathetic Innervation**

   a. Sympathetic innervation activity controls the **tonus**. Postganglionic sympathetic neurons release NE, which binds to α_1-adrenergic receptors to cause vasoconstriction of skin, skeletal muscle, and visceral blood vessels.

   b. **Doxazosin (Cardura), Prazosin (Minipress), and Terazosin (Hytrin) are α_1-adrenergic receptor antagonists** that cause vasodilation and are used to treat hypertension.

   c. **Propranolol is a nonselective β_1- and β_2-adrenergic receptor antagonist** that decreases heart rate and contractility directly by blocking β_1-adrenergic receptors in the SA node (which may lower blood pressure). Propranolol also decreases peripheral vascular resistance by blocking β_1-adrenergic receptors in the kidney, which leads to a decrease of renin, a decrease in the renin-angiotensin II system, and a decrease in angiotensin II, which causes peripheral vasodilation. Propranolol is used prophylactically not for acute cases of hypertension because its effects are more long-term modulatory effects.

2. **Prostaglandins (PGE$_1$, PGE$_2$), prostacyclin (PGI$_2$), bradykinins, histamine, and nitric oxide (NO)** are potent vasodilators.

3. **Thromboxane (TXA$_2$), endothelin 1, angiotensin II,** and **serotonin** are potent vasoconstrictors.

4. **Nifedipine (Procardia)** and **Nicardipine (Cardene)** are L-type Ca^{2+} channel blockers ("afterload-reducing drugs" used to treat hypertension and angina) that block Ca^{2+} entry into smooth muscle cells. This causes relaxation of **arterial** smooth muscle (i.e., vasodilation) and therefore decreases peripheral vascular resistance (PVR).

5. **Vasodilators (e.g., Hydralazine [Apresoline], Minoxidil [Loniten]).** These drugs ("afterload-reducing drugs" used to treat hypertension) relax predominately **arteriolar** smooth muscle (i.e., vasodilation), leading to a decrease in PVR. The action of hydralazine is uncertain but may involve NO. Minoxidil is a K^+ channel agonist that causes increased K^+ efflux, hyperpolarization, and relaxation of smooth muscle.

C. TUNICA ADVENTITIA consists of fibroblasts, type I collagen, and some elastic fibers.

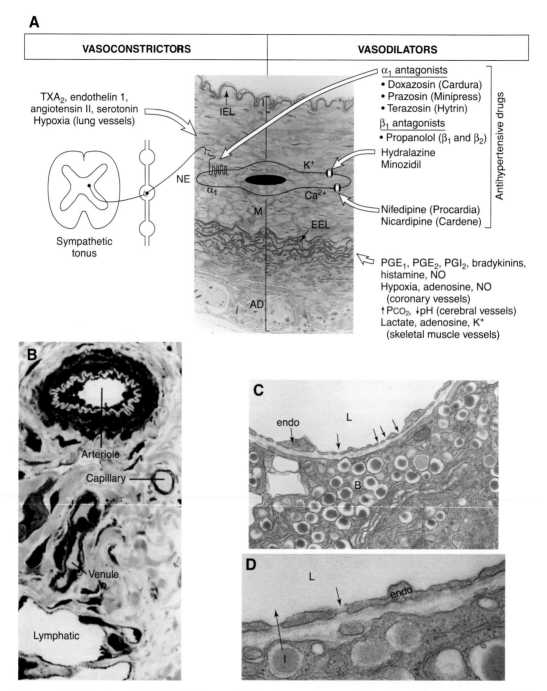

● **Figure 10-4 Blood vessels. A:** Light micrograph (LM) of a muscular artery. The tunica intima (I), tunica media (M), and tunica adventitia (AD) are indicated by the *brackets*. A typical smooth muscle cell with α_1-adrenergic receptors, K^+ channels, and Ca^{2+} channels is drawn within the tunica media. The various vasoconstrictors and vasodilators are indicated. The drugs that act as vasodilators are important clinically as antihypertensive drugs. EEL, external elastic lamina; IEL, internal elastic lamina; NE, norepinephrine; TXA_2, thromboxane A_2 PGE_1, prostaglandin E_1; PGE_2, prostaglandin E_2; PGI_2, prostaglandin I_2; NO, nitric oxide; P_{CO2}, partial pressure of carbon dioxide. **B:** LM of an arteriole, capillary, venule, and lymphatic vessel. **C:** Electron micrograph (EM) of a fenestrated capillary within the pancreatic islets of Langerhans (an endocrine gland) adjacent to a β cell. The fenestrae with diaphragms are indicated at the *arrows*. L, lumen of the capillary; B, β cell; endo, endothelial cell. **D:** High-magnification EM of a fenestrated capillary showing insulin (I) within a secretory granule and its route of release through the fenestrae (*large arrow*) into the lumen (L) of the capillary. The *small arrow* indicates fenestrae with diaphragm. endo, endothelial cell.

Types of Blood Vessels

A. ELASTIC (CONDUCTING) ARTERIES (e.g., pulmonary artery, aorta) have a tunica media with a prominent elastic fiber component that responds to the high systolic pressure generated by the heart.

B. MUSCULAR (DISTRIBUTING) ARTERIES have a tunica intima with a prominent internal elastic lamina and a tunica media with a prominent smooth muscle cell component.

C. ARTERIOLES have a tunica media that consists of only one to two layers of smooth muscle cells and play a major role in regulation of blood pressure.

D. METARTERIOLES are the smallest (or terminal) branches of the arterial system and flow directly into capillary beds. A **precapillary sphincter** plays a role in regulation of blood flow to capillary beds.

E. ARTERIOVENOUS ANASTOMOSES (AVAs) allow arteriolar blood to bypass the capillary bed and empty directly into venules. AVAs are found primarily in the skin to regulate body temperature. Constriction of the arteriolar component directs blood to the capillary bed, causing depletion of body heat. Dilation of the arteriolar component directs blood to the venules, causing conservation of body heat.

F. CAPILLARIES (FIGURE 10-4C, D) consist of a single layer of endothelial cells surrounded by a basal lamina and are the site of exchange (e.g., CO_2, O_2, water, glucose, amino acids, proteins) between blood and cells. Microvasculature damage associated with type 1 and Type 2 diabetes is due to **nonenzymatic glycosylation** of various proteins, which causes the release of harmful cytokines. The different types of capillaries include the following.

1. **Continuous capillaries** consist of a single layer of endothelial cells joined by a **zonula occludens** (a tight junction that extends around the entire perimeter of the cell) and contain no fenestrae (or pores). They are found in lung, muscle, and brain (blood-brain barrier).

2. **Fenestrated capillaries with diaphragms** consist of a single layer of endothelial cells joined by a **fascia occludens** (a tight junction that extends only partially around the perimeter of the cell, creating slitlike **intercellular spaces**) and contain **fenestrae (or pores) with diaphragms.** They are found in endocrine glands, intestine, and kidney.

3. **Fenestrated capillaries without diaphragms** are found solely within the kidney glomerulus.

4. **Discontinuous capillaries (sinusoids)** consist of a single layer of endothelial cells that are separated by wide gaps (i.e., no zonula occludens present) and contain fenestrae. They are found in the **liver, bone marrow,** and **spleen.**

 # Functions of Endothelium. Although endothelial cells (ECs) are fairly unremarkable microscopically, they are very active physiologically.

A. ECs maintain the subendothelial layer that prevents blood escape into the extravascular space by secretion of **basement membrane components, type III and IV collagen, elastin, mucopolysaccharides, vitronectin, fibronectin, proteases,** and **protease inhibitors.**

B. Normally, ECs act as a potent anticoagulant surface adjacent to blood by:
1. Expression of anticoagulant cell surface molecules: **glycosaminoglycans (GAGs), heparan sulfate–antithrombin III system, thrombin–thrombomodulin–protein C system,** and **plasminogen–plasmin activator system**

2. Secretion of **PGI$_2$ and endothelium-derived relaxing factor (EDRF)**, which cause vasodilation and inhibit platelet adhesion/aggregation
3. Secretion of **tissue plasminogen activator (TPA) and urokinase**, which stimulate the conversion of plasminogen → plasmin

C. Upon injury, ECs act as a potent procoagulation surface by the secretion of **tissue factor (TF), von Willebrand factor (vWF), factor V, plasminogen activator inhibitors (PAI-1, PAI-2), interleukin 1 (IL-1), tissue necrosis factor (TNF), and endothelin 1** (which affects smooth muscle cells of the tunica media and causes vasoconstriction).

D. ECs secrete vWF, which is stored in Weibel-Palade granules and promotes platelet adhesion to subendothelial collagen at an injury site and blood clotting. vWF combines with factor VIII secreted by hepatocytes to form a **factor VIII–vWF complex**. This complex circulates in the plasma as a unit and promotes blood clotting as well as platelet–vessel wall interactions necessary for blood clotting. **Von Willebrand disease is a common bleeding disorder in humans.**

E. ECs secrete **nitric oxide (NO)**, which affects smooth muscle cells of the tunica media and causes vasodilation.
   1. NO is synthesized by the reaction:

$$\text{Arginine} \xrightarrow{\text{NO synthase}} \text{NO} + \text{citrulline}$$

   2. NO activates guanylate cyclase in smooth muscle cells, causing **increased levels of cyclic guanosine monophosphate (cGMP) and vasodilation.**
   3. NO is involved in the vasodilation associated with penile erection. **Viagra**, used in the treatment of erectile dysfunction, is a cGMP phosphodiesterase inhibitor so that increased cGMP levels are maintained.
   4. **Nitroglycerin, Isosorbide Dinitrate (Isordil), and Amyl Nitrite (Aspirols, Vaporole)** are metabolized by smooth muscle cells to NO, which relaxes **venous (main effect)** and **arterial smooth muscle**, causing peripheral vasodilation. This results in decreased cardiac preload, decreased cardiac afterload, and decreased cardiac output. These drugs are used to treat **angina pectoris.**

F. ECs **convert** angiotensin I to angiotensin II **(predominately in lung capillaries) using the enzyme** angiotensin-converting enzyme (ACE), **which causes vasoconstriction and secretion of both aldosterone and ADH.**

G. ECs aid in the digestion of triacylglycerides (carried by very low-density lipoproteins [VLDLs] and chylomicrons) into fatty acids and glycerol catalyzed by **lipoprotein lipase** attached to ECs of skeletal muscle and adipose tissue capillaries.

H. ECs help in the passage of **lipid-soluble substances** (including O$_2$ and CO$_2$) by **diffusion** of **water-soluble substances** (including water, glucose, and amino acids) through the slitlike **intercellular spaces** and **large water-soluble substances** (e.g., proteins) by **pinocytosis.**

I. ECs exchange fluid between blood and cells, which is described by the **Starling equation.**

XII Clinical Considerations

A. CORONARY ARTERY WITH ATHEROSCLEROSIS (FIGURE 10-5)
   1. Atherosclerosis is considered an **intimal disease.**
   2. An atheromatous plaque may undergo many histologic changes, such as:
      a. **Plaque calcification**, which turns arteries into brittle pipes

    b.   **Hemorrhage into the plaque,** which induces focal rupture or ulceration

    c.   **Focal plaque rupture** at the luminal surface, which results in **thrombus formation,** whereby the thrombus may partially or completely occlude the lumen

3. Thrombus formation is initiated by platelet aggregation induced by **TXA₂.** TXA_2 is synthesized from arachidonic acid using the enzyme cyclooxygenase.

4. **Aspirin** covalently inhibits cyclooxygenase, and **nonsteroidal anti-inflammatory drugs (NSAIDs) such as ibuprofen and acetaminophen** reversibly inhibit cyclooxygenase and thereby block the synthesis of TXA_2. Consequently, low doses of aspirin and NSAIDs are effective in prevention of myocardial infarction.

5. **Thrombolysis** is stimulated by **TPA** treatment, which successfully decreases the extent of ischemic damage due to myocardial infarction. TPA stimulates the **conversion of plasminogen to plasmin.** Plasmin is a protease that digests fibrin within the thrombus.

B. KAPOSI SARCOMA (KS) (FIGURE 10-6)

1. KS is a malignant angioproliferative tumor derived from endothelial cells.

2. KS is a relatively rare vascular tumor endemic in parts of central Africa but has come to the forefront because of its high frequency of occurrence in **acquired immunodeficiency syndrome (AIDS) and immunosuppressed patients.**

3. KS is thought to be caused by the **human herpesvirus 8 (HHV-8).**

4. KS begins as painful purple to brown cutaneous nodules that most often appear on the hands and face.

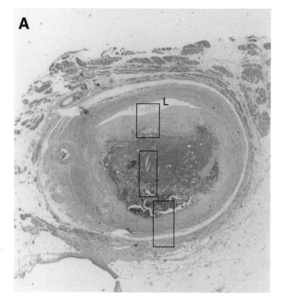

● **Figure 10-5 Atherosclerosis. A:** Coronary artery with atherosclerosis. The entire coronary artery is shown with an eccentric, narrow lumen (L) due to the presence of an atheromatous plaque (tunica intima thickening). (*continued*)

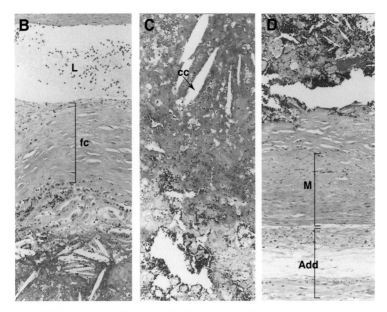

● **Figure 10-5** *Continued* **B–D:** High magnification of the *boxed areas* (shown in A) of the **atheromatous plaque.** The fibrous cap (fc) is composed of smooth muscle cells, a few leukocytes, and a relatively dense deposition of collagen. The deeper necrotic core (see C) consists of a disorganized mass of lipid material, cholesterol crystals (cc), cell debris, and foam cells (macrophages digesting modified LDL) of the fatty streak. Ad, tunica adventitia; M, tunica media.

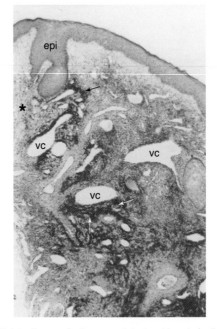

● **Figure 10-6 Kaposi sarcoma.** Light micrograph shows an intact epidermis (epi) of the skin covering the malignant vascular lesion in the dermis consisting of numerous vascular channels (vc), spindle-shaped neoplastic stromal cells (*), and extravasated red blood cells (*arrows*).

Chapter 11

Blood

① **Plasma** is the fluid portion of blood that contains many different proteins, including **albumin**, which maintains blood colloidal osmotic (oncotic) pressure; **γ-globulins**; **β-globulins**, which participate in the transport of hormones, metal ions, and lipids; and **fibrinogen**, which participates in blood clotting. Plasma without fibrinogen is called **serum**.

② **Red Blood Cells** (RBCs or erythrocytes)

A. CHARACTERISTICS

1. RBCs do not contain a nucleus or mitochondria.
2. RBCs use **glucose** as the primary fuel source (i.e., **glycolysis** or **hexose monophosphate shunt** during stress).
3. RBCs are biconcave-shaped disks (shape maintained by **spectrin**) and contain both **hemoglobin** and **carbonic anhydrase**.
4. Erythropoiesis (RBC formation) is regulated by **erythropoietin (EPO)**, which is a glycoprotein hormone secreted by endothelial cells of the peritubular capillary network of the kidney. Serum EPO levels can be extremely high (normal value: 4 to 16 IU/L) in patients with severe anemias (e.g., aplastic anemia, severe hemolytic anemia, and hematologic cancers).
5. RBCs have a lifespan of **100 to 120 days**.
6. The RBC membrane consists of a lipid bilayer anchored to a cytoskeletal network of proteins, which include the following (**Figure 11-1**).
   a. **Spectrin** maintains the biconcave shape of the RBC. The tail ends of spectrin bind to **actin** and **band 4.1 protein**.
   b. **Ankyrin** attaches to spectrin and **band 3 protein**.
   c. **Band 3 protein** is an anion transporter that allows HCO_3^- to cross the RBC membrane in exchange for Cl^-.
   d. **Band 4.2 protein (pallidin)** interacts with both ankyrin and band 3 protein.
   e. **RhAG (Rh-associated glycoprotein)** binds to ankyrin and targets RhD and RHCE antigens to the RBC surface.
   f. **Glycophorin** is highly glycosylated and imparts a strong negative charge on the RBC surface that reduces interaction between RBCs.
   g. **Band 4.1 protein** interacts with both spectrin and actin.
   h. **Actin** interacts with both spectrin and band 4.1 protein.
   i. **Glycophorins A, B, C, and D** are sialic-rich transmembrane glycoproteins that impart a strong negative charge to the RBC surface.

B. LAYERS. If blood is centrifuged (and clotting is prevented), three layers are separated:

1. **Top layer:** plasma
2. **Middle layer:** buffy coat containing leukocytes and platelets
3. **Bottom layer:** RBCs

C. HEMATOCRIT is the % volume of a blood sample occupied by RBCs. A normal hematocrit value = 45%. Hematocrit values less than 45% may indicate **anemia**.

D. ENVIRONMENT
1. **A hypotonic environment** causes RBCs to swell, rupture (thereby forming ghosts), and release hemoglobin. This process is called **hemolysis.**
2. **A hypertonic environment** causes RBCs to shrink so that spiny projections protrude from the surface. This process is called **crenation.**

E. ABO BLOOD GROUP SYSTEM (FIGURE 11-1). The A, B, and O blood group antigens are **neutral glycolipids.** Glycolipids are carbohydrate-containing sphingolipids linked to the outer leaflet of the RBC membrane. The ABO blood groups are defined by the presence of the immunodominant sugar: **N-acetylgalactosamine** for the A antigen and **D-galactose** for the B antigen. The four common blood groups in the ABO system are O (45%; **universal donor**), A (40%), B (11%), and AB (4%; **universal recipient**).

F. DUFFY BLOOD GROUP SYSTEM (FIGURE 11-1). The <u>D</u>uffy <u>a</u>ntigen/<u>r</u>eceptor for <u>c</u>hemokine (DARC) is an RBC surface transmembrane glycoprotein encoded by the *DARC* gene on chromosome 1q22.1. DARC acts as a multispecific receptor for **chemokines** of both the CC and CXC families and as a receptor of malaria parasites (*Plasmodium vivax* and *Plasmodium knowlesi*). People who lack DARC (FY*O allele) are resistant to malaria.

G. LEWIS BLOOD GROUP SYSTEM (FIGURE 11-1). The Lewis antigens (**Lewis a** and **Lewis b**) are RBC surface glycoproteins with <u>f</u>ucosyl<u>t</u>ransferase activity encoded by the *FUT2* gene and *FUT3* gene on chromosome 19p13.3. Lewis a and Lewis b are not produced by RBCs, but instead are secreted by exocrine epithelial cells and are subsequently adsorbed on the RBC surface. There is a link between Lewis antigens and the secretion of ABO blood group antigens. The presence of Lewis a antigens makes a person a **nonsecretor**, while the presence of Lewis b antigens makes a person a **secretor.**

H. KELL BLOOD GROUP SYSTEM (FIGURE 11-1). The <u>Kell</u> antigens are RBC surface transmembrane glycoproteins peptides encoded by the *KEL* gene on chromosome 7q33 for the **kell protein**. The Kell antigens are actually peptides found within the kell protein. The two most common alleles of the *KEL* gene are the K_1 (**Kell**) **allele** and K_2 (**Cellano**) **allele**. The Kell antigens normally associate with the Kx protein. In some people, the Kx protein is absent, resulting in **McLeod syndrome** characterized by acanthocytosis, reduced Kell antigen expression, disordered movements, psychological disturbances, and loss of reflexes. Kell antigens are important in **transfusion medicine, autoimmune hemolytic anemia, and hemolytic disease of the newborn.** People without Kell antigens (K_0) must be transfused with blood from K_0 donors in order to prevent hemolysis.

I. RHESUS (Rh) BLOOD GROUP SYSTEM (FIGURE 11-1)
1. The **Rhesus antigens** are RBC surface nonglycosylated transmembrane proteins encoded by the *RHD* gene on chromosome 1p36.2 for the **RhD antigen** and the *RHCE* gene on chromosome 1p36.11 for the **RhC antigen** and **RhE antigen**.
2. The Rh antigens commonly recognized on the RBC include D, C, c, E, and e.
3. The terms "**Rhesus factor**" and "**Rh factor**" are equivalent and refer to the **RhD antigen only**. The **RhD antigen** is highly immunogenic in persons who are not immunosuppressed.
4. RhD antigen probably acts as an **ion channel** for either CO_2 or **ammonium** (a toxic byproduct of energy metabolism) and possibly keeps the blood pH level balanced.
5. The Rh antigens play a role clinically in **compensated hemolytic anemia, hemolytic transfusion reactions, and hemolytic disease of the newborn.**

6. **Clinical Consideration: Hemolytic Disease of the Newborn (HDN)**
   a. **The Rh factor** is clinically important in pregnancy. If the mother is Rh−, she will produce Rh antibodies if the fetus is Rh+. This situation will not affect the first pregnancy, but will affect the second pregnancy with an Rh+ fetus. In the second pregnancy with an Rh+ fetus, a hemolytic condition of RBCs occurs known as **Rh-hemolytic disease of newborn (erythroblastosis fetalis).**
   b. Rh_0 **(D) Immune Globulin (RhoGAM, MICRhoGAM)** is a human immunoglobulin G (IgG) preparation that contains antibodies against Rh factor and prevents a maternal antibody response to Rh+ cells that may enter the maternal bloodstream of an Rh− mother. This drug is administered to Rh− mothers within 72 hours after the birth of an Rh+ baby to prevent erythroblastosis fetalis during subsequent pregnancies.

J. KERNICTERUS, which is a pathologic deposition of bilirubin in the basal ganglia, may develop due to the jaundice from the RBC hemolysis.

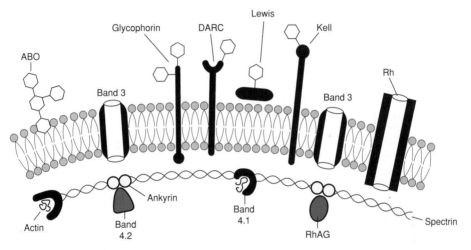

● Figure 11-1 **Diagram of the red blood cell (RBC) membrane.** Note the lipid bilayer anchored to a cytoskeletal network of proteins. In addition, the ABO, Duffy, Lewis, Kell, and Rhesus blood group antigens are shown. DARC, Duffy antigen/receptor for chemokine.

 Hemoglobin (Hb)

A. **CHARACTERISTICS**
   1. Hb is a globular protein consisting of **four subunits.**
      a. **Adult Hb (HbA)** consists of two **α-globin subunits** and two **β-globin subunits** designated Hb $\alpha_2\beta_2$.
      b. **Fetal Hb (HbF)** consists of two **α-globin subunits** and two **γ-globin subunits** designated Hb $\alpha_2\gamma_2$. HbF is the **major form of Hb during fetal development** since the O_2 affinity of HbF is higher than the O_2 affinity of HbA and thereby "pulls" O_2 from the maternal blood into fetal blood. The higher O_2 affinity of HbF is explained by **2,3-bisphosphoglycerate (BPG).** When 2,3-BPG binds HbA, the O_2 affinity of HbA is lowered. However, 2,3-BPG does not bind HbF, and therefore, the O_2 **affinity of HbF is higher.**
   2. Hb contains a **heme moiety,** which is an **iron (Fe)-containing porphyrin.** Fe^{2+} (ferrous state) binds O_2, forming **oxyhemoglobin.** Fe^{3+} (ferric state) does not bind O_2, forming **deoxyhemoglobin.** The heme moiety is synthesized partially in mitochondria and partially in cytoplasm.

3. The **Hb–O$_2$ dissociation curve** is **sigmoid shaped** because each successive O$_2$ that binds to Hb increases the affinity for the next oxygen (i.e., binding is cooperative). Therefore, the affinity for the fourth O$_2$ is the highest.
4. Concentration of Hb
    a. In males, the normal concentration of Hb is **13.5 to 17.5 g/dL.**
    b. In females, the normal concentration of Hb is **12.0 to 16.0 g/dL.**
5. **Types 1 and 2 diabetes.** The amount of **glycosylated Hb (HbA$_{1c}$)** is an indicator of blood glucose normalization over the previous 3 months (because the half-life of RBCs is 3 months) in patients with type 1 and type 2 diabetes. Long periods of elevated blood glucose levels result in an HbA$_{1c}$ = **12% to 20%,** whereas normal levels of HbA$_{1c}$ = **5%.**

IV Clinical Considerations (Figure 11-2)

A. HEREDITARY SPHEROCYTOSIS (HS)

1. HS is a genetic disorder caused by mutations in the *SPTA1* gene on chromosome 1q21 for **α-spectrin**, *SPTB* gene on chromosome 14q24.1 for **β-spectrin**, *ANK1* gene on chromosome 8p21.1 for **ankyrin (most common mutation)**, *SLC4A1* gene on chromosome 17q12 for **band 3 protein**, *EPB42* gene on chromosome 15q15 for **band 4.2 protein (pallidin)**, or *RHAG* gene on chromosome 6p21 for **Rh-associated glycoprotein.**
2. HS is the most common hemolytic anemia due to an RBC membrane defect and is often associated with **spectrin deficiency.**
3. **Clinical features include:** anemia, jaundice, and splenomegaly.

B. α-THALASSEMIA

1. α-Thalassemia is an autosomal recessive genetic disorder most commonly caused by a deletion of the *HBA1* gene and/or the *HBA2* gene on **chromosome 16p13.3** for the **α_1-globin subunit** of <u>hemoglo</u>bin and **α_2-globin subunit** of <u>hemoglo</u>bin, respectively. These deletions occur during unequal crossing over between homologous chromosomes during meiosis.
2. α-Thalassemia is defined by the reduced synthesis of α-globin subunits of hemoglobin. It should be noted that the clinical amount of α-globin subunits of hemoglobin is due to **four alleles.**
3. The deletions of the *HBA1* gene and/or the *HBA2* gene result in the **reduced amounts of HbF (Hb $\alpha_2\gamma_2$)** and **HbA (Hb $\alpha_2\beta_2$)** since there is reduced synthesis of α-globin subunits, which are common to both HbF and HbA.
4. There are two clinically significant forms of α-thalassemia:
    a. **Hb Bart hydrops fetalis syndrome (Hb Bart).** Hb Bart results from the inheritance of a deletion or dysfunction of all four α-globin alleles and is the most severe form of α-thalassemia. An **excess of γ-globin subunits** forms tetramers during fetal development that have extremely high affinity for oxygen but are unable to deliver oxygen to fetal tissues. **Clinical features include:** fetal onset of generalized edema, ascites, pleural and pericardial effusions, severe hypochromatic anemia, and death in the neonatal period.
    b. **Hemoglobin H (HbH) Disease.** HbH results from the inheritance of a deletion or dysfunction of three α-globin alleles. A relative **excess of β-globin subunits** forms insoluble inclusion bodies within mature red blood cells. **Clinical features include:** mild microcytic hypochromatic hemolytic anemia and hepatosplenomegaly.

C. β-THALASSEMIA

1. β-Thalassemia is an autosomal recessive genetic disorder caused by more than 200 missense or frameshift mutations in the *HBB* gene on **chromosome 11p15.5** for the **β-globin subunit of hemoglobin.**

2. β-Thalassemia is defined by the absence or reduced synthesis of β-globin subunits of hemoglobin. A $\boldsymbol{\beta^0}$ **mutation** refers to a mutation that causes the absence of β-globin subunits. A $\boldsymbol{\beta^+}$ **mutation** refers to a mutation that causes the reduced synthesis of β-globin subunits. It should be noted that the clinical amount of β-globin subunits of hemoglobin is due to **two alleles**.
3. The mutations in the *HBB* **gene** result in the **reduced amounts of HbA** (Hb $\boldsymbol{\alpha_2\beta_2}$) since there is reduced synthesis of β-globin subunits, which are found only in HbA.
4. Heterozygote carriers of β-thalassemia are often referred to as having **thalassemia minor**.
5. There are two clinically significant forms of β-thalassemia.
    a. **Thalassemia Major.** Thalassemia major results from the inheritance of a β^0 mutation of both β-globin alleles (β^0/β^0) and is the most severe form of β-thalassemia. An **excess of $\boldsymbol{\alpha}$-globin subunits** forms insoluble inclusion bodies within mature red blood cell precursors. **Clinical features include:** microcytic hypochromatic hemolytic anemia, abnormal peripheral blood smear with nucleated red blood cells, reduced amounts of HbA, severe anemia, hepatosplenomegaly, and failure to thrive; the individual becomes progressively pale, regular blood transfusion are necessary, and the individual usually comes to medical attention between 6 months and 2 years of age.
    b. **Thalassemia Intermedia.** Thalassemia intermedia results from the inheritance of a β^0 mutation of one β-globin allele (β^0/normal β) and is a less severe form of β-thalassemia. **Clinical features include:** a mild hemolytic anemia. Individuals are at risk for iron overload, regular blood transfusions are rarely necessary, and individuals usually come to medical attention at older than 2 years of age.

D. SICKLE CELL DISEASE (SCD)

1. SCD is an autosomal recessive genetic disorder caused by a missense mutation (G$\underline{A}$G $\rightarrow$ G$\underline{T}$G) at the second nucleotide of the sixth codon in the *HBB* **gene** on **chromosome 11p15.5**, which results in a normal **glutamic acid** $\rightarrow$ **valine** substitution (E6V) in the $\boldsymbol{\beta}$-**globin subunit** of h̲emoglob̲in.
2. SCD is defined by the presence of **E6V HbS** and accounts for 60% to 70% of SCD cases in the United States.
3. **Clinical features include:** infants appearing healthy at birth but becoming symptomatic later after fetal hemoglobin (HbF) levels decrease and HbS levels increase (note: HbF does not contain β-globin subunits); pain and/or swelling of hands and feet in infants and young children; varying degrees of hemolysis leading to chronic anemia, cholelithiasis, and delayed growth and sexual maturation; intermittent episodes of vascular occlusion in the brain, liver, lung or spleen; and acute and chronic organ dysfunction. In patients with osteomyelitis there is a disproportionate number of cases due to *Salmonella* infection. Functional asplenia usually results in adolescence after so-called autoinfarction of the spleen. Factors that induce sickling are PO_2 (e.g., high altitude) or a concentration of 60% HbS or greater in RBCs.

E. GLUCOSE-6-PHOSPHATE DEHYDROGENASE DEFICIENCY (G6PD)

1. G6PD is an X-linked genetic disorder caused by missense point mutations in the *G6PD* **gene** on **chromosome Xq28** for **glucose-6̲-p̲hosphate d̲ehydrogenase** enzyme.
2. G6PD enzyme converts glucose-6-phostphate to 6-phosphogluconolatone and reduces nicotinamide adenine dinucleotide (NADH) to NADHP, which is the initial step in the **hexose monophosphate (HMP) shunt**.
3. The main function of the HMP shunt is to protect RBCs from **oxidative injury** by the production of NADPH, which is an important cofactor in **glutathione** metabolism.

Glutathione is a sulfhydryl-containing tripeptide that functions as a reducing agent, thereby protecting against oxidative injury.

4. G6PD deficiency may confer a selective advantage against malaria.
5. **Clinical features include:** a wide spectrum of hemolytic syndromes; episodic anemia; a sudden destruction of older RBCs after exposure to high redox potential drugs (e.g., antimalarial drug primaquine, sulfa drugs), fava beans, or selected infections; and neonatal jaundice, which appears 2 to 3 days after birth.

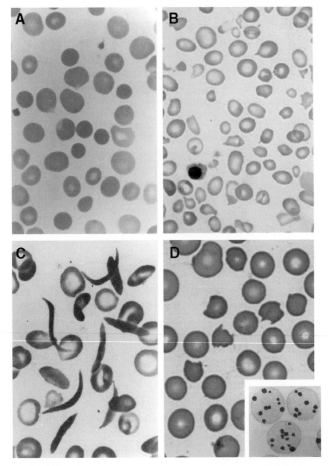

● **Figure 11-2 Red blood cell (RBC) disorders. A:** Hereditary spherocytosis. Hereditary spherocytosis results in anisocytosis (variation in size of RBCs) and spherocytes with no central pallor zone. The osmotic fragility test is the confirmatory test for hereditary spherocytosis. **B:** β-Thalassemia major. β-Thalassemia major is shown with some large, polychromatic RBCs that are newly released from the bone marrow in response to the anemia. However, most RBCs are small (microcytic) and colorless (hypochromic). Also apparent are many irregular-shaped RBCs (poikilocytes) that have been traumatized or damaged during passage through the spleen. **C:** Sickle cell anemia. Sickle cell anemia is shown with sickle RBCs (drepanocytes) due to the rod-shaped polymers of the inherited abnormal hemoglobin S (HbS). The RBC does not become sickled until it has lost its nucleus and has its full complement of HbS. Sickle cells are thin, elongated, and well filled with HbS. **D:** Glucose-6-phosphate dehydrogenase (G6PD) deficiency. G6PD deficiency leads to a denaturation of Hb, which forms Hb precipitates within the RBC (see inset) called **Heinz bodies.** As these RBCs percolate through the spleen, splenic macrophages "chew" the Heinz bodies so that RBCs have a "bite" of cytoplasm removed and are called bite cells. However, the majority of RBCs are normocytic and normochromatic.

White Blood Cells (WBCs or leukocytes)

A. NEUTROPHILS (POLYs, SEGs, OR PMNs)

1. Neutrophils are the most abundant leukocyte in the peripheral circulation (50% to 70%).
2. Neutrophils have a multilobed nucleus.
3. Neutrophils have neutral-staining granules that contain **lysozyme, lactoferrin, alkaline phosphatase**, and other **bacteriostatic and bacteriocidal substances**.
4. Neutrophils have azurophilic granules, which are primary lysosomes that contain **acid hydrolases** and **myeloperoxidase** (produces hypochlorite ions).
5. Neutrophils have **respiratory burst oxidase** (a membrane enzyme), which produces hydrogen peroxide (H_2O_2) and superoxide, which kill bacteria.
6. Neutrophils are the first to arrive at an area of tissue damage (within 30 minutes; **acute inflammation**), being attracted to the site by **complement C5a** and **leukotriene B$_4$**.
7. Neutrophils are highly adapted for **anaerobic glycolysis** with large amounts of **glycogen** to function in a devascularized area.
8. Neutrophils play an important role in **phagocytosis of bacteria and dead cells** by using **antibody receptors (Fc portion), complement factors**, and **bacterial polysaccharides** to bind to the foreign material. Neutrophils must bind to the foreign material to begin phagocytosis.
9. Neutrophils impart **natural (or innate) immunity** along with macrophages and natural killer (NK) cells.
10. Neutrophils have a lifespan of 6 to 10 hours, and 2 to 3 days in tissues.

B. EOSINOPHILS

1. Eosinophils make up 0% to 4% of the leukocytes in the peripheral circulation.
2. Eosinophils have a bilobed nucleus.
3. Eosinophils have highly eosinophilic-staining granules that contain **major basic protein, acid hydrolases**, and **peroxidase**.
4. Eosinophils have **immunoglobulin E (IgE) antibody receptors**.
5. Eosinophils play a role in **parasitic infection** (e.g., schistosomiasis, ascariasis, trichinosis).
6. Eosinophils play a role in **reducing the severity of allergic reactions** by secreting histaminase (which degrades histamine that is secreted by mast cells) and prostaglandin E$_1$ (PGE$_1$) and PGE$_2$ (which inhibit mast cell secretion).
7. Eosinophils have a lifespan of 1 to 10 hours, up to 10 days in tissues.

C. BASOPHILS

1. Basophils make up 0% to 2% of the leukocytes in the peripheral circulation (i.e., the least abundant leukocyte).
2. Basophils have highly basophilic-staining granules that contain **heparin, histamine, 5-hydroxytryptamine**, and **sulfated proteoglycans**.
3. Basophils have **IgE antibody receptors**.
4. Basophils play a role in immediate (type I) hypersensitivity reactions (anaphylactic reactions) causing **allergic rhinitis (hay fever), some forms of asthma, urticaria**, and **anaphylaxis**.
5. Basophils have a lifespan of 1 to 10 hours, variable in tissues.

D. MONOCYTES

1. Monocytes make up 2% to 9% of the leukocytes in the peripheral circulation.
2. Monocytes are members of the **monocyte–macrophage system**, which includes Kupffer cells in liver, alveolar macrophages, histiocytes in connective tissue, microglia in brain, Langerhans cells in skin, osteoclasts in bone, and dendritic antigen-presenting cells.

3. Monocytes have granules that are lysosomes that contain **acid hydrolases, aryl sulfatase, acid phosphatase,** and **peroxidase.**

4. Monocytes respond to dead cells, microorganisms, and inflammation by leaving the peripheral circulation to enter tissues and are then called macrophages.

5. Monocytes impart natural (innate) immunity along with neutrophils and NK cells.

6. Monocytes have a lifespan of **1 to 3 days, variable in tissue.**

E. NATURAL KILLER (NK) CELL is a member of the **null cell population** (i.e., lymphocytes that do not express the T-cell receptor or cell membrane immunoglobulins that distinguish lymphocytes as either T cells or B cells, respectively). NK cells are CD16$^+$ and capable of cytotoxicity without prior antigen sensitization. NK cells attack damaged cells, virus-infected cells, and tumor cells by release of **cytolysin** (a cytokine that causes cell membrane porosity) and endonuclease-mediated **apoptosis** (i.e., **cell-mediated cytotoxicity**). They impart natural (innate) immunity along with neutrophils and macrophages.

F. T LYMPHOCYTES (see Chapter 12)

G. B LYMPHOCYTES AND PLASMA CELLS (see Chapter 13)

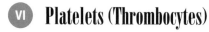

VI Platelets (Thrombocytes)

A. CHARACTERISTICS

1. Platelets are cell fragments derived from **megakaryocytes.**

2. Platelets are involved in **hemostasis (blood clotting).** Exposure of subendothelial collagen due to endothelial cell injury causes platelet adhesion mediated by von Willebrand factor (vWF). This stimulates platelet cell membrane phospholipases to free arachidonic acid, which is converted to thromboxane A_2 (TXA$_2$). TXA$_2$ contracts the platelet tubular system, which facilitates the release of platelet granules.

3. Platelets have α-granules that contain **platelet factor 4, platelet-derived growth factor (PDGF), factor V, and fibrinogen.**

4. Platelets have δ-granules that contain **serotonin, adenosine diphosphate (ADP),** and Ca^{2+}.

5. Platelets have a lifespan of **9 to 10 days.**

B. PHARMACOLOGY OF ANTIPLATELET DRUGS. These drugs increase bleeding time by inhibiting platelet aggregation.

1. **Aspirin (acetylsalicylic acid, Bayer, Bufferin)** is a nonsteroidal anti-inflammatory drug (NSAID) that irreversibly inhibits cyclooxygenase, thereby decreasing the production of TXA$_2$.

2. **Ticlopidine (Ticlid)** inhibits ADP-induced binding of fibrinogen to the platelet membrane.

3. **Dipyramidole (Dipridacot)** may increase adenosine levels, thereby inhibiting platelet aggregation. It is used clinically to prevent thromboemboli in patients with a prosthetic heart valve.

4. **Clopidogrel (Plavix)** irreversibly inhibits **ADP receptor subtype P2Y$_{12}$,** which prevents platelet aggregation by blocking the activation of the **platelet glycoprotein (GP) IIB/IIIA receptor** located on the surface of platelets. The platelet GP IIB/IIIA receptor plays a central role in platelet aggregation by binding to **fibrinogen,** fibronectin, von Willebrand factor, and vitronectin. Clopidogrel is used to inhibit blood clots in coronary artery disease, peripheral vascular disease, and cerebrovascular disease.

Hemostasis (Blood Clotting) (Figure 11-3)

A. TWO PATHWAYS

1. **Extrinsic pathway**
   a. Damaged tissue releases **thromboplastin**.
   b. Thromboplastin initiates a cascade involving **factors VII, X, and V and prothrombin activator**.
   c. Prothrombin activator converts **prothrombin (factor II)** → thrombin (factor IIa).
   d. Thrombin converts **fibrinogen (factor I)** → fibrin.
   e. Fibrin, along with RBCs, platelets, and plasma, forms a **blood clot (or thrombus)**.

2. **Intrinsic pathway**
   a. RBC trauma or RBC contact with subendothelial collagen initiates a cascade involving **factors XII, XI, IX, VIII, X, and V, and prothrombin activator**.
   b. Prothrombin activator converts **prothrombin (factor II)** → thrombin (factor IIa).
   c. Thrombin converts **fibrinogen (factor I)** → fibrin.
   d. Fibrin, along with RBCs, platelets, and plasma, forms a **blood clot (or thrombus)**.

B. VITAMIN K is essential for hemostasis because it acts as a cofactor for an enzyme involved in the posttranslational carboxylation of glutamic acid, forming **γ-carboxyglutamate residues** in certain blood factor proteins (e.g., factors X, IX, VII, II). This allows factor proteins to bind to cell membranes because γ-carboxyglutamate residues have a high affinity for Ca^{2+}. **Vitamin K deficiency** can result in hemorrhage. However, adult vitamin K deficiency is rare because intestinal bacteria produce 50% of the required vitamin K.

C. PHARMACOLOGY OF ANTICOAGULANTS

1. **Heparin** stimulates the proteolytic action of **antithrombin III**, which inactivates thrombin (factor IIa) and other blood factor proteins. It is used clinically as an anticoagulant during pregnancy since heparin does not cross the placenta, to treat deep vein thrombosis, and to treat pulmonary thromboembolism.

2. **Warfarin (Coumadin, Dicumarol)** inhibits the synthesis of **vitamin K**, thereby preventing the vitamin K–mediated formation of γ-carboxyglutamate residues in prothrombin (factor II) and other blood factor proteins. It is used clinically as an anticoagulant to treat deep vein thrombosis and pulmonary thromboembolism. It is contraindicated during pregnancy since it crosses the placenta and may interfere with fetal bone development.

D. PHARMACOLOGY OF THROMBOLYTICS

1. **Streptokinase (Streptase, Kabikinase)** is an indirect thrombolytic drug that combines with plasminogen to form an activator complex that converts plasminogen to plasmin.

2. **Tissue Plasminogen Activator (TPA, Alteplase) and Urokinase (Abbokinase)** are direct thrombolytic drugs that directly convert plasminogen to plasmin.

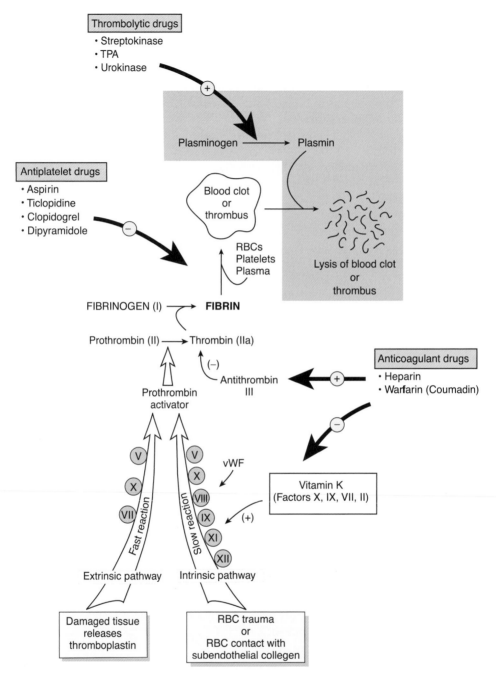

● **Figure 11-3 Diagram of hemostasis.** The extrinsic and intrinsic pathways are depicted, both of which lead to the production of prothrombin activator. Prothrombin activator converts prothrombin to thrombin. Thrombin subsequently converts fibrinogen to fibrin. Vitamin K is essential for hemostasis. The shaded box indicates the mechanism for lysis of the blood clot or thrombus. Plasmin initiates lysis. Note the action of thrombolytic, antiplatelet drugs, and anticoagulant drugs. TPA, tissue plasminogen activator; vWF, von Willebrand factor.

Clinical Considerations

A. HEMOPHILIA A (FACTOR VIII DEFICIENCY)

1. Hemophilia A is an **X-linked recessive** genetic disorder caused by a mutation in the **F8 gene** on **chromosome Xq28** for **coagulation factor VIII.**

2. Factor VIII participates in the **intrinsic pathway of hemostasis** (blood clotting).

3. Hemophilia A is defined by a reduced factor VIII clotting activity in the presence of normal vWF levels.

4. There are three clinically significant forms of hemophilia A.

    a. **Severe Hemophilia A.** Severe hemophilia A results from less than 1% of factor VIII clotting activity. **Clinical features include:** it usually being diagnosed before 1 year of age, prolonged oozing after injuries, renewed bleeding after initial bleeding has stopped, delayed bleeding, large "goose eggs" after minor head bumps, abnormal bleeding after minor injuries, deep muscle hematomas, frequent episodes of spontaneous joint bleeding, and two to five spontaneous bleeding episodes per month without adequate treatment.

    b. **Moderately Severe Hemophilia.** Moderately severe hemophilia A results from 1% to 5% of factor VIII clotting activity. **Clinical features include:** it usually being diagnosed before 5 to 6 years of age, prolonged oozing after injuries, renewed bleeding after initial bleeding has stopped, delayed bleeding, abnormal bleeding after minor injuries, rare episodes of spontaneous joint bleeding, and one bleeding episode per month to one bleeding episode per year.

    c. **Mild Hemophilia A.** Mild hemophilia A results from 6% to 35% of factor VIII clotting activity. **Clinical features include:** it usually being diagnosed later in life, prolonged oozing after injuries, renewed bleeding after initial bleeding has stopped, delayed bleeding, abnormal bleeding after major injuries, no episodes of spontaneous joint bleeding, and one bleeding episode per year to one bleeding episode per 10 years.

B. HEMOPHILIA B (FACTOR IX DEFICIENCY; CHRISTMAS DISEASE)

1. Hemophilia B is an X-linked recessive genetic disorder caused by a mutation in the **F9 gene** on **chromosome Xq27.1-q27.2** for **coagulation factor IX.**

2. Factor IX participates in the intrinsic pathway of hemostasis (blood clotting).

3. Hemophilia B is defined by a reduced factor IX clotting activity in the presence of normal vWF levels.

4. There are three clinically significant forms of hemophilia B.

    a. **Severe Hemophilia B.** Severe hemophilia B results from less than 1% of factor IX clotting activity. **Clinical features include:** it usually being diagnosed before 1 year of age, prolonged oozing after injuries, renewed bleeding after initial bleeding has stopped, delayed bleeding, large "goose eggs" after minor head bumps, abnormal bleeding after minor injuries, deep muscle hematomas, frequent episodes of spontaneous joint bleeding frequent, and two to five spontaneous bleeding episodes per month without adequate treatment.

    b. **Moderately Severe Hemophilia B.** Moderately severe hemophilia B results from 1% to 5% of factor IX clotting activity. **Clinical features include:** it usually being diagnosed before 5 to 6 years of age, prolonged oozing after injuries, renewed bleeding after initial bleeding has stopped, delayed bleeding, abnormal bleeding after minor injuries, rare episodes of spontaneous joint bleeding, and one bleeding episode per month to one bleeding episode per year.

    c. **Mild Hemophilia B.** Mild hemophilia B results from 5% to 30% of factor IX clotting activity. **Clinical features include:** it usually being diagnosed later in life, prolonged oozing after injuries, renewed bleeding after initial bleeding has stopped, delayed bleeding, abnormal bleeding after major injuries, no episodes of spontaneous joint bleeding, and one bleeding episode per year to one bleeding episode per 10 years.

C. VON WILLEBRAND DISEASE (vWD)

1. vWD is a genetic disorder caused by a mutation in the **VWF gene on chromosome 12p13.3** for **vWF.**

2. vWF participates in the intrinsic pathway of hemostasis (blood clotting). vWF acts as a carrier protein for factor VIII. vWF also forms a bridge between vascular subendothelial connective tissue and platelets by binding to the **platelet receptor Gp1b** at sites of endothelial damage.

3. vWD is defined by a reduced synthesis or reduced functionality of vWF.

4. There are three clinically significant forms of vWD.

   a. **Type 1 vWD.** Type 1 vWD is an autosomal dominant genetic disorder. Type 1 vWD results from a reduced synthesis of vWF. Type 1 vWD accounts for 75% of the cases (i.e., the most common type of vWD). **Clinical features include:** that it can be diagnosed at any age, lifelong easy bruising, nose bleeding (epistaxis), skin bleeding, prolonged bleeding from mucosal surfaces, heavy menstrual bleeding, and mild to moderately severe bleeding symptoms, although some patients are asymptomatic.

   b. **Type 2 vWD.** Type 2 vWD is an autosomal dominant or autosomal recessive genetic disorder. Type 2 vWD results from a reduced functionality of vWF. **Clinical features include:** that it can be diagnosed at any age, lifelong easy bruising, nose bleeding (epistaxis), skin bleeding, prolonged bleeding from mucosal surfaces, heavy menstrual bleeding, and moderate to moderately severe bleeding.

   c. **Type 3 vWD.** Type 3 vWD is an autosomal recessive genetic disorder. Type 3 vWD results from a reduced synthesis of vWF and factor VIII. Type 3 vWD is a rare disease but the most severe form of vWD. **Clinical features include:** nose bleeding (epistaxis), severe skin bleeding, severe bleeding from mucosal surfaces, muscle hematomas, and severe joint bleeding.

IX Red Bone Marrow (Myeloid Tissue)

A. The bone marrow is the main site of hemopoiesis, removes aged and defective RBCs by macrophage phagocytosis (along with the liver and spleen), and is the site of B-lymphocyte formation.

B. In the adult, red bone marrow is present in the vertebrae, sternum, ribs, skull, pelvis, and proximal femur. Bone marrow aspirates or biopsies are obtained from the superior iliac crest (posterior or anterior), sternum, or upper end of the tibia (in children).

C. The bone marrow consists of stromal (1%), myeloid (granulocytes; 65%), erythroid (RBC; 20%), and lymphoid (14%) components. The **myeloid/erythroid (M:E) ratio = 3:1 → 5:1** normally.

Selected Photomicrographs

A. Vitamin B_{12} deficiency, lead poisoning, iron deficiency, Howell-Jolly bodies (Figure 11-4)

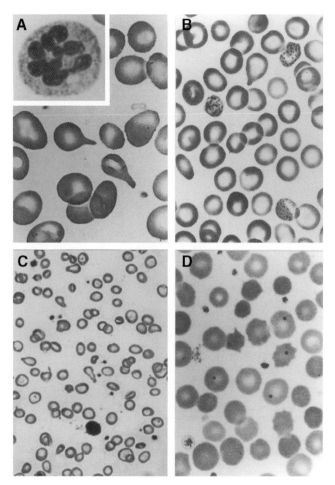

● **Figure 11-4 Red blood cell (RBC) disorders in deficiencies, poisoning, and splenectomy. A:** Pernicious anemia due to vitamin B_{12} deficiency caused by atrophic gastritis with decreased intrinsic factor production. Some RBCs are deformed as they pass through the splenic sinuses and appear teardrop shaped (dacryocytes), **macrocytic, and hyperchromic**. In addition, large neutrophils with a hypersegmented nucleus (five to six lobes) can be observed (inset). **B: Lead poisoning** is shown in which the RBCs are **microcytic and hypochromic** and show basophilic stippling, which probably represents breakdown of ribosomes. Lead denatures sulfhydryl (SH) groups in ferrochelatase within mitochondria that bind iron to protoporphyrin to form heme, thus inhibiting hemoglobin synthesis. As a result, unbound iron accumulates in mitochondria and forms ringed sideroblasts. **C:** Iron (Fe^{2+}) deficiency anemia is shown with RBCs that are **microcytic and hypochromic** with a thin rim of Hb at the periphery. Iron deficiency is probably the most common nutritional disorder in the world. Iron is transported in the body mainly by **transferrin**, which is synthesized by the liver. The main function of transferrin is to deliver iron to cells, particularly to RBC precursors, which need iron for Hb synthesis. **D:** Howell-Jolly bodies after splenectomy. Howell-Jolly bodies represent nuclear fragments that are normally removed from RBCs as they pass through the splenic sinuses. After splenectomy, increased numbers of RBCs with these inclusions are observed.

    B. Spur cells in alcoholic cirrhosis, burr cells in kidney failure, target cells (Figure 11-5)

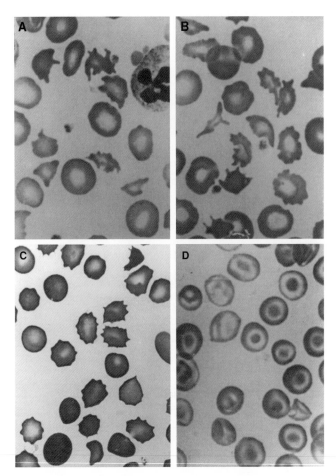

● **Figure 11-5 Red blood cells (RBCs) in various pathologies. A, B:** Hemolytic anemia associated with alcoholic cirrhosis shows RBCs with a periphery consisting of sharp points called **spur cells**. **C:** Anemia associated with kidney failure (or renal insufficiency) shows RBCs with a periphery consisting of bumps called burr cells. **D:** Target cells (or codocytes) have a central dark area of Hb that is surrounded by a colorless ring followed by a peripheral rim of Hb. Target cells can be found in a number of pathologic states, including thalassemia, obstructive liver disease, and iron deficiency.

C. Erythropoiesis (Figure 11-6)

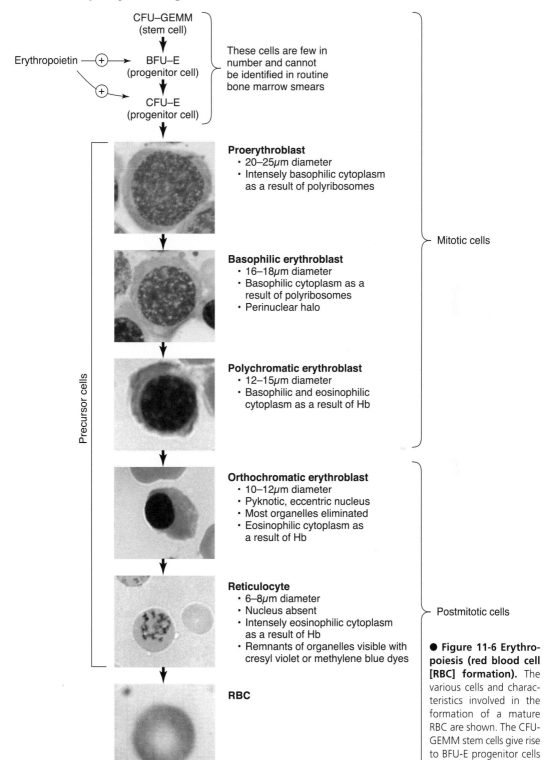

CFU–GEMM
(stem cell)

Erythropoietin ⟶ ⊕ ⟶ BFU–E
(progenitor cell)

⊕ ⟶ CFU–E
(progenitor cell)

These cells are few in number and cannot be identified in routine bone marrow smears

Precursor cells

Proerythroblast
• 20–25µm diameter
• Intensely basophilic cytoplasm as a result of polyribosomes

Basophilic erythroblast
• 16–18µm diameter
• Basophilic cytoplasm as a result of polyribosomes
• Perinuclear halo

Polychromatic erythroblast
• 12–15µm diameter
• Basophilic and eosinophilic cytoplasm as a result of Hb

Mitotic cells

Orthochromatic erythroblast
• 10–12µm diameter
• Pyknotic, eccentric nucleus
• Most organelles eliminated
• Eosinophilic cytoplasm as a result of Hb

Reticulocyte
• 6–8µm diameter
• Nucleus absent
• Intensely eosinophilic cytoplasm as a result of Hb
• Remnants of organelles visible with cresyl violet or methylene blue dyes

Postmitotic cells

RBC

● **Figure 11-6 Erythropoiesis (red blood cell [RBC] formation).** The various cells and characteristics involved in the formation of a mature RBC are shown. The CFU-GEMM stem cells give rise to BFU-E progenitor cells that form "bursts" of erythroid cells in culture. The BFU-E cells give rise to CFU-E progenitor cells. Note the action of erythropoietin. The CFU-E cells give rise to the various precursor cells leading to the mature RBC. Note the mitotic activity of the various cells. CFU-GEMM, colony-forming unit–granulocyte/erythroid/monocyte/megakaryocyte; BFU-E, burst-forming unit–erythroid; CFU-E, colony-forming unit–erythroid.

D. Granulopoiesis (neutrophilic) (Figure 11-7)

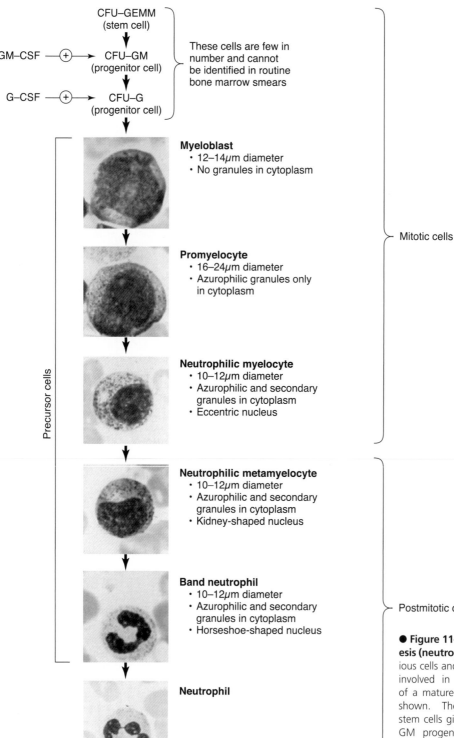

CFU–GEMM
(stem cell)

GM–CSF ——⊕——→ CFU–GM
(progenitor cell)

G–CSF ——⊕——→ CFU–G
(progenitor cell)

These cells are few in number and cannot be identified in routine bone marrow smears

Myeloblast
- 12–14μm diameter
- No granules in cytoplasm

Promyelocyte
- 16–24μm diameter
- Azurophilic granules only in cytoplasm

Neutrophilic myelocyte
- 10–12μm diameter
- Azurophilic and secondary granules in cytoplasm
- Eccentric nucleus

Mitotic cells

Neutrophilic metamyelocyte
- 10–12μm diameter
- Azurophilic and secondary granules in cytoplasm
- Kidney-shaped nucleus

Band neutrophil
- 10–12μm diameter
- Azurophilic and secondary granules in cytoplasm
- Horseshoe-shaped nucleus

Postmitotic cells

Neutrophil

Precursor cells

● **Figure 11-7 Granulopoiesis (neutrophilic).** The various cells and characteristics involved in the formation of a mature neutrophil are shown. The CFU-GEMM stem cells give rise to CFU-GM progenitor cells. The GFU-GM cells give rise to CFU-G progenitor cells. The CFU-G cells give rise to the various precursor cells leading to the mature neutrophil. Note the action of GM-CSF and G-CSF, which are glycoproteins secreted by the endothelial cells and macrophages within the bone marrow. Note the mitotic activity of the various cells. CFU-GEMM, colony-forming unit–granulocyte/erythroid/monocyte/megakaryocyte; CFU-GM, colony-forming unit–granulocyte/monocyte; CFU-G, colony-forming unit–granulocyte; GM-CSF, granulocyte/monocyte colony-stimulating factor; G-CSF, granulocyte colony-stimulating factor.

E. Various blood cells (Figure 11-8)

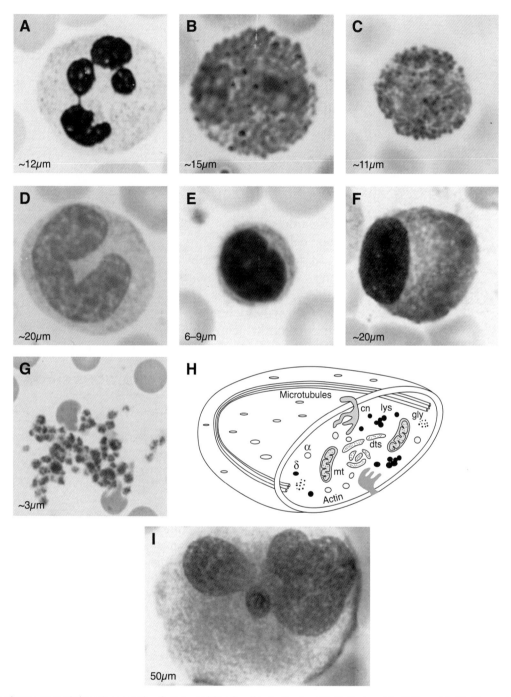

● **Figure 11-8 Light micrograph of various blood cells. A:** Neutrophil. **B:** Eosinophil. **C:** Basophil. **D:** Monocyte. **E:** Small lymphocyte. **F:** Plasma cell. B lymphocytes differentiate into plasma, whose main function is the synthesis and secretion of immunoglobulins. Plasma cells have an eccentric nucleus with a clock-face chromatin pattern, a perinuclear clear area (Hof area) corresponding to the Golgi, and a basophilic cytoplasm due to rough endoplasmic reticulum (rER) for protein synthesis. **G:** Platelets. **H:** Diagram of a platelet. Note the microtubules, actin cortex, membranous canalicular network (cn), dense tubular system (dts), lysosomes (lys), glycogen (gly), mitochondria (mt), α-granules, and δ-granules. **I:** Megakaryocyte.

Case Study 11-1

A 60-year-old man comes to your office complaining that "I've been feeling really tired lately and get out of breath just walking around the house." He also tells you that "my feet always go to sleep on me; they feel like pins and needles." After some discussion, he informs you that his tongue feels "kind of big and beefy" and that he has been falling down a lot. When questioned about his alcohol consumption, he emphatically denies being an alcoholic but admits that "I do like to have a glass of whiskey every day." In addition, you noticed that he walked very stiffly as he came into the examining room. What is the most likely diagnosis?

Differentials

• Beriberi, diabetes, folate deficiency due to alcoholism or poor diet, lead poisoning, uremia

Relevant Physical Examination Findings

• Conjunctiva and nail beds are pale.
• Skin is colored lemon yellow.
• Auscultation reveals a 2/6 systolic flow murmur over the left sternal border.
• A stiff, unsteady gait; hyperreflexia; loss of positional and vibratory sense in the lower limbs.

Relevant Lab Findings

• Blood chemistry: hemoglobin (Hgb) = 10.5 ug/L (low); mean corpuscular volume (MCV) = 120 fL (high); leukocyte count = 3,400/mm^3 (low); platelet count = 78,000/mm^3 (low); B_{12} = 85 pg/mL (low); methylmalonic acid = high; parietal cell autoantibodies = high; blood urea nitrogen (BUN) = normal; creatinine = normal
• Peripheral blood smear: megaloblastic anemia; neutrophils with hypersegmented nuclei
• Schilling test: positive

Diagnosis: Pernicious Anemia

• Pernicious Anemia. Pernicious anemia is an autoimmune disease that is associated with a predisposition to other autoimmune disorders (particularly of the adrenal and thyroid glands). Parietal cell autoantibodies develop, which causes a chronic fundal (type A) gastritis and parietal cell destruction. Parietal cells normally produce HCl and intrinsic factor (which is necessary for vitamin B_{12} absorption). The lack of intrinsic factor causes vitamin B_{12} deficiency, which leads to megaloblastic anemia and subacute combined degeneration of the posterior and lateral spinal tracts due to impairment of methylcobalamin-dependent methionine synthesis. Vitamin B_{12} deficiency may also be caused by surgical resection of the stomach or ileum, Crohn disease, strict vegan diet, bacterial overgrowth, or *Diphyllobothrium latum* infection.
• Beriberi. Beriberi is a disease caused by thiamine deficiency often due to alcoholism. Dry beriberi (first stage) is characterized by peripheral neuropathy. Wet beriberi (second stage) is characterized by high-output heart failure. Wernicke-Korsakoff syndrome (final stage) is characterized by confusion, ataxia, ophthalmoplegia, and confabulation.
• Diabetes. Clinical findings of diabetes include a diabetic peripheral neuropathy, gastroparesis, and the inability to regulate heart rate.
• Folate Deficiency. Folate deficiency may be caused by alcoholism, certain diets, pregnancy, celiac sprue, giardiasis, phenytoin, oral contraceptives, and antifolate chemotherapeutic agents. Clinical findings of folate deficiency include megaloblastic anemia but not subacute combined degeneration of the posterior and lateral spinal tracts.
• Lead Poisoning. Clinical findings of lead poisoning include motor neuropathy leading to wrist or foot drop; a microcytic, hypochromic anemia; basophilic stippling of RBCs; encephalopathy; Fanconi syndrome; and a lead line deposit in the gums.
• Uremia. Uremia is defined as elevated BUN and creatinine levels in the blood usually as a result of renal failure. Clinical findings of uremia include anemia, peripheral neuropathy, bleeding, heart failure, pericarditis, esophagitis, pruritus, and encephalopathy.

Case Study 11-2

A 16-year-old girl is sent to your office because she had a nose bleed during class and this was not the first time. The girl comes to your office saying that "I get these nosebleeds once in a while but they're no big deal because they stop after about 10 minutes. But, I think I bleed a lot more during my period than my girlfriends do." She also tells you that "my mother has some kind of bleeding problem, but she never speaks about it." After some discussion, she informs you that that her brother was in the Betty Ford Clinic for cocaine addiction. You ask her if she is using and she says, "I've tried it a few times but I'm no crackhead like my silly brother." What is the most likely diagnosis?

Differentials

- Coagulation disorders (secondary hemostasis), disorders with increased vascular fragility

Relevant Physical Examination Findings

- Physical examination is unremarkable.
- No history of vomiting blood (hematemesis), passage of bloody stools (hematochezia), or black, tarry stools (melena)
- No signs of ecchymoses (small hemorrhagic spots)

Relevant Lab Findings

- Blood chemistry: platelets = 250,000/μL (normal); prothrombin time (PT) = 13 seconds (normal); partial thromboplastin time (PTT) = 65 seconds (high); bleeding time = 10 minutes (high)
- Ristocetin assay = no aggregation of platelets

Diagnosis: Von Willebrand Disease

- Von Willebrand Disease (vWD). vWD is a type of primary hemostasis disorder and is the most common inherited bleeding disorder (autosomal dominant). vWD is due to low levels of vWF. Endothelial cells secrete vWF, which combines with factor VIII secreted by hepatocytes to form a factor VIII–vWF complex (this increases the half-life of factor VIII). This complex promotes blood clotting as well as platelet–subendothelial connective tissue interactions necessary for blood clotting. Platelets attach to the subendothelial connective tissue when the Gp1b glycoprotein receptor located on the cell membrane of the platelet binds to the factor VIII–vWF complex. Since vWF forms a complex with factor VIII, vWD patients have a qualitative (not quantitative) deficiency of factor VIII that leads to a prolonged PTT. Clinical findings of vWD include excessive bleeding from superficial cuts, bleeding from mucous membranes (e.g., gums, nasal mucosa), prolonged bleeding after dental work, menorrhagia, internal gastrointestinal bleeding, and easy bruising. Primary hemostasis disorders with a platelet count below 150,000/μL (quantitative) include bone marrow failure, Wiskott-Aldrich syndrome, idiopathic thrombocytopenic purpura, thrombotic thrombocytopenic purpura, hemolytic uremic syndrome, multiple transfusions, and splenic sequestering. Primary hemostasis disorders with a normal platelet count (qualitative) include vWD, Bernard-Soulier disease, Glanzmann thrombasthenia, aspirin overdose, and uremia. A prolonged bleeding time is diagnostic of a primary hemostasis disorder.
- Coagulation Disorders (Secondary Hemostasis). Coagulation disorders are clotting factor deficiencies involved in the coagulation cascade. Coagulation disorders include hemophilia A, hemophilia B (Christmas disease), and vitamin K deficiency. A prolonged PTT is diagnostic of a coagulation disorder. Clinical findings of coagulation disorders include severe bleeding from large blood vessels with hemarthrosis, large hematomas after trauma, and prolonged wound healing.
- Vascular Fragility. Diseases with increased vascular fragility include scurvy, Henoch-Schönlein purpura, rickettsial and meningococcal infections, Ehlers-Danlos syndrome, and Cushing syndrome. Clinical findings of disorders with increased vascular fragility include symptoms similar to primary hemostasis disorders but with a normal bleeding time.

Chapter 12

Thymus

I **General Features.** The thymus is derived embryologically from the **endodermal** pharyngeal pouch #3 which forms thymic epitheliocytes and becomes populated by T stem cells which migrate in from the **mesodermal** bone marrow. Therefore, the thymus has a dual embryological origin. At birth, the thymus weighs 10-15gms and increases to 20-40gms by puberty. Although the amount of lymphoid tissue decreases with age being replaced by adipose tissue, the thymus remains a source of T cells throughout life. In the adult, the thymus is a soft, bilobed, encapsulated gland that lies in the anterior mediastinum. The thymus is the main site of T cell differentiation. Histologically, the thymus is divided into the **cortex** and **medulla**.

II **Thymic Cortex (Figure 12-1)** consists of:

A. THYMIC EPITHELIOCYTES (endodermal origin; also called **thymic nurse cells**)
   1. Thymic epitheliocytes contain **cytokeratin** intermediate filaments and form a cellular meshwork joined by **desmosomes** into which thymocytes are tightly packed.
   2. They secrete:
      a. **Thymotaxin** which attracts T stem cells from the bone marrow into the thymus
      b. **Thymosin, Serum Thymic Factor, and Thymopoietin** all of which transform immature T cells into mature T cells.

B. THYMOCYTES (mesodermal origin) which include:
   1. **T stem cells**
   2. **Pre-T cells**
   3. **Immature T cells**

C. MACROPHAGES

D. THYMIC DENDRITIC CELLS located at the cortico-medullary junction.

III **Thymic Medulla (Figure 12-1)** consists of the following:

A. THYMIC EPITHELIOCYTES

B. MATURE T CELLS which include:
   1. **CD4$^+$ helper T cells**
   2. **CD4$^+$ or CD8$^+$ suppressor T cells**
   3. **CD8$^+$ cytotoxic T cells**

C. THYMIC (HASSALL'S) CORPUSCLES, which are whorl-like structures composed of keratinized thymic epitheliocytes

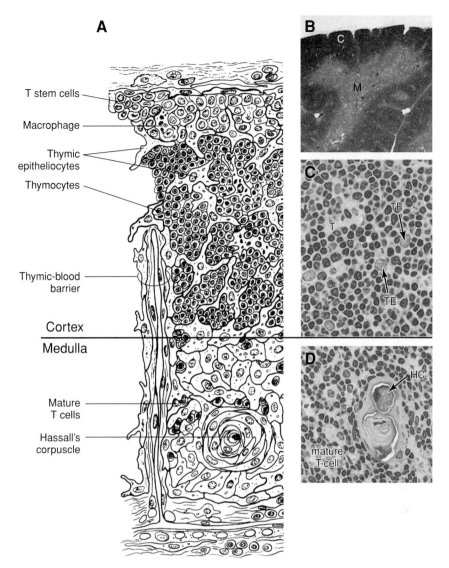

A

T stem cells

Macrophage

Thymic
epitheliocytes

Thymocytes

Thymic-blood
barrier

Cortex

Medulla

Mature
T cells

Hassall's
corpuscle

B

C

M

C

T

TE

TE

D

HC

mature
T-cell

● **Figure 12-1 LM Features of the Thymus. (A)** Diagram of the thymus. Note the various cell types within the cortex and medulla. **(B)** LM of thymus showing the darkly-stained cortex (C) and pale medulla (M). **(C)** LM of thymic cortex shows a large number of densely packed thymocytes (T) of various sizes. In addition, thymic epitheliocytes (TE;arrows) are apparent. **(D)** LM of thymic medulla showing the whorl-like Hassall's corpuscle (HC), which are keratinized thymic epitheliocytes surrounded by mature T cells.

Types of Mature T Cells

A. CD4⁺ HELPER T CELLS whose functions include:

   1. Recognition of antigen in association with **Class II MHC**
   2. Release of cytokines that stimulate proliferation of B lymphocytes and antibody production
   3. Proliferation of T cells
   4. Regulation of hematopoiesis
   5. Activation of macrophages

B. CD4⁺ OR CD8⁺ SUPPRESSOR T CELLS whose function is:

   1. Downregulation of the immune response.

C. CD8⁺ CYTOTOXIC T CELLS whose functions include:

   1. Recognition of antigen in association with **Class I MHC**
   2. Destruction of allogeneic cells, virus-infected cells, and fungi

3.   Release of **cytolysin** that causes membrane porosity and endonuclease-mediated apoptosis

V **Blood–Thymus Barrier.** This barrier is found **only in the thymic cortex** and assures that immature T cells undergo positive and negative selection in an antigen-free environment. This barrier consists of: **tight junctions between nonfenestrated endothelial cells, basal lamina, and thymic epitheliocytes.**

VI **T Cell Lymphopoiesis (T Cell Formation) (Figure 12-2)**

A. **HEMOPOIETIC STEM CELLS** differentiate into **lymphoid progenitor cells** which form **T stem cells** within the bone marrow.

B. Under the influence of **thymotaxin**, T stem cells leave the bone marrow and enter the thymic cortex where they differentiate into **pre-T cells**. Pre-T cells begin T cell receptor (TcR) gene rearrangement and express TcR.

C. **IMMATURE T CELLS** express TcR, CD4, and CD8 and undergo positive or negative selection under the influence of thymosin, serum thymic factor, and thymopoietin.
   1. **Positive selection** is a process whereby CD4$^+$ CD8$^+$ T cells bind with a certain affinity to MHC proteins expressed on thymic epitheliocytes such that the CD4$^+$ CD8$^+$ T cells become "**educated**"; all other CD4$^+$ CD8$^+$ T cells undergo apoptosis. This means that a mature T-cell will respond to antigen only when presented by a MHC protein that it encountered at this stage in its development. This is known as **MHC restriction of T cell responses**.
   2. **Negative selection** is a process whereby CD4$^+$ CD8$^+$ T cells interact with thymic dendritic cells at the cortico-medullary junction of the thymus such that CD4$^+$ CD8$^+$ T cells that recognize "self" antigens undergo apoptosis (or are somehow inactivated) leaving only CD4$^+$ CD8$^+$ T cells that recognize only foreign antigens.

D. **MATURE T CELLS** downregulate CD4 or CD8 to form either: **CD4$^+$ helper T cells, CD4$^+$ or CD8$^+$ suppressor T cells, or CD8$^+$ cytotoxic T cells.**

E. Mature T cells migrate to the **paracortex (thymic-dependent zone) of all lymph nodes, peri-arterial lymphatic sheath (PALS) in the spleen, and gut-associated lymphatic tissue (GALT)** to await antigen exposure.

F. **EXOGENOUS ANTIGENS** (circulating in the bloodstream)
   1. Exogenous antigens are internalized by **antigen-presenting cells (APCs)** and then undergo lysosomal degradation in **endolysosomes** to form antigen peptide fragments.
   2. The antigen peptide fragments become associated with **Class II MHC**, transported, and exposed on the cell surface of the APC.
   3. The antigen peptide fragment + MHC Class II on the surface of the APC is recognized by **CD4$^+$ helper T cells** which secrete **IL-2** (stimulates proliferation of B and T cells), **IL-4** and **IL-5** (activate antibody production by causing B cell differentiation into plasma cells and promote isotype switching and hypermutation), **TNF-α** (activates macrophages), and **IFN-γ** (activate macrophages and natural killer cells).

G. **ENDOGENOUS ANTIGENS** (virus or bacteria within a cell)
   1. Endogenous antigens undergo proteosomal degradation in **proteosomes** within the infected cell to form antigen peptide fragments.
   2. The antigen peptide fragments become associated with **Class I MHC**, transported, and exposed on the cell surface of the infected cell.
   3. The antigen peptide fragment + Class I MHC on the surface of the infected cell is recognized by **CD8$^+$ cytotoxic T cells**, which secrete **perforins, cytolysins, lymphotoxins,** and **serine esterases** which cause membrane porosity and endonuclease-mediated apoptosis of the infected cell.

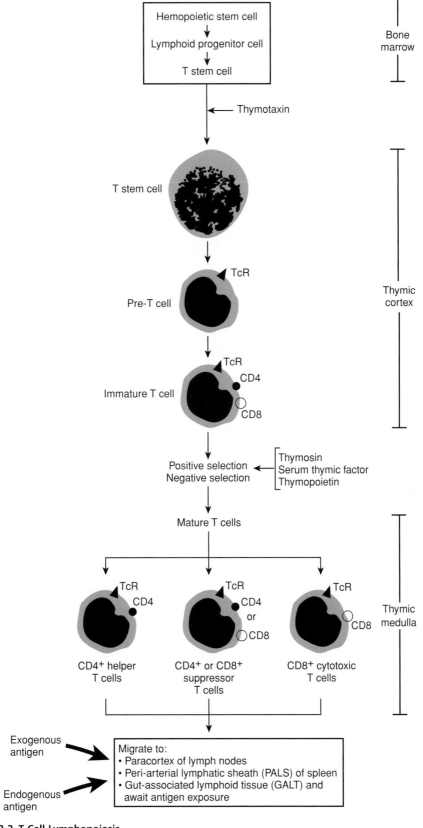

● **Figure 12-2 T Cell Lymphopoiesis.**

VII Clinical Considerations

A. **INVOLUTION OF THE THYMUS** can be accelerated by: stress, adrenocorticotrophic hormone (ACTH), or steroids.

B. **HYPERTROPHY OF THE THYMUS** can be caused by: T_3, prolactin, or growth hormone.

C. **NEONATAL THYMECTOMY** severely impairs cell-mediated immunity and also somewhat diminishes humoral immunity because $CD4^+$ helper T cell function is compromised. The lymph nodes and spleen are **reduced in size** because the thymic-dependent zone of the lymph nodes and periarterial lymphatic sheath of the spleen, respectively, do not become populated with T cells.

D. **ADULT THYMECTOMY** causes less severe impairment of cell-mediated immunity and humoral immunity because the lymph nodes and spleen are already well populated with long-lived T cells.

E. **CONGENITAL THYMIC APLASIA (DiGEORGE SYNDROME)** is a disorder characterized by hypocalcemia and recurrent infections with viruses, bacteria, fungi, and protozoa. It occurs in infants when pharyngeal **pouches #3 and #4** fail to develop embryologically which results in the absence of the **thymus** and **parathyroid glands**. These infants have **no T cells**. Many infants even fail to mount an immunoglobulin response which requires $CD4^+$ helper T cells.

F. **ACQUIRED IMMUNE DEFICIENCY SYNDROME (AIDS)** is a disorder that slowly weakens the immune system through selective destruction of **$CD4^+$ helper T cells.**

VIII Selected Photomicrographs

A. **THYMOMA (FIGURE 12-3)**

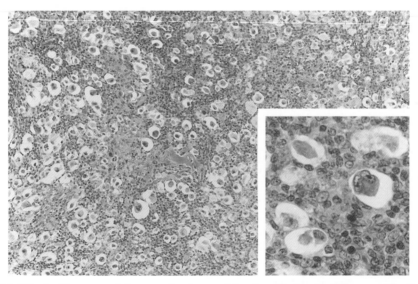

● **Figure 12-3 LM of a Thymoma.** A thymoma is a tumor of thymic epitheliocytes. A huge proliferation of thymic epitheliocytes is shown (compare with normal thymus in Figure 12-1C). Inset shows high magnification of thymic epitheliocytes.

Chapter 13

Lymph Node

① **General Features (Figure 13-1).** A lymph node is a small, encapsulated, ovoid to bean-shaped gland that lies in the course of lymphatic vessels draining various anatomic regions. Histologically, a lymph node is divided into the **cortex** and **medulla**.

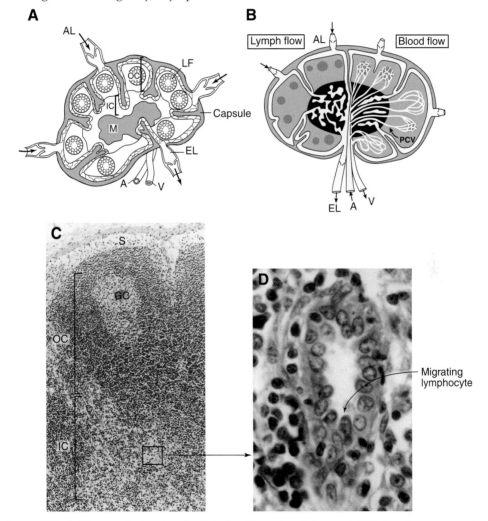

● **Figure 13-1 A:** Diagram of a lymph node. Note the afferent lymphatic vessels (AL) along the convex surface; efferent lymphatic vessel (EL), artery (A), and vein (V) at the hilus; outer cortex (OC) with lymphatic follicles (LF), many of which contain germinal centers; inner cortex (IC); and medulla (M). **B:** Diagram showing the flow of lymph and blood through the lymph node. PCV, postcapillary venule. **C:** Light micrograph of a normal lymph node showing the subcapsular sinus (S), outer cortex (OC), inner cortex (IC), and germinal center (GC) of a lymphatic follicle. **D:** Electron micrograph of the *boxed area* in C showing a postcapillary venule within the inner cortex. Note the lymphocytes exiting the bloodstream to repopulate the lymph node.

II **Outer Cortex** consists of:

A. MATURE (VIRGIN) B CELLS. Mature B cells are organized into **lymphatic follicles** that may contain **germinal centers**. Germinal centers are evidence of activated B cells that begin the transformation into plasma cells.

B. FOLLICULAR DENDRITIC CELLS. Follicular dendritic cells have an antigen-presenting function. Not acc. to Ross & Pawlina.

C. MACROPHAGES

D. FIBROBLASTS (RETICULAR CELLS). Fibroblasts secrete **type III collagen** (reticular fibers) that form a stromal meshwork.

III **Inner Cortex** (also called the **paracortex** or **thymic-dependent zone**) consists of:

A. MATURE T CELLS

B. DENDRITIC CELLS. Dendritic cells have an antigen-presenting function.

C. MACROPHAGES

D. FIBROBLASTS (RETICULAR CELLS). Fibroblasts secrete **type III collagen** (reticular fibers) that form a stromal meshwork.

IV **Medulla** consists of:

A. LYMPHOCYTES

B. PLASMA CELLS. Plasma cells increasingly populate the medulla of antigen-stimulated lymph nodes so that the medulla becomes a **major site of immunoglobulin secretion.**

C. MACROPHAGES. Macrophages are very numerous in the medulla so that the medulla becomes a **major site of phagocytosis.**

D. FIBROBLASTS (RETICULAR CELLS). Fibroblasts secrete **type III collagen** (reticular fibers) that form a stromal meshwork.

V **Flow of Lymph** occurs through afferent lymphatic vessels with valves entering at the convex surface → subcapsular (marginal) sinus → cortical sinuses → medullary sinuses → efferent lymphatic vessel with valves exiting at the hilum. Sinuses contain sinus macrophages, veiled cells, and reticular fibers that crisscross the lumen in a haphazard fashion.

VI **Flow of Blood** occurs through arteries that enter at the hilum → a capillary network within the outer and inner cortex → postcapillary (high endothelial) venules within the inner cortex → veins that leave at the hilum. **Postcapillary (high endothelial) venules** have **lymphocyte homing receptors** and are the major site where B cells and T cells exit the bloodstream to repopulate their specific portion of the lymph node. Lymphocytes leave the lymph node by entering a nearby sinus, which drains into an efferent lymphatic vessel.

VII **B-Cell Lymphopoiesis (B-cell Formation) (Figure 13-2).** In early fetal development, B-cell lymphopoiesis occurs in the **fetal liver**. In later fetal development and throughout the rest of adult life, B-cell lymphopoiesis occurs in the bone marrow. In humans, the **bone marrow is considered the primary site of B-cell lymphopoiesis.**

A. **HEMOPOIETIC STEM CELLS** originating in the bone marrow differentiate into **lymphoid progenitor cells**, which later form **B stem cells**.

B. B stem cells form **pro–B cells**, which begin heavy chain gene rearrangement.

C. **PRE–B CELLS** continue heavy chain gene rearrangement.

D. **IMMATURE B CELLS** (immunoglobulin M [IgM]$^+$) begin light chain gene rearrangement and express **antigen-specific IgM** (i.e., will recognize only one antigen) on its cell surface.

E. **MATURE (OR VIRGIN) B CELLS** (IgM$^+$/IgD$^+$) express **antigen-specific IgM and IgD** on their cell surface. Mature B cells migrate to the **outer cortex of lymph nodes, lymphatic follicles in the spleen**, and **gut-associated lymphoid tissue (GALT)** to await antigen exposure.

F. **EARLY IMMUNE RESPONSE**
   1. Early in the immune response, mature B cells bind antigen using IgM and IgD.
   2. As a consequence of antigen binding, two transmembrane proteins (**CD79a and CD79b**) that function as signal transducers cause proliferation and differentiation of B cells into **plasma cells that secrete either IgM or IgD**.

G. **LATER IMMUNE RESPONSE**
   1. Later in the immune response, **antigen-presenting cells (APCs; macrophages)** phagocytose the antigen where it undergoes lysosomal degradation in **endolysosomes** to form antigen peptide fragments.
   2. The **antigen peptide fragments** become associated with the **class II major histocompatibility complex (MHC)** and are transported and exposed on the cell surface of the APC.
   3. The antigen peptide fragment + class II MHC on the surface of the APC is recognized by **CD4$^+$ helper T cells**, which secrete **interleukin 2 (IL-2**; stimulates proliferation of B and T cells), **IL-4 and IL-5** (activate antibody production by causing B-cell differentiation into plasma cells and promote isotype switching and hypermutation), **tumor necrosis factor-α (TNF-α**; activates macrophages), and **interferon-γ (IFN-γ**; activates macrophages and natural killer cells).
   4. Under the influence of IL-4 and IL-5, mature B cells undergo **isotype switching** and **hypermutation**.
      a. **Isotype Switching** is a gene rearrangement process whereby the μ (mu; M) and δ (delta; D) **constant segments** of the heavy chain (C_H) are spliced out and replaced with either γ (gamma; G), ε (epsilon; E), or α (alpha; A) C_H segments. This allows mature B cells to differentiate into **plasma cells that secrete IgG, IgE, or IgA**.
      b. **Hypermutation** is a mutation process whereby a high rate of mutations occurs in the **variable segments** of the heavy chain (V_H) and light chain (V_κ or V_λ). This allows mature B cells to differentiate into plasma cells that secrete IgG, IgE, or IgA that will bind antigen with greater and greater affinity.

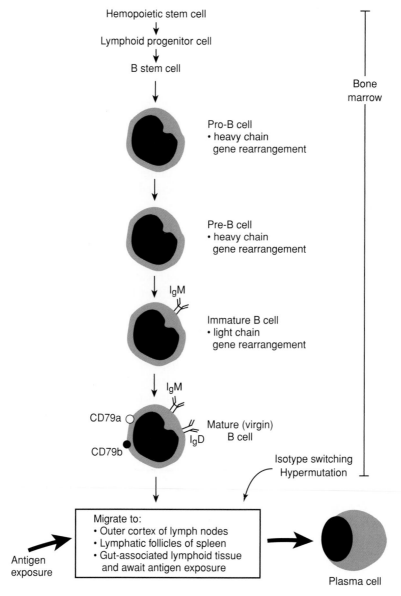

● **Figure 13-2 B-cell lymphopoiesis.**

VIII **Cytokines (Table 13-1)**

A. **PROPERTIES**

1. Cytokines are small, soluble, secreted proteins that enable immune cells to communicate with each other and therefore play an integral role in the initiation, perpetuation, and downregulation of the immune response.

2. Cytokine activity demonstrates **redundancy** and **pleiotropy**. Cytokine redundancy means that many different cytokines may elicit the same activity. Cytokine pleiotropy means that a single cytokine can cause multiple activities.

3. Cytokines act in an **autocrine manner** (i.e., they act on cells that secrete them) or a **paracrine manner** (i.e., they act on nearby cells).

4. Cytokines are often produced in a **cascade** (i.e., one cytokine stimulates its target cell to produce additional cytokines).

5. Cytokines may act **synergistically** (i.e., two or more cytokines acting with one another) or **antagonistically** (i.e., two or more cytokines acting against one another).

B. CYTOKINE RECEPTORS. Cytokines elicit their activity by binding to **high-affinity cell surface receptors** on target cells, thereby initiating an intracellular **signal transduction pathway**. Cytokine receptors have been grouped into several families.

1. **Hematopoietin Family of Receptors.** This family of receptors is characterized by four conserved cysteine residues and a conserved Trp-Ser-X-Trp-Ser sequence in the extracellular domain. These receptors generally have two subunits, an **α-subunit** for cytokine binding and a **β-subunit** for signal transduction. Cytokine binding promotes **dimerization** of the α-subunit and β-subunit. This family of receptors binds IL-2, IL-3, IL-4, IL-5, IL-6, IL-7, erythropoietin, and granulocyte–monocyte colony-stimulating factor (GM-CSF).

2. **Interferon (IFN) Family of Receptors.** This family of receptors is characterized by four conserved cysteine residues but does not have a conserved Trp-Ser-X-Trp-Ser sequence in the extracellular domain. This family of receptors binds IFN-α, IFN-β, and IFN-γ.

3. **Tumor Necrosis Factor (TNF) Family of Receptors.** This family of receptors is characterized by four extracellular domains. This family of receptor binds TNF-α, TNF-β, membrane-bound CD40, and Fas (which signals a cell to undergo apoptosis).

4. **Seven-Pass Transmembrane Helix Family of Receptors.** This family of receptors is characterized by seven transmembrane domains and the interaction with G proteins. This family of receptors binds IL-8, macrophage inflammatory protein (MIP-1), and monocyte chemotactic protein (MCP-1), which are chemokines.

C. CHEMOKINES. Chemokines are chemotactic cytokines that promote chemotaxis (migration) of leukocytes to inflammatory sites. Chemokines are divided into two groups:

1. **Chemokines-α or C-X-C Chemokines.** These chemokines have their first two cysteine residues separated by one amino acid.

2. **Chemokines-β or C-C Chemokines.** These chemokines have two adjacent cysteine residues. This family of receptors is characterized by four conserved cysteine residues and a conserved Trp-Ser-X-Trp-Ser sequence in the extracellular domain.

TABLE 13-1		SELECTED CYTOKINES AND THEIR ACTIVITY	
Cytokine	Producing Cell	Target Cell	Activity
IL-1	Monocytes Macrophages B cells Dendritic cells	T cells B cells Endothelial cells CNS Hepatocytes	Activation of T cells Maturation and proliferation of B cells Increased cell adhesion Fever, sickness behavior Synthesis and release of acute-phase proteins
IL-2	T cells	T cells B cells NK cells	Proliferation and differentiation of T cells Proliferation and differentiation of B cells Proliferation and activation of NK cells
IL-4	Th2 cells Mast cells	T cells B cells Macrophages	Proliferation of T cells Isotype switch to IgE by B cells Inhibits IFN-γ activation
IL-6	Th2 cells Macrophages Bone marrow stromal cells Dendritic cells	B cells Plasma cells Hepatocytes Hemopoietic cells	Differentiation into plasma cells Stimulation of antibody secretion Synthesis and release of acute-phase proteins Differentiation of hemopoietic cells
IL-8	Macrophages Endothelial cells	All immune cells Endothelial cells	Chemotaxis of all migratory immune cells Activation and chemotaxis of neutrophils Inhibition of histamine release by basophils Inhibition of IgE production by B cells Promotion of angiogenesis
TNF-α	Th1 cells Macrophages Dendritic cells NK cells Mast cells	Virtually all cells in the body	Proinflammatory actions Proliferation of cells Differentiation of cells Cytotoxic for transformed cells

TGF-β	T cells
	Monocytes
		Monocytes
		Macrophages
		B cells
		Various cells of
		  the body
			Chemotaxis of monocytes
			Chemotaxis of macrophages and promotion of
			  IL-1 synthesis
			Promotion of IgA synthesis
			Proliferation of various cells of the body

IFN-γ	Th1 cells
	Cytotoxic T cells
	NK cells
		T cells
		B cells
		Macrophages
			Development of Th1 cells and proliferation of
			  Th2 cells
			Isotype switch to IgG by B cells
			Activation and expression of MHC by
			  macrophages

MCP	Endothelial cells Fibroblasts Smooth muscle cells	Monocytes T cells NK cells Macrophages Basophils Eosinophils	Chemotaxis of monocytes Chemotaxis of T cells Chemotaxis of NK cells Activation of macrophages Promotion of histamine release Activation of eosinophils
MIP	Macrophages	Neutrophils T cells Hematopoietic precursor cells	Chemotaxis of neutrophils Chemotaxis of T cells Inhibition of hematopoiesis
GM-CSF	Th cells	Granulocytes Monocytes Hematopoietic precursor cells	Proliferation and differentiation of granulocytes Proliferation and differentiation of monocytes Proliferation of hematopoietic precursor cells

IL, interleukin; CNS, central nervous system; NK, natural killer; Th, T helper cells; Ig, immunoglobulin; IFN, interferon; TNF, tumor necrosis factor; MHC, major histocompatability complex; MCP, monocyte chemotactic protein; MIP, macrophage inflammatory protein; GM-CSF, granulocyte–macrophage colony-stimulating factor.

IX   Clinical Consideration (Figure 13-3). The population of lymphocytes within lymph nodes changes in certain clinical states, such as **agammaglobulinemia, DiGeorge syndrome, severe combined immunodeficiency (SCID), adenosine deaminase deficiency (ADA; "bubble boy" disease),** and **late-stage acquired immunodeficiency syndrome (AIDS).**

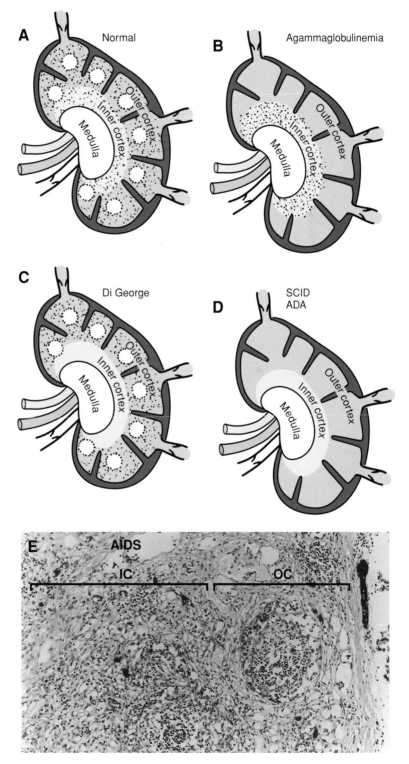

● **Figure 13-3 Diagram of lymph nodes in various clinical states. A:** Normal lymph node. Diagram shows a normal lymph node with B cells (outer cortex) and T cells (inner cortex) that impart a humoral immune response and cell-mediated immune response to the individual, respectively. **B:** X-linked infantile (Bruton) agammaglobulinemia. Diagram shows a lymph node in X-linked infantile (Bruton) agammaglobulinemia with B cells absent but T cells present, so that humoral immune response is absent but cell-mediated immune response is present. **C:** DiGeorge syndrome. Diagram shows a lymph node in DiGeorge syndrome with B cells present but T cells absent, so that humoral immune response is present but cell-mediated immune response is absent. **D:** Severe combined immunodeficiency disease (SCID) or adenosine deaminase deficiency (ADA; "bubble boy" disease). Diagram shows a lymph node in SCID or ADA with B cells and T cells absent, so that both humoral immune response and cell-mediated immune response are absent. **E:** Acquired immunodeficiency syndrome (AIDS). Lymph node in late-stage AIDS shows a marked reduction of lymphocytes, especially in the inner cortex (IC). OC, outer cortex.

Case Study 13-1

A 38-year-old woman who is a manicurist comes to your office complaining that "My back hurts real bad especially when I bend over or turn to the side. I bought a new chair with a lumbar support for work but it hasn't helped." She also tells you that she has always worked very hard (6 days a week) because she had a lot of energy and loves her job, but lately she feels very fatigued and can't work as much. After some discussion, she informs you that she has had recent bouts of confusion, weakness, polyuria, and constipation, and has smoked cigarettes (2 packs a day) for 24 years. The woman is clearly worried and says, "If I don't get better, I will lose my business and I have three kids to support all by myself." What is the most likely diagnosis?

Differentials

- Herniated disc, metastatic bone lesions, osteoarthritis, fibromyalgia

Relevant Physical Examination Findings

- Tenderness to palpation in the thoracic and lumbar spine
- Limited range of motion due to pain

Relevant Lab Findings

- Blood chemistry: pancytopenia; red blood cell (RBC) rouleaux formation; monoclonal M spike on electrophoresis; Ca^{2+} = 15 mg/dL (high); RBC sedimentation rate = 50 mm/h (high)
- Bone marrow sample: atypical plasma cells
- Urinalysis: Bence Jones proteins
- Radiograph: diffuse lytic lesions of the skull, vertebrae, and long bones

Diagnosis: Multiple Myeloma

- **Multiple myeloma** is a disorder characterized by malignant monoclonal plasma cells that proliferate in the bone marrow and produce immunoglobulins (usually IgG or IgA). The plasma cell proliferation causes a space-occupying lesion in the marrow, resulting in myelo-suppressive anemia and pancytopenia. Clinical findings of multiple myeloma include osteolytic lesions, pathologic fractures, anemia, renal insufficiency, and recurrent bacterial infections.
- A herniated disc will produce a sharp, localized pain at a specific dermatome.
- A metastatic bone lesion due to breast cancer or lung cancer is a possibility, but the bone marrow sample showed no infiltration of metastatic cancer cells.
- Osteoarthritis is a noninflammatory, "wear and tear" disease caused by mechanical injury and affects the interphalangeal joints in the hand. Clinical findings of fibromyalgia include widespread musculoskeletal pain, stiffness, paresthesia, fatigue, sleep problems, and multiple tender points.

Chapter 14

Spleen

I **General Features.** The spleen is the largest lymphoid organ, weighing about 150 g, and is covered by a connective tissue **capsule** that sends a **trabecular network** into the parenchyma of the gland. The parenchyma is divided into the **white pulp** and **red pulp**, each of which have different functions. On the cut surface of the fresh spleen, the unaided eye can distinguish white pulp, which appears as small, pale islands of lymphoid tissue, and red pulp, which appears bright red due to the large number of red blood cells (RBCs). The splenic artery, splenic vein, and efferent lymphatics (the spleen has **no afferent lymphatics**) are found at the **hilus**.

II **White Pulp (Figure 14-1).** The white pulp immunologically monitors the blood (unlike lymph nodes, which monitor lymph) where T cells and B cells interact to form a large number of plasma cells that migrate to the red pulp and produce immunoglobulins. The white pulp consists of the following:

A. MATURE (VIRGIN) B CELLS. Mature B cells are organized into **lymphatic follicles** that are closely associated with the **central artery.**

B. MATURE T CELLS. Mature T cells are organized into a sheath around a central artery called the **periarterial lymphatic sheath (PALS)**, which is a thymic-dependent zone similar to the inner cortex of a lymph node.

III **Marginal Zone.** The marginal zone is located between the white pulp and red pulp. The marginal zone is the **site where the immune response is initiated** (which occurs in the spleen as foreign antigens encounter antigen-presenting cells) and where **lymphocytes exit the bloodstream** to repopulate the spleen. The marginal zone consists of the following:

A. MACROPHAGES

B. ANTIGEN-PRESENTING CELLS (APCS)

IV **Red Pulp.** The red pulp removes senescent, damaged, or genetically altered (e.g., sickle cell disease) RBCs and particulate matter from the circulation by macrophages. The iron (Fe^{2+}) portion of hemoglobin is stored as ferritin and eventually recycled. The heme moiety of hemoglobin is broken down into bilirubin, is transferred to the liver, and becomes a component of bile. The red pulp also stores platelets and is the site of immunoglobulin production released from plasma cells. The red pulp is organized into **splenic (Billroth) cords**, which are separated by **splenic venous sinusoids.**

A. SPLENIC (BILLROTH) CORDS consist of the following:
1. **Macrophages**
2. **Plasma cells**
3. **Lymphocytes**
4. **RBCs**

5. **Fibroblasts** (reticular cells), which secrete **type III collagen** (reticular fibers) that form a stromal meshwork

B. SPLENIC VENOUS SINUSOIDS

1. These sinusoids are lined by specialized endothelial cells that are long and narrow and have wide gaps between their lateral margins with connecting rings of basement membrane for support. This microanatomy resembles the metal hoops (i.e., basement membrane) that support the wooden staves (i.e., endothelial cells) of a barrel.

2. These cells provide an effective **filter** between the splenic cords and lumen of the sinusoids.

3. Defective RBCs, dead leukocytes, senescent platelets, and particulate matter are phagocytosed by macrophages as they try to negotiate the filter.

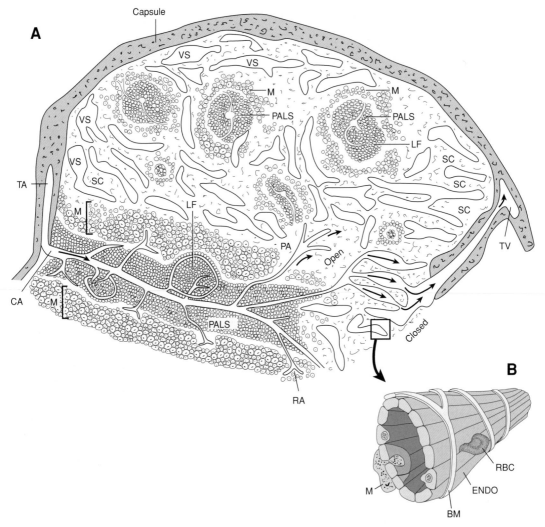

● **Figure 14-1 General features of the spleen. A:** Diagram of normal splenic architecture and vascular pattern. The trabecular artery (TA) branches into a central artery (CA) that becomes ensheathed by T cells, forming the periarterial lymphatic sheath (PALS). Some branches of the CA terminate in the marginal zone (M) where the immune response in the spleen is initiated and where lymphocytes exit the bloodstream to repopulate the spleen. The CA branches into penicillar arterioles (PA) that may open directly into the red pulp, forming an extensive extravascular compartment of blood (open circulation), or empty directly into splenic venous sinusoids (VS; closed circulation). Splenic venous sinusoids empty into trabecular veins (TV). Along the central artery, lymphatic follicles (LF) consisting of B cells are apparent. **B:** A closer view of a venous sinusoid (*boxed area* in A). The venous sinusoid consists of long, narrow endothelial cells (endo) with wide gaps at the lateral margins. Connecting rings of basement membrane (BM) are present. A red blood cell (RBC) is shown migrating from the splenic cord through the wide gaps between the endothelial cells. Macrophages (M) in close association with the venous sinusoids will phagocytose defective RBCs or particulate matter.

V **Blood Flow** through the spleen involves the splenic artery → trabecular arteries → central arteries → penicillar arterioles (open or closed circulation) → splenic venous sinusoids → trabecular veins → and splenic vein.

VI **Clinical Considerations**

A. **HOWELL-JOLLY BODIES** are found after splenectomy and represent nuclear fragments that are normally removed from RBCs as they pass through the splenic sinuses. After splenectomy, increased numbers of RBCs with Howell-Jolly bodies are observed.

B. **OVERWHELMING POSTSPLENECTOMY SEPSIS.** Postsplenectomy patients (especially children) are at great risk for **bacterial septicemia** because of decreased opsonic production, decreased immunoglobulin M (IgM) levels, and decreased clearance of bacteria from blood. The most commonly involved pathogens are *Streptococcus pneumoniae*, *Haemophilus influenzae*, and *Neisseria meningitidis*, which are encapsulated bacteria. Patients with **sickle cell anemia** usually undergo "autosplenectomy" due to multiple infarcts caused by stagnation of abnormal RBCs and are therefore prime targets for postsplenectomy sepsis. Clinical features include: influenzalike symptoms, which progress to high fever, shock, and death.

C. **CONGESTIVE SPLENOMEGALY** is usually due to portal hypertension caused by cirrhosis. The spleen is frequently covered by a "sugar-coated" capsule and focal areas of fibrosis containing iron and calcium called Gandy-Gamna nodules.

D. **FELTY SYNDROME** is a syndrome with the combined features of **rheumatoid arthritis**, **splenomegaly**, and **neutropenia**.

VII **Hypersensitivity Reactions.** The thymus, lymph nodes, and spleen are the major organs of the immune system. In addition to providing protection, the immune system may also produce deleterious reactions called **hypersensitivity or allergic reactions**, which include the following.

A. **TYPE I ANAPHYLACTIC REACTIONS** are mediated by IgE (i.e., antibody mediated), which binds to antibody receptors on basophils and mast cells. When cross-linked by antigens, IgE triggers basophils and mast cells to release their contents. Reaction occurs within **minutes**. Clinically, this type of reaction occurs in a wide spectrum ranging from **rashes and wheal-and-flare reactions to anaphylactic shock**.

B. **TYPE II CYTOTOXIC REACTIONS** are mediated by IgG or IgM (i.e., antibody mediated), which bind to antigen on the surface of a cell and kill the cell through complement activation. Clinically, this type of reaction occurs in **blood transfusion reactions, Rh incompatibility, transplant rejection via antibodies, drug-induced thrombocytopenia purpura, hemolytic anemia, and autoimmune diseases**.

C. **TYPE III IMMUNE COMPLEX REACTIONS** are mediated by **antigen–antibody complexes** (i.e., **antibody mediated**) that activate complement, which in turn activates neutrophils and macrophages to cause tissue damage. Reaction occurs within **hours**. Clinically, this type of reaction occurs in **serum sickness, chronic glomerulonephritis, poststreptococcal glomerulonephritis, rheumatoid arthritis, systemic lupus erythematosus, polyarteritis nodosa, Farmer lung, and the Arthus reaction**.

D. TYPE IV DELAYED-TYPE REACTIONS are mediated by **T cells** (i.e., **cell mediated**). This type of reaction takes longer to mount (**1 to 2 days**) than antibody-mediated reactions (types I through III) due to the time it takes to mobilize T cells through a cascade of activation events. Clinically, this type of reaction occurs in **poison ivy dermatitis (contact sensitivity)**, whereby Langerhans cells (antigen-presenting cells) in the skin respond to urushiol (an oil); **transplant rejection via cells; tuberculin reaction** (*Mycobacterium tuberculosis;* **purified protein derivative skin test**); **sarcoidosis; Crohn disease; and ulcerative colitis.**

Chapter 15

Esophagus and Stomach

Esophagus

I General Features. The esophagus is a continuous muscular tube that begins at the cricoid cartilage and ends at the gastroesophageal junction. The esophagus consists of a **mucosa, submucosa, muscularis externa**, and **adventitia**.

II Mucosa

A. The mucosa consists of a **nonkeratinized stratified squamous epithelium** (except the distal 2 cm at the gastroesophageal junction, which is lined by simple columnar epithelium), **lamina propria, and muscularis mucosae**.

B. Within the lamina propria, **mucosal glands (esophageal cardiac glands)** are found concentrated in the terminal portion of the esophagus near the gastroesophageal junction. The esophageal cardiac glands secrete neutral **mucus** that protects the distal esophagus from damage due to gastric acid reflux.

III Submucosa. The submucosa contains **submucosal glands** that are found throughout the esophagus but concentrated more in the **proximal portion** of the esophagus. The submucosal glands secrete **acidic mucus** that lubricates the lumen of the esophagus.

IV Muscularis Externa

A. The **distal 50%** of the esophagus consists of smooth muscle only. In this area, the smooth muscle is organized into an **inner circular layer** and **outer longitudinal layer**.

B. The **lower esophageal sphincter (LES)** separates the esophagus from the stomach and prevents **gastroesophageal reflux**, which is the reflux of acidic gastric contents into the esophagus (i.e., gastroesophageal reflux disease [GERD]). The LES is composed of smooth **muscle** with the inner circular layer of smooth muscle the major determinant of LES tone.

V Gastroesophageal (GE) Junction. The histologic GE junction does NOT correspond to the gross anatomic GE junction. The mucosal lining of the cardiac portion of the stomach **extends about 2 cm into the esophagus** such that the distal 2 cm of the esophagus is lined by a simple columnar epithelium. The junction where stratified squamous epithelium changes to simple columnar epithelium (or the mucosal GE junction) can be seen macroscopically as a **zig-zag line** (called the **Z-line**). This distinction is clinically very important. especially when dealing with Barrett esophagus.

Clinical Considerations

A. GERD

1. **General features.** GERD is described as the symptoms or mucosal damage produced by the abnormal reflux of gastric contents through the LES into the esophagus.

2. **Pathologic findings.** Pathologic findings include: hyperemia (engorgement of blood); superficial erosions and ulcers, which appear as vertical linear streaks; squamous epithelium that shows hydropic changes; and increased lymphocytes, eosinophils, and neutrophils.

3. **Clinical findings.** Clinical features include: **heartburn (or pyrosis)**, which may worsen when bending or lying down; **regurgitation**; and **dysphagia (difficulty in swallowing)**. Heartburn is typically described as a retrosternal burning discomfort that radiates toward the neck most commonly experienced in the postprandial period. Regurgitation is the effortless return of gastric contents into the pharynx without nausea, retching, or abdominal contractions. Dysphagia is common in the setting of long-standing heartburn. The most dreaded cause of dysphagia is esophageal cancer (e.g., either adenocarcinoma arising from Barrett metaplasia or squamous cell carcinoma). Alcohol, chocolate, fatty foods, and cigarette smoking accentuate the reflux.

B. BARRETT ESOPHAGUS

1. Barrett esophagus can be defined as the replacement of esophageal stratified squamous epithelium with metaplastic "intestinalized" simple columnar epithelium with goblet cells extending **at least 3 cm** into the esophagus. This metaplastic invasion is most commonly caused by GERD. The clinical importance of this metaplastic invasion is that virtually all lower esophageal adenocarcinomas occur as sequelae.

2. The mucosal lining of the cardiac portion of the stomach **extends about 2 cm into the esophagus** such that the distal 2 cm of the esophagus is lined by a simple columnar epithelium, instead of stratified squamous epithelium. The junction where stratified squamous epithelium changes to simple columnar epithelium (or the mucosal GE junction) can be seen macroscopically as a **zig-zag line** (called the **Z-line**). This distinction is clinically very important, especially when dealing with Barrett esophagus.

Stomach

General Features. The function of the stomach is to macerate, homogenize, and partially digest the swallowed food to produce a semisolid paste called **chyme**. The stomach is organized into a **mucosa** (consisting of an epithelium, glands, lamina propria, and muscularis mucosae), **submucosa** (connective tissue containing blood vessels, nerves, and Meissner plexus), **muscularis externa** (smooth muscle randomly arranged containing Auerbach plexus), and **serosa**. The inner luminal surface of the stomach contains longitudinal ridges of mucosa and submucosa called **rugae** and is dotted with millions of openings called **gastric pits or foveolae**.

Gastric Mucosa (Figure 15-1). The epithelium of the gastric mucosa lines the lumen of the stomach and consists of **surface mucous cells** that are attached to each other by juxtaluminal tight junctions. Surface mucous cells secrete **mucus and HCO_3^-** to protect the mucosa from the acid pH and hydrolytic enzymes contained in the gastric juice.

Gastric Glands (Figure 15-1). The epithelium of the gastric mucosa also invaginates to form gastric glands, which contain the following cell types.

A. STEM CELLS demonstrate a high rate of **mitosis**. They migrate upward to replace surface mucous cells every 4 to 7 days and downward to replace other cell types.

B. **MUCOUS NECK CELLS** secrete **mucus.**

C. **PARIETAL CELLS** secrete the following:
1. **HCl (gastric acid)** into the gastric lumen. HCl is produced through the action of carbonic **anhydrase** and H^+-K^+ **adenosine triphosphatase (ATPase;** a H^+ pump). Since Cl^- is secreted along with H^+, the secretion product of parietal cells is HCl.
2. HCO_3^- into the bloodstream, causing a rise in the pH called the "**alkaline tide.**"
3. **Intrinsic Factor,** which is necessary for **vitamin B_{12}** absorption. **Pernicious anemia** may result due to vitamin B_{12} deficiency caused by atrophic gastritis with decreased intrinsic factor production (see Figure 11-4A).

D. **CHIEF CELLS** secrete **pepsinogen** (inactive), which is converted to **pepsin** (active) upon contact with the acid pH of the gastric juice. Chief cells also secrete **lipase.**

E. **ENTEROENDOCRINE CELLS**
1. **G cells** secrete **gastrin (in response to a meal),** which stimulates HCl secretion from parietal cells, stimulates histamine release from enterochromaffinlike cells, and promotes growth of the gastric mucosa. They are found predominately in the antrum of the stomach so that, in the case of ulcers, the antrum may be resected in order to reduce the amount of HCl secretion.
2. **Enterochromaffinlike (ECL) Cells** secrete **serotonin,** which increases gut motility, and **histamine,** which stimulates HCl secretion.
3. **D cells** secrete **somatostatin,** which inhibits secretion of nearby enteroendocrine cells.

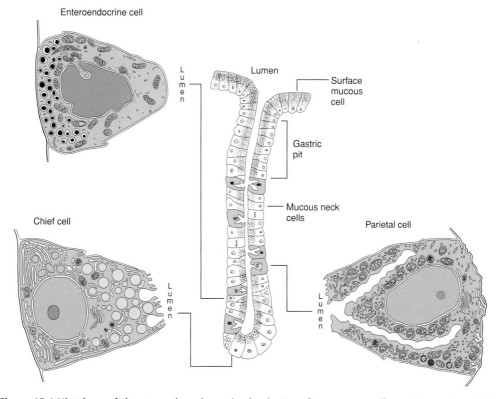

● **Figure 15-1 Histology of the stomach and gastric glands.** A **surface mucous cell** contains rough endoplasmic reticulum (rER), a well-developed Golgi, and numerous mucus-containing granules that are oriented toward the lumen of the stomach. A **mucous neck cell** is a flower bouquet–shaped cell that contains rER, a well-developed Golgi, and large, spherical mucus-containing granules oriented toward the gastric gland lumen. A **parietal cell** is a large, triangular-shaped, acidophilic cell that contains numerous mitochondria and an **intracellular canalicular system** that is continuous with the cell membrane and related to an elaborate tubulovesicular **network**. An **enteroendocrine cell** contains rER, Golgi, and numerous secretory granules that are oriented toward capillaries within the lamina propria (i.e., away from the gastric gland lumen). A **chief cell** is an intensely basophilic cell that contains extensive rER, Golgi, and granules that are oriented toward the gastric gland lumen.

Clinical Considerations

A. **GASTRIC ULCERS (FIGURE 15-2)**

1. Ulcers are a breach in the mucosa that extends into the submucosa or deeper.

2. They occur where exposure to the aggressive action of gastric juice is high (e.g., stomach, duodenum, or esophagus). **Sucralfate (Carafate or Sulcrate)** is a drug that forms a polymer in an acidic environment, which protects ulcers from further irritation and damage.

3. The bacteria *Helicobacter pylori* play a causative role in ulcers. The antibiotic regimens of **bismuth subsalicylate (Pepto-Bismol), tetracycline, and metronidazole** or **amoxicillin and clarithromycin** are effective in eradication of *H. pylori*.

4. Other treatment of ulcers includes ways to reduce HCl secretion.
   a. **Surgical resection of the pyloric antrum** removes G cells that secrete gastrin (which stimulates HCl secretion).
   b. **Omeprazole (Losec)** is an irreversible H^+-K^+ ATPase inhibitor that inhibits HCl secretion from parietal cells.
   c. **Atropine** is a muscarinic acetylcholine receptor (mAChR) antagonist that blocks the stimulatory effects of ACh released from postganglionic parasympathetic neurons (cranial nerve [CN] X) on HCl secretion.
   d. **Cimetidine (Tagamet), Ranitidine (Zantac), Nizatidine (Axid), and Famotidine (Pepcid)** are H_2-receptor antagonists that block the stimulatory effects of histamine released from ECL cells or mast cells upon HCl secretion. The H_2 receptor is a G protein–linked receptor that increases cyclic adenosine monophosphate (cAMP) levels.
   e. **Misoprostol (Cytotec)** is a prostaglandin E_1 (PGE_1) analog that inhibits HCl secretion and stimulates secretion of mucus and HCO_3^-.

B. **GASTRINOMA (ZOLLINGER-ELLISON SYNDROME)**

1. A gastrinoma is a malignant tumor consisting of G cells and is generally associated with the multiple endocrine neoplasia type 1 (MEN 1) syndrome.

2. A gastrinoma secretes **excess gastrin**, thereby producing hyperacidity (HCl) and peptic ulcer disease.

3. In most cases, a single peptic ulcer is observed but multiple ulcers may also occur. A gastrinoma should always be suspected if a peptic ulcer is found in an unusual site.

4. **Clinical features include:** abdominal pain caused by peptic ulcer, diarrhea (malabsorption since enzymes cannot work in an acid pH), markedly increased basal acid output (BAO) test, confirmatory secretin test (secretin administration results in an elevation of gastrin levels in patients with a gastrinoma), and serum gastrin levels greater than 600 pg/mL.

5. Other causes of elevated serum gastrin levels include use of H_2 blockers (e.g., Tagamet, Zantac, etc.), which decreases HCl production and thereby elevates gastrin, and atrophic gastritis, which decreases HCl production (by destruction of parietal cells) and thereby elevates gastrin.

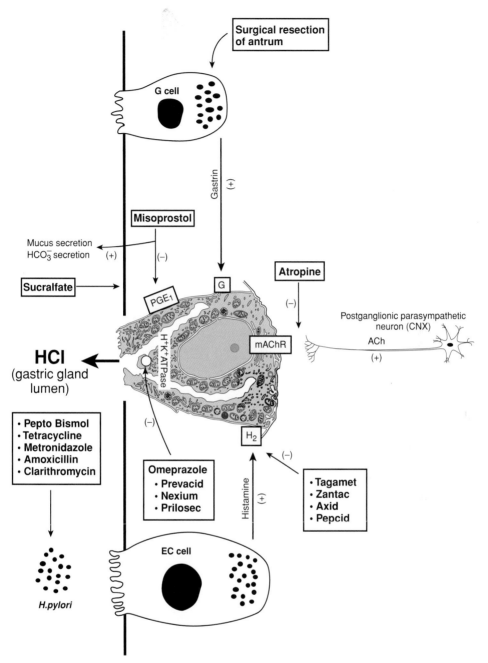

● **Figure 15-2 Control of HCl secretion from the parietal cell and its role in gastric ulcers.** Note the site of action of the various drugs used to treat a gastric ulcer. ACh, acetylcholine; mAChR, muscarinic acetylcholine receptor; H_2, histamine receptor; G, gastrin receptor; PGE_1, prostaglandin E_1.

Chapter 16

Small Intestine

I   General Features. The function of the small intestine is **to continue digestion of the chyme** received from the stomach using enzymes of the glycocalyx, pancreatic enzymes, and liver bile and **to absorb the nutrients** derived from the digestive process. The small intestine is organized into a **mucosa** (consisting of an epithelium, glands, lamina propria, and muscularis mucosae), **submucosa** (connective tissue containing blood vessels, nerves, and Meissner plexus), **muscularis externa** (smooth muscle arranged as an inner circular layer and outer longitudinal layer and containing Auerbach plexus), and **serosa**. The inner luminal surface of the small intestine contains semilunar ridges of mucosa and submucosa called **plica circulares (or valves of Kerckring)**, is dotted with millions of openings where the intestinal glands open to the surface, and contains fingerlike projections of the epithelium and lamina propria called **villi**.

II   Intestinal Mucosa (Figure 16-1). The epithelium of the intestinal mucosa covers the villi and consists of the following cell types:

A. **SURFACE ABSORPTIVE CELLS (ENTEROCYTES)** are joined by juxtaluminal tight junctions and possess **microvilli** that are coated by filamentous glycoproteins called the **glycocalyx**. The glycocalyx contains important enzymes, which include **maltase, α-dextrinase, sucrase, lactase, trehalase, aminopeptidases,** and **enterokinase** (which converts the inactive form [e.g., trypsinogen] of pancreatic enzymes to the active form [e.g., trypsin]). Enterocytes absorb carbohydrates, protein, lipids, vitamins, Ca^{2+}, and Fe^{2+} from the intestinal lumen and transport them to the blood or lymph.

1. **Carbohydrates** are digested to monosaccharides (glucose, galactose, fructose; only monosaccharides can be absorbed). Glucose and galactose enter enterocytes by secondary active transport using the **Na^+-dependent glucose cotransporter**. Fructose enters enterocytes by facilitated diffusion using the **GLUT5 transporter**. Glucose, galactose, and fructose exit enterocytes by facilitated diffusion using the **GLUT2 transporter** and are delivered to portal **blood**.

2. **Proteins** are digested to amino acids, dipeptides, and tripeptides. Most amino acids, dipeptides, and tripeptides enter enterocytes by secondary active transport using **Na^+–amino acid cotransporters** (there are four separate cotransporters for neutral, basic, acidic, and imino amino acids). Dipeptides and tripeptides are then further digested to amino acids by **cytoplasmic peptidases**. Amino acids exit enterocytes by facilitated diffusion and are delivered to portal **blood**.

3. **Triacylglycerols** (the main fat in a human diet) are emulsified by bile salts and digested to fatty acids and monoacylglycerols.

    a. Long-chain fatty acids (>12 carbons), monoacylglycerols, cholesterol, and fat-soluble vitamins (A, D, E, and K) are packaged into **micelles** and enter enterocytes by diffusion assisted by **fatty acid–binding proteins (FABPs)**. Within the enterocyte, **resynthesis of triacylglycerols** occurs in the **smooth endoplasmic**

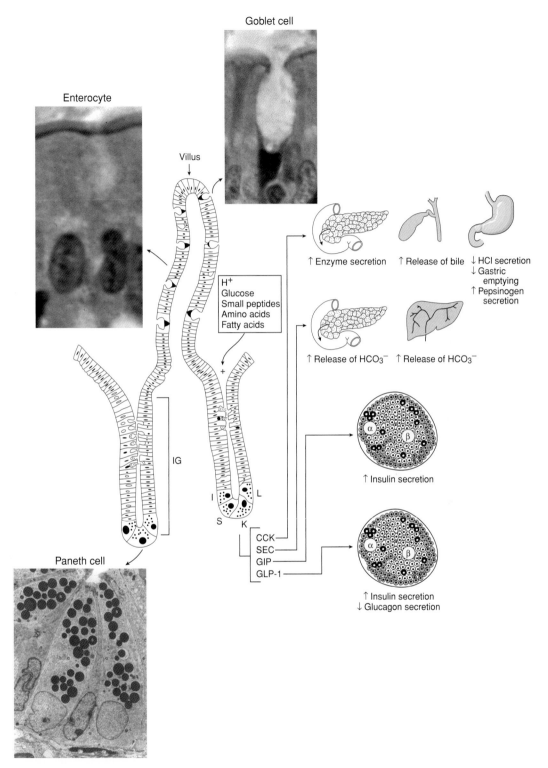

Goblet cell

Enterocyte

Villus

H+
Glucose
Small peptides
Amino acids
Fatty acids

↑ Enzyme secretion   ↑ Release of bile   ↓ HCl secretion
                                           ↓ Gastric
                                             emptying
                                           ↑ Pepsinogen
                                             secretion

↑ Release of HCO₃⁻   ↑ Release of HCO₃⁻

α   β

↑ Insulin secretion

IG

I   L
S   K

CCK
SEC
GIP
GLP-1

α   β

↑ Insulin secretion
↓ Glucagon secretion

Paneth cell

● **Figure 16-1 Histology of the small intestine.** The diagram shows a villus and intestinal gland (IG) along with photomicrographs of a goblet cell, surface absorptive cell (enterocyte), and Paneth cell. The hormonal secretion from intestinal glands and their actions are also indicated. Note that H+, glucose, small peptides, amino acids, and fatty acids within the lumen of the intestinal gland stimulate I cells (I), S cells (S), K cells (K), and L cells (L) to secrete cholecystokinin (CCK), secretin (SEC), gastric inhibitory peptide (GIP), and glucagonlike peptide 1 (GLP-1), respectively. Note the action of various hormones.

reticulum (sER), which contains acyl-coenzyme A (CoA) synthetase and acyl-transferases. Subsequently, the triacylglycerols, cholesterol, and fat-soluble vitamins are packaged by the **Golgi** with **apoproteins** into **chylomicrons**, which are delivered to lymph via **lacteals.**

    b.   Short- and medium-chain fatty acids (<12 carbons) and glycerol enter the enterocyte directly by diffusion (no micelle packaging), exit the enterocyte by diffusion (no chylomicron packaging), and are delivered to **portal blood.**

    c.   **Xenical** is a drug used in the treatment of morbid obesity that blocks about 30% of dietary fat from being absorbed.

  4. **Water-soluble vitamins** enter the enterocyte by diffusion, although some require a Na^+-dependent cotransporter. **Vitamin B_{12}** is absorbed in the **ileum** and requires **intrinsic factor** secreted by parietal cells of the stomach.

  5. **Ca^{2+}** is absorbed and requires $1,25(OH)_2$-vitamin D, which is produced by the kidney.

  6. **Fe^{2+}** enters the enterocyte as "**heme Fe^{2+}**" (Fe^{2+} bound to hemoglobin or myoglobin) or as **free Fe^{2+}**. Within the enterocyte, heme Fe^{2+} is degraded to release free Fe^{2+}. Free Fe^{2+} is released into the blood and circulates in the blood bound to **transferrin.**

B. **GOBLET CELLS** synthesize **mucinogen**, which is stored in membrane-bound granules.

Ⅲ Intestinal Glands (Crypts of Lieberkühn; Figure 16-1)

A. **STEM CELLS** demonstrate a high rate of mitosis and replace enterocytes and goblet cells every 3 to 6 days.

B. **PANETH CELLS** are found at the base of the intestinal glands and secrete the following.

  1. **Lysozyme** is a proteolytic enzyme that degrades the peptidoglycan coat of bacteria, thereby increasing membrane permeability of bacteria so that they swell and rupture.

  2. **Tumor necrosis factor-α (TNF-α)** is a proinflammatory substance.

  3. **Defensins (cryptdins)** increase the membrane permeability of bacteria and other parasites by formation of ion channels.

C. **ENTEROENDOCRINE CELLS**

  1. **I Cells** secrete **cholecystokinin (CCK)** in response to small peptides, amino acids, and fatty acids within the gut lumen. CCK **stimulates enzyme secretion** from pancreatic acinar cells, **stimulates release of bile** from the gallbladder (by contraction of gallbladder smooth muscle and relaxation of the sphincter of Oddi), decreases HCl secretion and gastric emptying, and increases pepsinogen secretion from the stomach.

  2. **S Cells** secrete **secretin (called nature's antacid)** in response to H^+ and fatty acids within the gut lumen. Secretin **stimulates release of HCO_3^-** from the pancreas and the liver biliary tract.

  3. **K Cells** secrete **gastric inhibitory peptide (GIP)** in response to orally administered glucose, amino acids, and fatty acids in the gut lumen. GIP **stimulates insulin secretion** from pancreatic islets. This explains why an oral glucose load produces higher serum insulin levels than an intravenous glucose load.

  4. **L Cells** secrete **glucagonlike peptide 1 (GLP-1)** in response to orally administered glucose, amino acids, and fatty acids in the gut lumen. GLP-1 **stimulates insulin secretion in the presence of hyperglycemia** and **inhibits postprandial glucagon secretion** from pancreatic islets. GLP-1 may be an effective therapeutic agent for **type 2 diabetes** since the stimulatory effect of GLP-1 on insulin secretion is preserved in type 2 diabetic patients.

  5. **Mo Cells** secrete **motilin.**

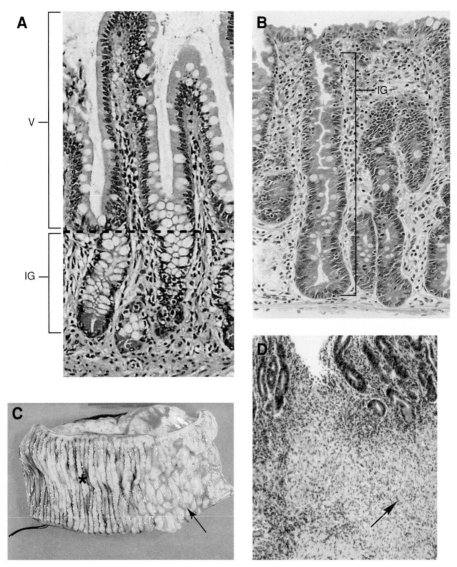

● **Figure 16-2 Normal and pathologic features of the small intestine. A:** Light micrograph (LM) of normal small intestine showing villi (V) and intestinal glands (IG). *Dotted line* indicates boundary of villi and intestinal glands. Compare to celiac disease in B and note the loss of villi in celiac disease. **B:** LM pathology of celiac disease (sprue). Note the chronic inflammation of the lamina propria adjacent to intestinal glands along with the loss of villi (compare to normal in A). Inflammation is generally confined to the mucosa. A gluten-free diet will eliminate the inflammation and allow villi to return to normal. **C, D:** Crohn disease. **C:** Gross specimen of ileum from a patient with Crohn disease. Note the prominent cobblestoning (*arrow*) due to multiple transverse and linear ulcers. The other portion of the ileum is normal (*). **D:** LM pathology of Crohn disease showing a submucosal granuloma (*arrow*) that may extend into the muscularis externa.

IV **Gut-Associated Lymphatic Tissue (GALT; Peyer Patches)** are lymphatic follicles found in the intestinal mucosa and submucosa that are covered by an epithelial lining containing **M cells.** M cells are **antigen-transporting cells,** which have **microfolds** on their luminal surface.

A. M cells endocytose antigens into protease-containing vesicles at their apical domain. These vesicles are transported across the M cell to the basolateral domain where the antigen is discharged into the intercellular space in close vicinity to **mature (or virgin) B lymphocytes** (see Chapter 13, Figure 13-2).

B. Under the influence of CD4$^+$ helper T cells and IL-2, mature B lymphocytes differentiate into **plasma cells** that secrete antigen-specific **immunoglobulin A (IgA)** into the lamina propria.

C. IgA within the lamina propria binds to the **poly-Ig receptor** on the basal domain of the enterocyte to form an **IgA + poly-Ig receptor complex,** which is endocytosed and transported across the enterocyte. At the apical domain, the complex is cleaved such that IgA is released into the intestinal lumen joined with the **secretory piece** of the receptor and is known as **secretory IgA (sIgA).**

D. A significant amount of IgA also enters the bloodstream and is processed by hepatocytes in the liver using the same mechanism as enterocytes mentioned previously. The secretory IgA is released into bile canaliculi and travels to the intestinal lumen with bile.

E. sIgA binding to microorganisms/antigens reduces their ability to penetrate the epithelial lining.

Ⓥ Clinical Considerations

A. CELIAC DISEASE (GLUTEN-SENSITIVE ENTEROPATHY)

1. **General features.** Celiac disease is a hypersensitivity to **gluten** and **gliadin** protein found in wheat, barley, and rye grains. Celiac disease is characterized by a generalized malabsorption, mucosal lesions within the small intestine, and prompt reversal of clinical symptoms when gluten-containing foods are removed from the diet.

2. **Pathologic findings.** Pathologic findings include: blunting or disappearance of villi; damage of mucosal epithelial cells; accumulation of a large number of lymphocytes, plasma cells, macrophages, and eosinophils within the lamina propria of the intestinal mucosa upon ingestion of gluten-containing foods; and detection of gliadin antibodies in the blood. Most severe histologic abnormalities are found in the duodenum and proximal jejunum.

3. **Clinical findings.** Clinical findings include: generalized malabsorption, chronic diarrhea, flatulence, weight loss, and fatigue.

B. CROHN DISEASE (CD)

1. **General features.** CD is a chronic inflammatory bowel disease that usually appears in teenagers and young adults. CD most commonly affects the **ileum and the ascending right colon.** The etiology of CD is unknown, although epidemiologic studies have indicated a **strong genetic predisposition** and immunologic studies have indicated a role of **cytotoxic T cells** in the damage to the intestinal wall.

2. **Pathologic findings.** Pathologic findings include: transmural nodular lymphoid aggregates; noncaseating epithelioid granulomas; neutrophilic infiltration of the intestinal glands, which ultimately destroys the glands, leading to ulcers; and coalescence of the ulcers into **long, serpentine ulcers** ("**linear ulcers**") oriented along the long axis of the bowel. A classic feature of Crohn disease is the clear demarcation between diseased bowel segments located directly next to uninvolved normal bowel and a **cobblestone appearance** that can be seen grossly and radiographically.

3. **Clinical findings.** Clinical findings include: recurrent right lower quadrant colicky abdominal pain, intermittent bouts of diarrhea, weight loss associated with malabsorption and malnutrition, recurrent fever, weakness, strictures of the intestinal lumen, formation of fistulas, and perforation.

C. CHOLERA

1. **General features.** *Vibrio cholerae* (O1 or O139 strains of the El Tor biotype) causes cholera. Clinical findings include sudden onset of profuse watery diarrhea with mucous flecks but no blood ("rice-water stools"), and no fever. There may be vomiting. Hypovolemic shock will occur (fatal within 8 hours) if electrolytes and fluids are not replaced. The incubation period is 2 to 3 days, and a long-lasting immunity to the serotype occurs.

2. **Causative Agent (*V. cholerae*).** The genus *Vibrio* is **gram-negative bacilli.** *V. cholerae* is a gram-negative bacillus, facultative anaerobic, oxidase positive, and a slow lactose fermenter; does not produce H_2S gas; prefers an alkaline environment; has a single flagellum; and is comma shaped.

3. **Reservoir.** *V. cholerae* is transmitted by contaminated food and water. There are no known animal reservoirs or vectors. Human fecal contamination of coastal sea waters has caused epidemics associated with eating raw or undercooked sea food.

4. **Virulence factors.** *V. cholerae* does not enter enterocytes but instead remains in the intestinal lumen and secretes an enterotoxin called **cholera toxin (choleragen).** Cholera toxin consists of **one A subunit (with an A1 and A2 component) and five B subunits (an A-B component toxin).** The B subunits bind to the GM_1 **ganglioside** on the cell membrane. The A2 component facilitates entry into the cell membrane. The A1 component (an adenosine diphosphate [ADP]-ribosyl transferase) ADP-ribosylates a G_S protein (**ADP ribosylation**), which in turn stimulates adenylate cyclase.

D. LACTOSE INTOLERANCE (LI; LACTASE NONPERSISTENCE; ADULT-TYPE HYPOLACTASIA)

1. LI is an autosomal recessive genetic disorder associated with short tandem repeat polymorphisms (STRPs) in the promoter region that affects transcriptional activity of the *LCT* **gene** on **chromosome 2q21** for **lactase-phlorizin hydrolase,** which catalyzes the reaction lactose $\rightarrow$ glucose + galactose.

2. These STRPs in the human population lead to two distinct phenotypes: **lactase persistent** individuals and **lactase nonpersistent** individuals.

3. All healthy newborn children up to the age of $\approx$5 to 7 years have high levels of lactase-phlorizin hydrolase activity so that they can digest large quantities of lactose present in milk.

4. Northern European adults (particularly Scandinavian) retain high levels of lactase-phlorizin activity and are known as **lactase persistent** and therefore **lactose tolerant.**

5. However, a majority of the world's adults (particularly Africa and Asia) lose the high levels of lactase-phlorizin activity and are known as **lactase nonpersistent** and therefore **lactose intolerant.**

6. **Clinical findings include:** diarrhea; crampy abdominal pain localized to the periumbilical area or lower quadrant; flatulence; nausea; vomiting; audible borborygmi; stools that are bulky, frothy, and watery; and bloating after milk or lactose consumption.

Case Study 16-1

A 22-year-old man comes to your office complaining that "I have bouts of diarrhea in the morning that come and go, and I have a fever and pain on the lower right side near my appendix." After some discussion, he informs you that he has not noticed any blood in the diarrhea and that he has lost 20 pounds this past year. What is the most likely diagnosis?

Differentials

- Acute appendicitis, irritable bowel syndrome, ulcerative colitis

Relevant Physical Examination Findings

- Middle Eastern heritage
- Fever
- Palpable, tender mass in the lower right quadrant
- Guarding is not present
- Psoas and obturator signs are negative
- Rectal examination: negative for occult blood

Relevant Lab Findings

- Blood chemistry: hemoglobin (Hgb) = 10g/dL (low); hematocrit (Hct) = 32% (low); white blood cells (WBCs) = 15,000/mm^3 (high); albumin = 3g/L (low)
- Stool sample: culture = negative; occult blood = negative
- Barium enema radiograph: reflux of barium into terminal ileum, luminal narrowing ("string sign"), cobblestone pattern, wall thickening
- Colonoscopy: ulceration; strictures in the colonic mucosa

Diagnosis: Crohn Disease

- Crohn disease (CD). See discussion in IV.B of this chapter.
- Acute appendicitis is most often caused by inflammation of the lymphoid tissue or the presence of a fecalith. Clinical findings of acute appendicitis include diffuse periumbilical pain that migrates to the lower right quadrant; anorexia; guarding of the lower right quadrant present; tenderness at the McBurney point; positive psoas sign (passive extension of right hip is painful); positive obturator sign (passive flexion and inward rotation of right hip is painful).
- Irritable bowel syndrome (IBS) is the most common gastrointestinal tract disease in the general population and involves an abnormality in colonic motility that is precipitated by stress or high-fat meals. Clinical findings of IBS include cramps, constipation, alternating bouts of constipation and diarrhea, or chronic diarrhea. IBS is more common in females and occurs before 30 years of age.
- Ulcerative colitis is a type of idiopathic inflammatory bowel disease. Ulcerative colitis always involves the rectum and extends proximally for varying distances. The inflammation is continuous (i.e., there are no "skip areas" as in Crohn disease). The etiology of ulcerative colitis is unknown. Clinical signs of ulcerative colitis include bloody diarrhea with mucus and pus, malaise, fever, weight loss, and anemia; it may lead to toxic megacolon.

Case Study 16-2

A 60-year-old man comes to your office complaining that "I have real bad watery diarrhea that seems to be getting worse over the last 6 months; sometimes when I have diarrhea I feel nauseated and vomit a lot." He also tells you that "I'm getting hot flashes just like my wife did during menopause and a while back I remember having black, tarry stools." After some discussion, he informs you that he has been trying to lose a few pounds and started the Atkins high-carbohydrate diet. What is the most likely diagnosis?

Differentials

- Crohn disease, infectious diarrhea, irritable bowel syndrome, VIPoma

Relevant Physical Examination Findings

- Auscultation reveals diffuse wheezes over both lungs and a pulmonic ejection murmur over the right sternal border at intercostal space 2.
- Liver is palpable well below the costal margin.
- Hyperactive bowel sounds are apparent.

Relevant Lab Findings

- Blood chemistry: WBCs = 7000/μL (normal); Hgb = 14 g/dL (normal); hematocrit = 42% (normal); platelet count = 153,000/mm^3 (normal); K$^+$ = 4.2 mEq/L (normal); pH = 7.42 (normal)
- Stool sample showed positive for heme and no evidence of parasites.
- Urinalysis: positive for 5-hydroxyindoleacetic acid (5-HIAA)
- Computed tomography scan: nodular masses in the duodenum and liver

Diagnosis: Carcinoid Tumor

- Carcinoid tumor (CAR). CARs account for $\approx$50% of all malignant tumors of the small intestine and arise from neuroendocrine cells, which are most numerous in the appendix and terminal ileum. CARs found in the appendix almost never metastasize. However, CARs found in other regions of the small intestine may metastasize to the liver. CARs secrete serotonin (5-HT), which is broken down by monoamine oxidase to 5-HIAA. 5-HT in the systemic circulation causes carcinoid syndrome. Clinical findings of CARs include diarrhea, episodic flushing, bronchospasm, cyanosis, telangiectasia, and fibrosis of the valves on the right side of the heart. CARs are composed of small, round cells containing cytoplasmic granules arranged in nests, cords, or rosettes located within the submucosa.
- Crohn disease (CD). See discussion in IV.B.
- Infectious diarrhea may be caused by *Giardia lamblia* or *Entamoeba histolytica*, which can be identified in a stool sample. Infectious diarrhea rarely lasts for 6 months (except in the cases of certain parasites).
- Irritable bowel syndrome (IBS) is the most common gastrointestinal tract disease in the general population and involves an abnormality in colonic motility that is precipitated by stress or high-fat meals. Clinical findings of IBS include cramps, constipation, alternating bouts of constipation and diarrhea, or chronic diarrhea. IBS is more common in females and occurs before 30 years of age.
- VIPoma is a rare tumor of the pancreatic islets. Clinical findings of VIPoma include watery diarrhea, hypokalemia, and achlorhydria. The Atkins high-carbohydrate has nothing to do with his condition.

Chapter 17

Large Intestine (Colon)

I **General Features.** The function of the large intestine is to absorb Na^+, Cl^-, and H_2O from the lumen; to soften fecal matter by addition of mucus; and to eliminate fecal matter. The large intestine is organized into a **mucosa** (consisting of an epithelium, glands, lamina propria, and muscularis mucosae), **submucosa** (connective tissue containing blood vessels, nerves, and Meissner plexus), **muscularis externa** (smooth muscle arranged as an inner circular layer and three outer longitudinal bands called **teniae coli** and containing Auerbach plexus; contraction of teniae coli forms sacculations called **haustra**), and **serosa** (contains fatty tags called **appendices epiploicae**). The inner luminal surface is smooth (i.e., no rugae, plicae circulares, no villi) and is dotted with millions of openings where intestinal glands open to the surface.

II **Large Intestinal Mucosa.** The epithelium of the mucosa consists of the following cell types.

A. **ABSORPTIVE CELLS (ENTEROCYTES)** absorb Na^+, Cl^-, and H_2O by facilitated diffusion using ion channels under the regulation of aldosterone. Aldosterone increases the number Na^+ ion channels, thereby increasing the amount of Na^+ absorbed. **Sedatives, anesthetics, and steroids** are also absorbed, which is clinically important when medication cannot be delivered orally.

B. **GOBLET CELLS** synthesize mucinogen, which is stored in membrane-bound granules.

III **Intestinal Glands** contain:

A. **ABSORPTIVE CELLS (ENTEROCYTES)**

B. **GOBLET CELLS**

C. **STEM CELLS,** which demonstrate a high rate of mitosis and replace surface absorptive cells and goblet cells every 5 to 6 days

D. **ENTEROENDOCRINE CELLS**

IV **GUT-Associated Lymphatic Tissue (GALT)** is prominent within the lamina propria throughout the large intestine.

V **Anal Canal (Figure 17-1)** is divided into the upper and lower anal canal by the **pectinate line.**

A. **UPPER ANAL CANAL.** The mucosa extends into longitudinal folds called the **anal columns (or columns of Morgagni).** The base of the anal columns defines the **pectinate** line. The anal columns are connected at their bases by transverse folds of mucosa called the **anal valves**. Behind the anal valves are small, blind pouches called the **anal sinuses** into which mucous **anal glands** open. The upper anal canal is lined by a typical simple columnar epithelium (colonic epithelium) and intestinal glands. The colonic epithelium undergoes a transition to a stratified squamous epithelium in an area near the pectinate line called the **transitional zone**. The upper anal canal is derived embryologically from the **hindgut (endoderm)**.

B. LOWER ANAL CANAL. The lower anal canal is lined by a **nonkeratinized stratified squamous epithelium** called the squamous zone. The lower anal canal is derived embryologically from the **proctodeum (ectoderm)**.

C. ANAL VERGE is the point where the perianal skin begins and is lined by a **keratinized stratified squamous epithelium.**

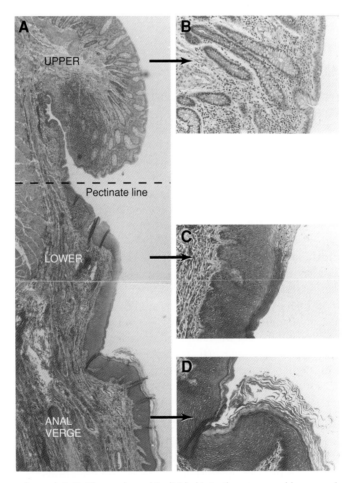

● **Figure 17-1 The anal canal A–D:** The anal canal is divided into the upper and lower anal canal by the pectinate line. The upper anal canal is lined by a typical simple columnar (colonic) epithelium arranged as intestinal glands (see **B**). The colonic epithelium undergoes a transition at the pectinate line to a nonkeratinized stratified squamous epithelium lining the lower anal canal (see **C**). The anal verge is lined by a keratinized stratified squamous epithelium (see **D**). The upper anal canal is derived embryologically from the hindgut, whereas the lower anal canal is derived embryologically from the proctodeum. This dual embryologic origin has important clinical considerations as indicated. (*continued*)

Upper Anal Canal	Venous drainage is by the superior rectal vein → portal vein. Varicosities of the superior rectal vein are called **internal hemorrhoids.** Tumors will drain to **deep** lymphatic nodes (not palpable). Sensory innervation is for stretch sensation. No pain sensation is present. Therefore, internal hemorrhoids or tumors in this area will **not** be accompanied by patient complaints of pain. Motor innervation involves autonomic control of the internal anal sphincter (smooth muscle).
Lower Anal Canal	Venous drainage is by the inferior rectal vein → inferior vena cava. Varicosities of the inferior rectal vein are called **external hemorrhoids.** Tumors will drain to **superficial** lymphatic nodes (palpable). Sensory innervation is for pain, temperature, and touch. Therefore, external hemorrhoids or tumors in this area will be accompanied by patient complaints of pain. Motor innervation involves voluntary control of the external anal sphincter (skeletal muscle).

● **Figure 17-1** *Continued*

Ⓥ Clinical Considerations

A. NONSYNDROMIC CONGENITAL INTESTINAL AGANGLIONOSIS (HIRSCHSPRUNG DISEASE; HSCR)

1. Nonsyndromic HSCR is an autosomal dominant genetic disorder caused by a mutation (≈90% of HSCR cases) in the *RET* (**re**arranged during **t**ransfection) gene on chromosome 10q11.2 for a **receptor tyrosine kinase**. The mutations in the *RET* gene are **loss-of-function mutations.**

2. RET protein is expressed by enteric neuronal precursor cells after they leave the neural tube and throughout their colonization of the gut tube. RET ligands are **GDNF (glial cell line–derived neurotrophic factor)** and NRTN (**neurturin**), which are expressed by nearby mesenchymal cells.

3. **Clinical features include:** arrest of the caudal migration of neural crest cells resulting in the absence of ganglionic cells in the myenteric and submucosal plexuses, abdominal pain and distention, **inability to pass meconium within the first 48 hours of life,** gushing of fecal material upon a rectal digital examination, constipation, emesis, a loss of peristalsis in the colon segment distal to the normal innervated colon, and the failure of internal anal sphincter to relax following rectal distention (i.e., abnormal rectoanal reflex); 80% of HSCR-affected individuals have aganglionosis restricted to the rectosigmoid colon ("short-segment disease"), and 15% to 20% of HSCR-affected individuals have aganglionosis that extends proximal to the sigmoid colon ("long-segment disease").

B. FAMILIAL ADENOMATOUS POLYPOSIS (FAP)

1. FAP is an autosomal dominant genetic disorder caused by a mutation in the *APC* gene on chromosome 5q21-q22 for the **a**denomatous **p**olyposis **c**oli protein. The mutations in the APC gene are **loss-of-function mutations.**

2. The APC protein binds **glycogen synthase kinase 3b (GSK-3b),** which targets **β-catenin.** APC protein maintains normal apoptosis and inhibits cell proliferation through the **Wnt signal transduction pathway** so that the *APC* gene belongs to the family of **tumor suppressor genes.**

3. A majority of colorectal cancers develop slowly through a series of histopathologic changes, each of which has been associated with mutations of specific proto-oncogenes and tumor suppressor genes, as follows:

   a. Normal epithelium → a small polyp involves mutation of the *APC* **tumor suppressor gene.**

b. Small polyp → large polyp involves mutation of *RAS* **proto-oncogene.**

c. Large polyp → carcinoma → metastasis involves mutation of the *DCC* (<u>d</u>eleted in <u>c</u>olon <u>c</u>ancer) **tumor suppressor gene** and the *TP53* **tumor suppressor gene.**

4. **Clinical features include:** the following: colorectal adenomatous polyps appear at 7 to 35 years of age, inevitably leading to colon cancer; thousands of polyps can be observed in the colon; gastric polyps may be present; and patients are often advised to undergo prophylactic colectomy early in life to avert colon cancer.

C. **GARDNER SYNDROME** is a variation of FAP whereby patients demonstrate adenomatous polyps and multiple osteomas.

D. **TURCOT SYNDROME** is a variation of FAP whereby patients demonstrate adenomatous polyps and gliomas.

E. **HEREDITARY NONPOLYPOSIS COLORECTAL CANCER (HNPCC; OR WARTHIN-LYNCH SYNDROME)**

1. HNPCC is an autosomal dominant genetic disorder caused most commonly by mutations in the *hMSH2* **gene** on **chromosome 2p** or the *hMLH1* **gene** on **chromosome 3p,** which encode for **DNA mismatch repair enzymes.** These DNA repair enzymes recognize single nucleotide mismatches or loops that occur in microsatellite repeat areas.

2. In HNPCC, there is a germline mutation in one allele of the *hMSH2* gene or the *hMLH1* gene and then a somatic "second hit" occurs in the other allele.

3. **Clinical features include:** onset of colorectal cancer at a young age, high frequency of carcinomas proximal to the splenic flexure, multiple synchronous or metachronous colorectal cancers, and presence of extracolonic cancers (e.g., endometrial and ovarian cancer; adenocarcinomas of the stomach, small intestine, and hepatobiliary tract). HNPCC accounts for 3% to 5% of all colorectal cancers.

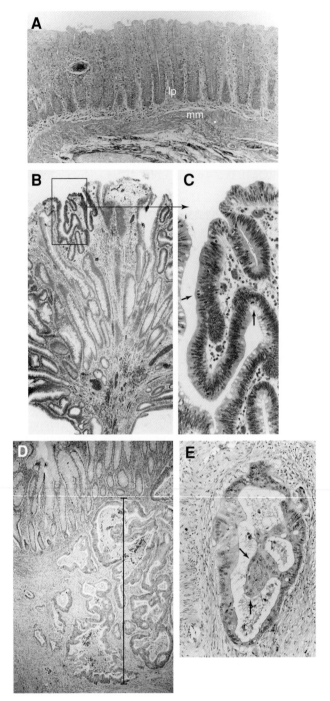

● **Figure 17-2 Normal and pathologic features of the colon. A:** Light micrograph (LM) of normal colon. The mucosa shows typical simple columnar (colonic) epithelium arranged as intestinal glands, lamina propria (lp), and muscularis mucosa (mm). Note the straight, regular arrangement of the intestinal glands that terminate at the basement membrane intact at the muscularis mucosa. **B, C:** LM of an adenomatous polyp. A polyp is a tumorous mass that extends into the lumen of the colon. Note the convoluted, irregular arrangement of the intestinal glands with the basement membrane intact. The epithelium is transformed into a pseudostratified epithelium with mitotic figures apparent (*arrows*; C is a high magnification of the *boxed area* in B). **D, E:** LM of an adenocarcinoma of the colon. Note the convoluted, irregular arrangement of the intestinal glands that have breached the basement membrane to extend deep into the submucosa and/or muscularis externa (*bracket*). The epithelium is transformed into a pseudostratified epithelium that grows in a disorderly pattern extending into the lumen of the gland (*arrows*; E is a high magnification of a typical area in D).

Chapter 18

Liver and Gallbladder

I **Hepatocytes.** Hepatocytes contain the Golgi complex, rough endoplasmic reticulum (rER), smooth endoplasmic reticulum (sER), mitochondria, lysosomes, peroxisomes, lipid, and glycogen. The functions of hepatocytes include:

A. Degradation of ammonia (NH_3). NH_3, which is produced from protein and nucleic acid catabolism, is highly neurotoxic and is therefore converted to nontoxic **urea** in hepatocytes by the **urea cycle.** The urea is released from the liver into the blood and excreted in the urine by the kidneys.

B. Production of 50% of the lymph found within the thoracic duct

C. Production of bile. The cell membrane of the hepatocytes lining the bile canaliculus contains the:
   1. **Multidrug resistance 1 transporter (MDR1),** which transports **cholesterol** into the bile canaliculus
   2. **Multidrug resistance 2 transporter (MDR2),** which transports **phospholipids (mainly lecithin)** into the bile canaliculus
   3. **Multidrug resistance-related protein (MRP-2),** which transports **bilirubin glucuronide (bile pigment)** and **glutathione conjugates** into the bile canaliculus
   4. **Biliary acid transporter (BAT),** which transports **bile salts** (cholic acid and chenodeoxycholic acid conjugated to glycine or taurine) into the bile canaliculus
   5. **Ion exchanger,** which allows passage of HCO_3^- and Cl^- into the bile canaliculus
   6. **Ectoenzymes,** which generate nucleosides and amino acids, which enter the bile canaliculus
   7. **Tight junctions** surrounding the bile canaliculus are relatively "leaky," which allows passage of H_2O and Na^+ into the bile canaliculus.
   8. **Secretory IgA** is also released into the bile canaliculus.

D. CONJUGATION OF BILIRUBIN
   1. Bilirubin (water insoluble) is derived from the breakdown of hemoglobin (i.e., senescent red blood cells [RBCs]) by macrophages and in the spleen and Kupffer cells.
   2. Bilirubin travels in the blood as an **albumin–bilirubin complex** (note: free bilirubin is toxic to the brain [e.g., **kernicterus**]).
   3. Bilirubin is endocytosed by hepatocytes and conjugated to glucuronide by **uridine 5′-diphospho (UDP)-glucuronosyltransferase** in the sER to form **bilirubin-glucuronide** (a water-soluble bile pigment), which is released into bile canaliculi.
   4. Within the distal small intestine and colon, bilirubin-glucuronide is broken down to **free bilirubin** by intestinal bacterial flora. Free bilirubin is reduced to **urobilinogen** and excreted in feces.
   5. Abnormalities in bilirubin metabolism result in **hyperbilirubinemia,** in which there is either an elevation in unconjugated bilirubin alone or of both unconjugated and conjugated bilirubin. Clinical considerations include:

a. **Gilbert Syndrome.** Gilbert syndrome is an autosomal recessive genetic disorder caused by a mutation in the **promoter region** of the *UGT1A1* gene on **chromosome 2q37**, which encodes **UDP-glucuronosyltransferase.** This results in reduced **amounts** of UDP-glucuronosyltransferase. **Clinical features include: unconjugated hyperbilirubinemia** and jaundice. Most patients are asymptomatic; some patients complain of malaise, abdominal discomfort, or fatigue. No specific therapy is required.

b. **Crigler-Najjar Syndrome.** Crigler-Najjar syndrome is a rare autosomal recessive genetic disorder caused by a mutation in the *UCT1A1* **gene** on **chromosome 2q37**, which encodes **UDP-glucuronosyltransferase.** This results in reduced **activity** of **UDP-glucuronosyltransferase.** Crigler-Najjar syndrome is divided into type I and type II forms. **Clinical features of type I include: unconjugated hyperbilirubinemia,** severe jaundice, and neurologic impairment due to bilirubin encephalopathy that may result in permanent neurologic sequelae (i.e., kernicterus). **Clinical features of type II include: unconjugated hyperbilirubinemia (< type I levels)**; patients survive into adulthood without neurologic impairment.

c. **Dubin-Johnson Syndrome.** Dubin-Johnson syndrome is an autosomal recessive genetic disorder caused by a mutation in the *MRP-2* **gene** on **chromosome 10q23**, which encodes for **m**ultidrug **r**esistance-related **p**rotein. This results in decreased transport of conjugated bilirubin into the bile canaliculi. **Clinical features include: conjugated hyperbilirubinemia** and mild jaundice; it is a benign condition, and no treatment is necessary.

E. Maintenance of blood glucose levels by glucose uptake and glycogen synthesis

F. Glycogen storage and degradation to glucose

G. Gluconeogenesis (i.e., conversion of amino acids and lipids into glucose)

H. Synthesis of cholesterol. The synthesis of cholesterol occurs mainly in the liver and intestine. Two molecules of **acetyl-coenzyme A (CoA;** derived mainly from glucose) condense to produce **acetoacetyl-CoA** using **thiolase.** All 27 carbon atoms of cholesterol are derived from acetyl-CoA. Acetoacetyl-CoA reacts with another **acetyl-CoA** to form **hydroxymethylglutaryl-CoA (HMG-CoA)** using **HMG-CoA synthetase.** HMG-CoA is reduced to **mevalonic acid** using **HMG-CoA reductase.** The synthesis of mevalonic acid is the committed step in cholesterol synthesis.

I. Synthesis of plasma proteins (e.g., albumin, fibrinogen, prothrombin, vitamin K–dependent clotting factors)

J. **UPTAKE AND RELEASE OF IMMUNOGLOBULIN A (IGA).** IgA binds to the **poly-Ig receptor** on hepatocytes to form an IgA + poly-Ig receptor complex, which is endocytosed and transported toward the bile canaliculus. At the bile canaliculus, the complex is cleaved such that IgA is released into the bile canaliculus joined with the secretory piece of the receptor and is known as **secretory IgA (sIgA).** sIgA binding to microorganisms/antigens/toxins within the lumen of the gastrointestinal (GI) tract reduces their ability to penetrate the epithelial lining of the GI tract.

K. **STORAGE OF VITAMIN A.** The hepatic stellate cells (fat-storing cells; Ito cells) store vitamin A (retinol) as **retinyl ester.** When vitamin A levels in the blood are low, retinyl ester is hydrolyzed to form retinol. Retinol binds to **retinal-binding protein** and is released into the blood. Vitamin A is necessary for the light reaction of vision, growth of bone at the epiphyseal growth plate, reproduction, and differentiation and maintenance of epithelial tissues.

L. Uptake and inactivation of steroids, lipid-soluble drugs (e.g., phenobarbital), vitamins A and D, triiodothyronine (T_3) and thyroxine (T_4) by removal of iodine, and nonpolar carcinogens by enzymes in the sER

   1. Phase I Reactions (Oxidation). The enzymes that catalyze **cytochrome P_{450}-dependent phase I reactions** are **heme protein monooxygenases** of the **cytochrome P_{450} class** (also called the **microsomal mixed function oxidases**), which catalyze the biotransformation of drugs by hydroxylation, dealkylation, oxidation, desulfuration, and epoxide formation. In addition, there are **cytochrome P_{450}-independent phase I reactions**, which allow local hydrolysis of ester-containing and amide-containing drugs (e.g., local anesthetics) at their site of administration and allow the oxidation of amine-containing compounds (e.g., catecholamines, tyramine) using **monoamine oxidase.**

   2. Phase II Reactions (Conjugation). The enzymes that catalyze phase II reactions are transfer enzymes that catalyze the biotransformation of drugs by glucuronidation (using **UDP-glucuronyl transferase** and **UDP-glucuronic acid** as the glucuronide donor), acetylation, glycine conjugation, sulfate conjugation, glutathione conjugation, and methylation.

M. Metabolism of ethanol. After absorption in the stomach, most ethanol is metabolized in the liver by **alcohol dehydrogenase (ADH pathway)** to produce **acetaldehyde** and **excess H^+** in the cytoplasm. An excess of acetaldehyde is toxic, causing mitochondrial damage, microtubule disruption, and protein alterations that induce an autoimmune response. With chronic ethanol intake, ethanol is metabolized in the liver by the **microsomal ethanol-oxidizing system (MEOS)** to produce **acetaldehyde** and **excess oxygen free radicals** in the cytoplasm. Free radical causes lipid peroxidation, resulting in cell membrane damage.

N. SYNTHESIS OF BILE SALTS. Bile salts are synthesized from cholesterol when an α-OH group is added to carbon 7 of cholesterol to form **7α-hydroxycholesterol** using **7α-hydroxylase** (the rate-limiting step). This results in the formation of **chenocholic acid** and **cholic acid.** Chenocholic acid and cholic acid can conjugate with either glycine or taurine amino acids, forming **glycochenocholic acid, taurochenocholic acid, glycocholic acid,** or **taurocholic acid.**

O. 25-Hydroxylation of vitamin D

P. STORAGE OF IRON. The hepatocytes store iron bound to **ferritin**, which is a very large protein that can bind up to 4500 atoms of iron. In iron overload, ferritin undergoes lysosomal digestion and iron aggregates as **hemosiderin** (a golden brown hemoglobin-derived pigment). The more extreme accumulation of iron is called **hemochromatosis**, which is associated with liver and pancreas damage.

Q. SYNTHESIS OF THE 11 NONESSENTIAL AMINO ACIDS. Of the 20 amino acids commonly found in proteins, the hepatocytes can synthesize 11 amino acids (hence the term nonessential): glycine, alanine, asparagine, serine, glutamine, proline, aspartic acid, glutamic acid, cysteine, tyrosine, and arginine. The remaining nine amino acids (essential amino acids) must be consumed in the diet: valine, leucine, isoleucine, threonine, phenylalanine, tryptophan, methionine, histidine, and lysine.

R. SYNTHESIS OF KETONE BODIES (acetoacetate and 3-hydroxybutyrate)

S. Secretion of angiotensinogen

T. Secretion of **α_1-antitrypsin**, which is a serum protease inhibitor. Methionine 358 in the reactive center of α_1-antitrypsin acts as a "bait" for elastase where elastase is trapped and inactivated. This protects the physiologically important **elastic fibers** present in the lung from destruction.

1. **α_1-Antitrypsin Deficiency.** α_1-Antitrypsin deficiency is an autosomal recessive genetic disorder caused by a missense mutation in the *SERPINA1* gene on chromosome 14q32.1 for the <u>serpin</u> peptidase inhibitor <u>A1</u> (also called α_1-antitrypsin). In this missense mutation, methionine 358 is replaced with arginine (i.e., the **Pittsburgh variant**), which destroys the affinity for elastase. This results in **pulmonary emphysema** because tissue-destructive elastase is allowed to act in an uncontrolled manner in the lung.

U. Maintenance of blood lipid levels by fatty acid uptake, fatty acid esterification to triglycerides in the sER, and combination of triacylglycerides with protein in the Golgi to form **lipoproteins**, which include:

1. **VLDL (very low-density lipoprotein)** is rich in triacylglycerides and travels to adipose tissue and skeletal muscle where the triacylglycerides are hydrolyzed by lipoprotein lipase to fatty acids.

2. **LDL (low-density lipoprotein)** is rich in cholesterol and distributes cholesterol to cells throughout the body that have specific LDL receptors. LDL is called "**bad cholesterol**" and is the target in lipid-lowering therapy.

3. **HDL (high-density lipoprotein)** plays a role in the hydrolysis of triacylglycerides in chylomicrons and VLDL by providing **apoprotein C** for the activation of lipoprotein lipase. HDL facilitates the flow of excess plasma triacylglycerides and cholesterol back to the liver; hence, HDL is called "**good cholesterol.**" The enzyme **lecithin-cholesterol acyl transferase (LCAT)** is associated with HDL and converts cholesterol → cholesterol ester (i.e., cholesterol + a fatty acid).

II **Kupffer Cells** are **macrophages** derived from circulating monocytes that are found in the liver sinusoids. These cells secrete proinflammatory cytokines: **tumor necrosis factor-α** (TNF-α; causes a slowdown in bile flow called cholestasis), **interleukin-6** (causes synthesis of acute-phase proteins by hepatocytes), and **transforming growth factor-β** (TGF-β; causes synthesis of type I collagen by hepatic stellate cells).

III **Hepatic Stellate Cells (Fat-Storing Cells; ITO Cells)** are found in the perisinusoidal space (space of Disse). These cells contain **fat**, **store and metabolize vitamin A**, and secrete **type I collagen**. In liver cirrhosis, increased deposition of type I collagen (along with laminin and proteoglycans) in the perisinusoidal space narrows the diameter of the sinusoid, causing **portal hypertension.**

IV **Classic Liver Lobule (Figure 18–1).** The classic liver lobule is roughly hexagon shaped with a **central vein** at its center and six **portal triads** at its periphery. A portal triad consists of:

A. **HEPATIC ARTERIOLE.** The hepatic arterioles (terminal branches of the **right and left hepatic arteries**) carry oxygen-rich blood and contribute 20% of the blood within the liver sinusoids. The blood flows from the periphery to the center of the lobule (i.e., **centripetal flow**).

B. **PORTAL VENULE.** The portal venules (terminal branches of the **portal vein**) carry nutrient-rich blood and contribute 80% of the blood within the liver sinusoids. The blood flows from the periphery to the center of the lobule (i.e., **centripetal flow**).

C. **BILE DUCTULE.** Bile follows this route: bile canaliculi → cholangioles → canals of Hering → bile ductules in the portal triad → right and left hepatic ducts → common hepatic duct → common bile duct. Bile flows from the center of the lobule to the periphery (i.e., **centrifugal flow**). **Cholestasis** is a general term that defines the:

1. Impaired production of bile at the level of the hepatocyte, called **intrahepatic cholestasis**

2. Impaired excretion of bile due to a blockage (e.g., tumor of pancreas or presence of gallstones [**cholelithiasis**]), called **extrahepatic cholestasis**

D. LYMPHATIC VESSEL. Lymph follows this route: space of Disse → lymphatic vessels in the portal triad → lymphatic vessels that parallel the portal vein → thoracic duct. Lymph flows from the center of the lobule to the periphery of a liver lobule (i.e., **centrifugal flow**).

Ⓥ Liver Acinus (Figure 18-1). The liver acinus is divided into **zone 1**, **zone 2**, and **zone 3** based on the location of hepatocytes to incoming blood. Hepatocytes within each zone have specific characteristics as indicated in the table in Figure 18-1.

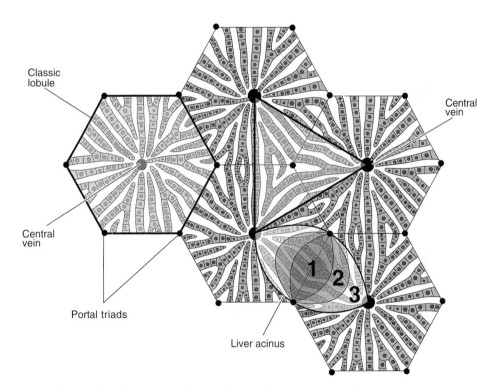

VARIOUS TYPES OF LIVER DAMAGE DUE TO DRUGS/CHEMICALS

Morphologic Appearance	Drug/Chemical
Acute Hepatitis	Isoniazid (10%–20% liver damage; acetyl hydrazine is the active metabolite); salicylate, halothane (symptoms occur after 1 week, fever precedes jaundice, and metabolites form via action of P_{450} system); methyldopa (positive Coombs test), phenytoin, and ketoconazole
Chronic Active Hepatitis	Methyldopa, acetaminophen (Tylenol), aspirin, isoniazid, nitrofurantoin, and halothane

● **Figure 18-1 Diagram of a classic liver lobule and liver acinus.** The classic liver lobule contains a central vein at its center with six portal triads at the periphery. The liver acinus defines three zones (zones 1, 2, and 3) based on the location of hepatocytes to incoming blood. Hepatocytes in zone 1 are nearest the incoming blood, hepatocytes in zone 2 are intermediate, and hepatocytes in zone 3 are farthest from the incoming blood. (*continued*)

VARIOUS TYPES OF LIVER DAMAGE DUE TO DRUGS/CHEMICALS

Morphologic Appearance	Drug/Chemical
Zonal Necrosis	**Zone 1:** Undergo necrosis in poisoning due to yellow phosphorus, manganese, ferrous sulphate, allyl alcohol, and endotoxin of *Proteus vulgaris* Undergo necrosis due to **chronic hepatitis**, primary biliary cirrhosis, bile duct occlusion, and preeclampsia/eclampsia (Note: Hepatic disease is very common in preeclamptic women and monitoring of platelet count and serum liver enzymes is standard practice.) Are exposed to blood high in nutrients and oxygen; synthesize glycogen and plasma proteins actively **Zone 2:** Undergo necrosis due to **yellow fever** Are exposed to blood intermediate in nutrients and oxygen **Zone 3:** Undergo necrosis due to **ischemic injury**, **right-sided cardiac failure**, and bone marrow transplantation Undergo necrosis in poisoning due to **carbon tetrachloride**, chloroform, L-amanitin, pyrrolizidine alkaloids (bush tea), tannic acid, copper, **acetaminophen** (free radicals formed; acetylcysteine therapy replaces glutathione to neutralize free radicals)
Intrahepatic Cholestasis	**Noninflammatory:** oral contraceptives and anabolic steroids **Inflammatory:** erythromycin estolate, amoxicillin-clavulanic acid, chlorpromazine, and thiazides
Fatty Change	**Single droplet:** ethanol, corticosteroids, amiodarone (looks like alcoholic hepatitis) **Microvesicular:** tetracycline, valproic acid
Fibrosis	Methotrexate, hypervitaminosis A
Vascular Lesions	**Budd-Chiari syndrome:** oral contraceptives **Peliosis hepatis:** oral contraceptives, anabolic steroids **Angiosarcoma:** vinyl chloride, arsenic, Thorotrast
Tumors	**Nodular hyperplasia:** azathioprine, anticancer agents **Benign tumors:** oral contraceptives **Malignant tumors:** oral contraceptives
Granulomatous Hepatitis	Allopurinol, hydralazine, sulfonamides, phenylbutazone

● **Figure 18-1** *Continued*

VI **Repair (Regeneration).** Hepatocytes are a relatively stable cell population under normal circumstances (i.e., not under continual renewal). Upon partial surgical removal or damage by toxic substances, hepatocytes demonstrate a high rate of mitosis.

VII **Clinical Considerations**

A. **VIRAL HEPATITIS** is a term used to describe infection of the liver by a group of viruses that have a particular affinity for the liver, which include the following.

 1. **Hepatitis A virus (HAV).** HAV belonging to the Picornaviridae virus family is a **nonsegmented, single-stranded, positive sense RNA (ss+RNA) virus**. HAV infection is commonly called "**infectious hepatitis**." HAV never pursues a chronic course and has **no carrier state**, and infection provides lifelong immunity. HAV is transmitted by the fecal–oral route because HAV is released into the stool in high concentrations. **Clinical features include:** acute, self-limiting disease; fatigue; malaise; nausea; vomiting; anorexia; fever; right upper quadrant pain; dark urine;

acholic stools (light-colored stools lacking bilirubin pigment); jaundice; pruritus; and marked elevation of serum alanine aminotransferase (ALT) and serum aspartate aminotransferase (AST). HAV IgM is the first detectable antibody in the serum and is the gold standard for acute illness detection; HAV IgG is detectable in the serum during the early convalescent period and remains detectable for decades. The incubation period is 2 to 6 weeks, and there is no predominant season of infection.

2. **Hepatitis B virus (HBV).** HBV belonging to the Hepadnavirus family is a **small, circular, partially double-stranded DNA virus.** HBV infection is commonly called **"serum hepatitis."** Humans are the only significant reservoir for HBV. HBV is transmitted through **blood** (e.g., accidental needle sticks, intravenous drug users who share needles, tattooing, etc.), from **mother to baby,** or **sexually.** HBV infection results in two major clinical syndromes called **acute hepatitis B** and **chronic hepatitis B.** Acute hepatitis B is an acute, self-limiting disease (similar to hepatitis A) in which complete recovery and lifelong immunity generally occur. Acute hepatitis B may progress to fulminant hepatitis, which can be fatal in 7 to 10 days. Chronic hepatitis B is the presence of necrosis and inflammation in the liver along with the persistence of HBsAg in the serum for longer than 6 months. **Clinical features of chronic hepatitis B include:** the following: many patients are asymptomatic (unless they progress to cirrhosis or extrahepatic manifestations); some patients experience nonspecific symptoms like fatigue; extrahepatic manifestations are caused by circulating immune complexes and include polyarteritis nodosa and a membranous nephropathy; a **carrier state** may result; a **chronic persistent** type demonstrates minimal necrosis and is associated with a favorable outcome; and a **chronic active** type demonstrates piecemeal necrosis and bridging necrosis, which can lead to cirrhosis and/or hepatocellular carcinoma.

3. **Hepatitis C virus (HCV).** HCV virus belonging to the **Flaviviridae virus family** is a **nonsegmented, single-stranded, positive sense RNA (ss+RNA) virus.** HCV is a global health problem with more than 170 million carriers. HCV is the most common indication for liver transplantation and accounts for 50% of patients on the waiting list. HCV is transmitted through **blood** (e.g., accidental needle sticks, intravenous drug users who share needles, tattooing, etc.), from **mother to baby,** or **sexually.** HCV infection results in two major clinical syndromes called **acute hepatitis C** and **chronic hepatitis C.** Acute hepatitis C is an acute, self-limiting disease and rarely progresses to fulminant hepatitis. Chronic hepatitis C occurs very frequently after acute hepatitis C infection ($\approx$50% to 70% of cases). Chronic hepatitis C often progresses to chronic active hepatitis within 10 to 15 years, cirrhosis (20% of chronic cases), and liver failure (20% of chronic cases). **Clinical features of chronic hepatitis C include:** malaise; nausea; anorexia; myalgia; arthralgia; weakness; weight loss; and extrahepatic manifestations including essential mixed cryoglobulinemia, membranoproliferative glomerulonephritis, type 1 diabetes, non-Hodgkin lymphoma, porphyria cutanea tarda, lichen planus, arthralgia, and sicca syndrome; also, a **carrier state** may result.

B. **PRIMARY BILIARY CIRRHOSIS** is caused by a granulomatous destruction of medium-sized **intrahepatic bile ducts** with cirrhosis appearing late in the course of the disease. It is characterized by **mitochondrial pyruvate dehydrogenase autoantibodies,** the role of which is not clear.

C. **PRIMARY SCLEROSING CHOLANGITIS** is caused by inflammation, fibrosis, and segmental dilatation of both **intrahepatic and extrahepatic bile ducts.** It is characterized by **antineutrophil cytoplasmic autoantibodies.** It is frequently seen in association with chronic **ulcerative colitis** of the bowel.

Ⅷ Selected Photomicrographs

A. Electron micrographs of hepatocytes, Kupffer cell, space of Disse, and bile canaliculus and light micrograph of portal triad (Figure 18-2)

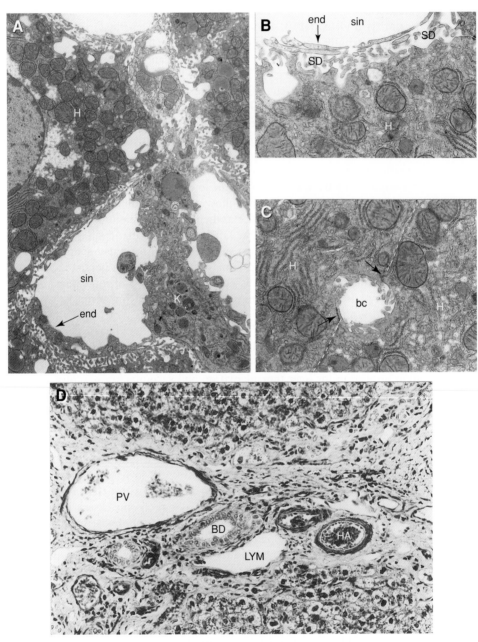

● **Figure 18-2 General features of the liver. A–C:** Electron micrograph of the liver. **A:** A Kupffer cell (K) is shown within the lumen of a hepatic sinusoid (sin). The sinusoid is lined by a discontinuous endothelium (endo). H, hepatocyte. **B:** The basolateral border of a hepatocyte (H) is shown projecting microvilli into the space of Disse (SD). The space of Disse is separated from the hepatic sinusoid (sin) by a discontinuous endothelium (endo). **C:** Two adjacent hepatocytes (H) are shown abutting each other (*dotted lines*) to form a bile canaliculus (bc) that is bounded by tight junctions (*arrows*) that serve to contain the bile. **D:** Light micrograph of the liver showing the components of a portal tract: hepatic arteriole (HA), portal venule (PV), bile ductule (BD), and a lymphatic vessel (LYM).

B. Light micrograph of normal liver and alcoholic liver cirrhosis (Figure 18-3)

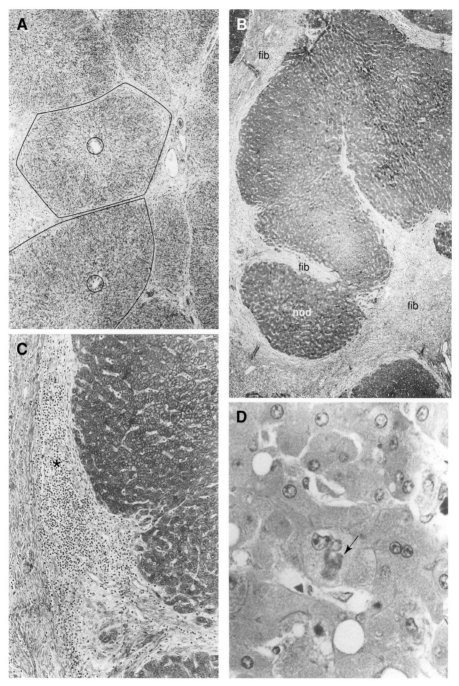

● **Figure 18-3 Normal liver and liver cirrhosis. A:** Light micrograph (LM) of normal liver. The classic liver lobules (*outlined*) with central vein (*circle*) are clearly dealinated. **B–D:** LM of alcoholic liver cirrhosis. **B:** Broad bands of fibrous septae (fib) are present in alcoholic liver cirrhosis that bridge regions of the liver from central vein to portal triad and from portal triad to portal triad. This fibrotic activity will entrap sections of hepatic parenchyma that undergo regeneration to form nodules (nod). **C:** Neutrophil, lymphocyte, and macrophage infiltration (*) is prominent at the periphery of the liver lobule. **D:** Some hepatocytes accumulate tangled masses of cytokeratin intermediate filaments within the cytoplasm known as **Mallory bodies** (*arrow*). Alcoholism results in a **fatty liver, steatohepatitis** (fatty liver plus inflammation), **cirrhosis** (collagen proliferation and fibrosis), and **hepatocellular carcinoma.**

C. Light micrograph of normal gallbladder and cholecystitis (Figure 18-4)

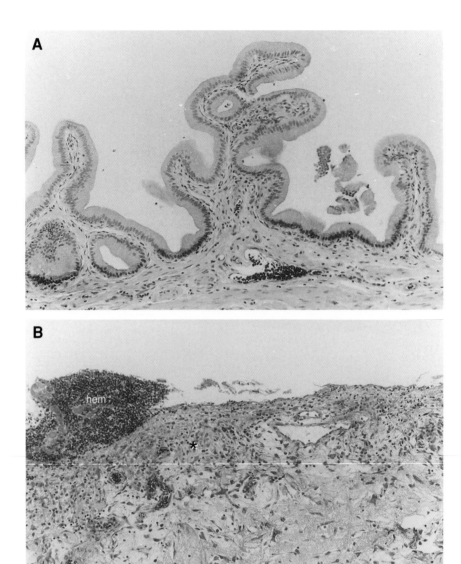

● **Figure 18-4 Normal gallbladder and cholecystitis. A:** Light micrograph (LM) of normal gallbladder. The main function of the gallbladder is storage, concentration, and release of bile. The gallbladder consists of a mucosa, muscularis externa, and adventitia. There is no submucosa in the gallbladder. Numerous mucosal folds lined by a simple columnar epithelium are shown that project into the lumen of the gallbladder. These mucosal folds flatten out as the gallbladder is distended. At times, the mucosa may penetrate deep into the muscularis externa to form **Rokitansky-Aschoff sinuses,** which are early indicators of pathologic changes within the mucosa. **B:** LM of cholecystitis (inflammation of the gallbladder). Acute or chronic cholecystitis is generally associated with the presence of gallstones. In this case, the mucosal epithelium is completely obliterated, and there is focal hemorrhage (hem) and lymphocyte infiltration (*) of the lamina propria.

Chapter 19

Exocrine Pancreas and Islets of Langerhans

I. Exocrine Pancreas

A. The functional unit of the exocrine pancreas is the pancreatic **acinus**, which consists of **acinar cells** that contain rough endoplasmic reticulum (rER), Golgi, and zymogen granules. Acinar cells secrete digestive enzymes, which include **trypsinogen, chymotrypsinogen, procarboxypeptidase, lipase, amylase, elastase, ribonuclease, deoxyribonuclease, cholesterol esterase**, and **phospholipase**. The secretion of digestive enzymes is stimulated by cholecystokinin (CCK) released by I cells of the small intestine.

B. The exocrine pancreas also contains a **network of ducts**: centroacinar cells of the intercalated duct → intralobular duct → interlobular duct → main pancreatic duct (duct of Wirsung) → joins the common bile duct at the hepatoduodenal ampulla (ampulla of Vater) → duodenum. The duct network delivers digestive enzymes to the duodenum and secretes HCO_3^-. Secretion of HCO_3^- by the intercalated and intralobular ducts is stimulated by secretin (SEC) released by S cells of the small intestine.

C. CLINICAL CONSIDERATION. Pancreatitis is the inflammation of the pancreas that is almost always associated with acinar cell injury. **Chronic pancreatitis** is the relapsing inflammation of the pancreas causing pain and eventually irreversible damage in which **pancreatic calcifications** (pathognomonic) are frequently diagnosed by imaging procedures. **Acute pancreatitis** is an acute condition associated with abdominal pain and raised levels of pancreatic enzymes in the blood and urine (Figure 19-1). Increased levels of amylase in the pleural fluid are pathognomonic of acute pancreatitis. About 80% of acute pancreatitis cases are associated with **biliary tract disease** or **alcoholism**. Its most severe form is known as **acute hemorrhagic pancreatitis**. The ultimate pathologic process is the destructive effect of pancreatic enzymes released from damaged acinar cells, resulting in the **autodigestion** of the pancreas.

II. Endocrine Pancreas (Figure 19-1).
The endocrine pancreas makes up only 2% of the entire pancreas and consists of the **islets of Langerhans** that are scattered throughout the pancreas. The islets of Langerhans consist mainly of the following cell types:

A. ALPHA (α) CELLS (20% of the islet) secrete **glucagon** (29 amino acids) in response to hypoglycemia, which will elevate blood glucose, free fatty acid, and ketone levels. Glucagon binds to the **glucagon receptor**, which is a G protein–linked receptor present on hepatocytes and adipocytes. Glucagon is derived from a large precursor protein called **preproglucagon** encoded by the *GCG* gene on chromosome 2q36. About 30% to 40% of glucagon within the blood is derived from α cells; the remainder is derived from cells within the gastrointestinal tract called **enteroglucagon**.

B. BETA (β) CELLS (75% of the islet) secrete **insulin** (51 amino acids consisting of **chain A** [21 amino acids] and **chain B** [30 amino acids] held together by **disulfide bonds**) in

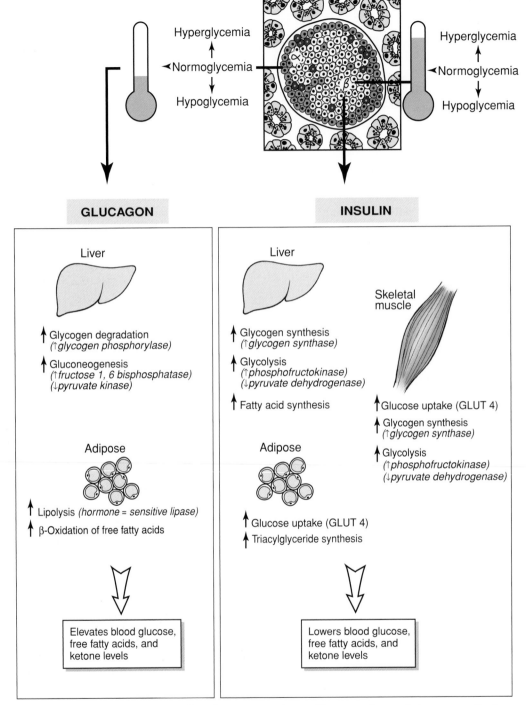

● **Figure 19-1 Effect of glucagon and insulin on target tissues.** The target tissues of glucagon are the liver and adipose. The target tissues of insulin are liver, adipose, and skeletal muscle. The main biochemical pathways and enzyme (*in parentheses*) that are affected by glucagon and insulin are indicated. The alpha (α) cells (*shaded*), beta (β) cells (*white*), and delta (δ) cells (*black*) are shown with the islet of Langerhans.

response to hyperglycemia, which will lower blood glucose, free fatty acid, and ketone levels. Insulin binds to the **insulin receptor**, which is a **receptor tyrosine kinase** present on hepatocytes, skeletal muscle cells, and adipocytes. Insulin is derived from a large precursor protein called **preproinsulin** encoded by the *INS* gene on chromosome 11p15. Preproinsulin is converted to proinsulin by removal of the **signal sequence** in the rER. **Proinsulin** (86 amino acids; consists of the **C-peptide** connecting chain A and chain B together) is transferred to the Golgi where it is packaged into secretory granules. Within secretory granules, proinsulin is cleaved by a protease to release the C peptide (35 amino acids) from insulin. Insulin secretion is triggered when glucose enters the β cell via **glucose transporter 2 (GLUT2)**. The β cell possesses K^+/adenosine triphosphate (ATP) ion channels (which consist of **Kir6.2** and **SUR1** subunits) and **voltage-gated Ca^{2+} ion channels**, both of which are involved in insulin secretion.

C. **DELTA (δ) CELLS** (5% of the islet) secrete **somatostatin** (14 amino acids), which inhibits hormone secretion from nearby cells in a paracrine manner. Somatostatin binds to the **somatostatin receptor**, which is a **G protein–linked receptor**.

Clinical Considerations

A. **TYPE 1 DIABETES (POLYGENIC)**

1. **Characteristics.** Type 1 diabetes is marked by **autoantibodies** and an **insulitis reaction** that results in the **destruction of pancreatic β cells**. Clinical features include: hyperglycemia, ketoacidosis, and exogenous insulin dependence. Long-term clinical effects include neuropathy, retinopathy leading to blindness, and nephropathy leading to kidney failure.

2. **Genetic studies.** Type 1 diabetes is a **multifactorial inherited disease**, which means that many genes that have a small, equal, and additive effect (genetic component) and an environmental component are involved. If one considers only the genetic component of a multifactorial disease, the term **polygenic** is used. Type 1 diabetes shows an association with HLA (human leukocyte antigen complex) loci named **HLA-DR3** and **HLA-DR4** located on chromosome 6p. It is hypothesized that genes closely linked to HLA-DR3 and HLA-DR4 loci somehow alter the immune response such that the individual has an immune response to an environmental antigen (e.g., virus). The immune response "spills over" and leads to the destruction of pancreatic β cells, whereby **glutamic acid decarboxylase (GAD$_{65}$)**, insulin, and tyrosine phosphatases **IA-2 and IA-2β** autoantibodies may play a role. The insulitis reaction is characterized mainly by infiltration of islets by **CD8$^+$ T lymphocytes**.

B. **TYPE 2 DIABETES (POLYGENIC)**

1. **Characteristics.** Type 2 diabetes is marked by **insulin resistance of peripheral tissues** and **abnormal β-cell function**. It is often detected during routine screening by detection of hyperglycemia or by patient complaints of polyuria. Before the onset of frank symptoms, individuals pass through phases, which include (a) hyperinsulinemia is present and euglycemia is maintained, (b) hyperinsulinemia is present but postprandial hyperglycemia is observed, or (c) insulin secretion declines in the face of persistent insulin resistance of peripheral tissues.

2. **Genetic studies.** Type 2 diabetes is a **multifactorial inherited disease**. At this time, genetic studies show no association with a major susceptibility gene. Instead, type 2 diabetes may involve multiple genes that convey limited degrees of susceptibility.

C. **PHARMACOLOGY OF DIABETES.** Oral hypoglycemics are used to treat type 2 diabetes.

1. **Tolbutamide (Orinase), Acetohexamide (Dymelor), Tolazamide (Tolinase), Chlorpropamide (Diabinese), Glyburide (Micronase), and Glipizide (Glucotrol)** are sulfonylurea derivatives that **block K^+/ATP ion channels** (by binding to the SUR1 subunit). The resulting depolarization **activates voltage-gated Ca^{2+} ion channels**, which allows an influx of Ca^{2+}. Ca^{2+} mediates the fusion of insulin secretory granules with the cell membrane, triggering insulin secretion. The second-generation sulfonylureas (glyburide and glipizide) are more potent that their first-generation counterparts.

2. **Metformin (Glucophage)** is an oral antidiabetic drug used in the treatment of type 2 diabetes, particularly in obese patients. Metformin is a biguanide that reduces hyperglycemia primarily by **suppression of hepatic gluconeogenesis** through the **activation of adenosine monophosphate (AMP)-activated protein kinase (AMPK)**.

3. **Acarbose and Miglitol** are α-glucosidase inhibitors that slow down carbohydrate absorption from the intestine.

4. **Byetta** (which is a glucagonlike peptide 1 [GLP-1]) increases insulin secretion in both normal physiology and type 2 diabetes. Byetta is the first in a new class of drugs called **incretin mimetics** for the treatment of type 2 diabetes. **Incretins** are gut peptides that stimulate insulin secretion. Incretin mimetics are drugs that mimic the insulin stimulatory activity of the two gut peptides, gastric inhibitory peptide (GIP) and GLP-1. Incretins are quickly inactivated by **dipeptidyl peptidase-4 (DPP-4)**.

5. **Januvia and Galvus** inhibit the enzyme DPP-4, which quickly inactivates both GIP and GLP-1.

D. ISLET CELL TUMORS

1. **Insulinoma.** An insulinoma (most common islet cell tumor) is a benign tumor consisting of islet β cells and is generally associated with the multiple endocrine neoplasia type 1 (MEN 1) syndrome. An insulinoma secretes **excess insulin and C peptide**, thereby producing a fasting hypoglycemia. Clinical findings include neuroglycopenia (brain without glucose), hypoglycemia, increased serum insulin levels, and increased serum C-peptide levels. The differential diagnosis is **factitious hypoglycemia** caused by surreptitious insulin injections. In factitious hypoglycemia, there are hypoglycemia and increased serum insulin levels, but decreased serum C-peptide levels due to the suppression of endogenous insulin secretion by hypoglycemia.

2. **Glucagonoma.** A glucagonoma is a malignant tumor consisting of islet α cells. A glucagonoma secretes **excess glucagon**, thereby producing a fasting hyperglycemia (i.e., diabetes). Clinical findings include a characteristic rash called **necrolytic migratory erythema**.

3. **Somatostatinoma.** A somatostatinoma is a malignant tumor consisting of islet δ cells. A somatostatinoma secretes **excess somatostatin**. Clinical findings include achlorhydria (lack of HCl production due to the inhibition of gastrin by somatostatin), cholelithiasis (formation of gallstones due to the inhibition of CCK by somatostatin), diabetes (increased blood glucose levels due to inhibition of GIP by somatostatin), and steatorrhea (excessive amount of fat in the feces due to inhibition of secretin and CCK by somatostatin).

Ⅳ Selected Photomicrographs

A. Normal exocrine pancreas and pancreatitis (Figure 19-2)

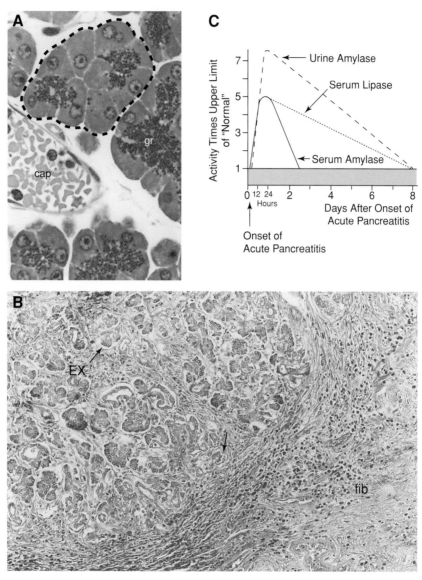

● **Figure 19-2 Normal pancreas and pancreatitis. A:** Light micrograph (LM) of normal exocrine pancreas. Acinar cells containing numerous granules (gr) are arranged in an acinus (*dotted lines*). A small capillary (cap) can be observed. **B:** LM of pancreatitis. A large area of exocrine pancreas (ex) is shown surrounded by thick fibrous bands (fib) that are highly infiltrated with lymphocytes (inflammatory response). Acinar cells undergoing autolysis are shown (*arrows*). **C:** Enzyme panel following acute pancreatitis.

B. A normal islet of Langerhans and an islet of Langerhans in type 1 diabetes and type 2 diabetes (Figure 19-3)

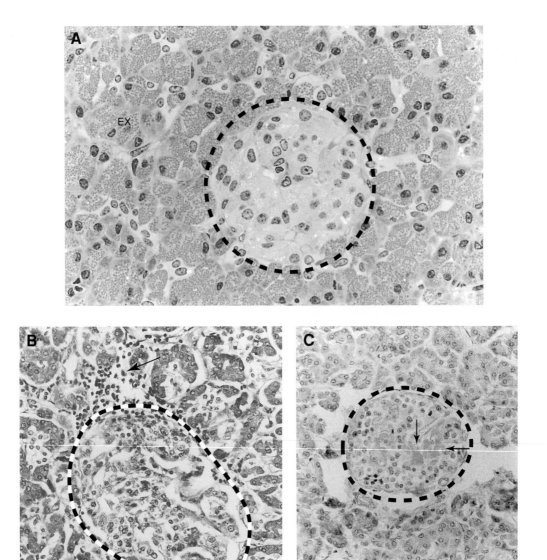

● **Figure 19-3 A:** Light micrograph (LM) of a normal islet of Langerhans. A normal islet of Langerhans (*dotted circle*) is shown surrounded by exocrine pancreas (ex). **B:** LM of an islet of Langerhans in type 1 diabetes. The islet (*dotted circle*) is shown with conspicuous lymphocytic infiltration (insulitis reaction; *arrow*) that probably leads to the destruction of the β cells within the islet. **C:** LM of an islet of Langerhans in type 2 diabetes. The islet (*dotted circle*) is shown with conspicuous amyloid deposition (*arrows*).

Case Study 19-1

A father brings his 10-year-old daughter into your office complaining that "she is always thirsty and drinks a heck of a lot of water." He also tells you that "she doesn't want to eat or drink today because she says she feels sick to her stomach and is vomiting. But, she is still urinating a lot." After some discussion, he informs you his daughter had a high fever about 2 weeks ago and he took her to the emergency room. The father is obviously concerned about his daughter but you sense a deeper level of worry and you ask him about it. He tells you, "Doc, I lost my wife last year because of kidney failure and I am afraid my daughter has the same thing. I can't lose my daughter, too. She is all I got left." What is the most likely diagnosis?

Differentials

- Gastroenteritis, hypoglycemic coma, metabolic acidosis, nonketotic hyperglycemic hyperosmolar coma (NHHK)

Relevant Physical Examination Findings

- Breathing is rapid and deep (Kussmaul respirations)
- Sweet smell on her breath
- Dry skin and oral mucosa

Relevant Lab Findings

- Blood chemistry: glucose = 490 mg/dL (high); ketone bodies = high; Na^+ = 128 mEq/L (low); K^+ = 6.2 mEq/L (high); HCO_3^- = 9.8 mEq/L (low); pH = 7.1 (low); anion gap 22 (high); osmolarity = 330 mOsm/kg (high); blood urea nitrogen (BUN) = 25 mg/dL (high); creatinine = 1.0 mg/dL (normal); lactate = normal
- Urinalysis: ketones = >80 (high); glucose = >1000 mg/dL (high)

Diagnosis: Diabetic Ketoacidosis

- **Diabetic Ketoacidosis (DKA).** DKA occurs secondary to infection or lack of insulin therapy in type 1 diabetics (who lack endogenous circulating insulin). Therefore, the metabolic breakdown of fat stores in adipose tissue into fatty acids causes an increase in ketone body formation. Note: One of the functions of insulin is to inhibit the metabolic breakdown of fat stores in adipose tissue into fatty acids. The lack of insulin in type 1 diabetics also results in a rise of counterregulatory hormones (e.g., glucagon, epinephrine, cortisol, and growth hormone), which causes increased glycogen breakdown, increased gluconeogenesis in the liver, inhibition of glycolysis, and decreased peripheral utilization of glucose, all of which lead to hyperglycemia. The increased levels of glucose and ketone bodies in the glomerular filtrate (due to exceeding the transport maximum [T_M]) results in an osmotic diuresis, which provokes hypovolemia, dehydration, and loss of electrolytes in the urine. The dehydration activates the renin-angiotensin system, which causes the release of aldosterone. Aldosterone acts on the principal cells of the cortical collecting duct and causes increased K^+ secretion (plasma → tubular fluid), and thereby increases K^+ excretion in the urine. The hyperkalemia results from the movement of K^+ out of the cells in exchange for H^+ that is prevalent in the serum due to the metabolic acidosis. Metabolic acidosis causes Kussmaul respirations in response to a ↓ serum pH. The elevated anion gap acidosis results from the production of excess organic acids (e.g., ketone bodies) and the body's inability to neutralize the excess acid.
- Gastroenteritis is a viral or bacterial infection of the stomach or small bowel. Clinical findings of gastroenteritis include a profuse vomiting that results in a metabolic alkalosis (i.e., loss of H^+ and Cl^- from the stomach).
- Hypoglycemic Coma. Clinical findings of hypoglycemic coma include low blood glucose levels, pallor, sweating, hunger, tremors, and increased heart rate due to increased levels of epinephrine.

- Metabolic acidosis ($\downarrow$ serum pH and HCO_3^- levels) has several causes beside DKA. A normal gap metabolic acidosis may be caused by diarrhea, renal tubular acidosis, and acetazolamide overdose. An elevated gap metabolic acidosis may be caused by chronic renal failure, uremia, lactic acidosis, DKA, salicylate overdose, methanol ingestion, and ethylene glycol ingestion. The normal creatinine levels rule out chronic renal failure. The normal lactate levels rule out lactic acidosis.
- NHHK is a condition that occurs in older adults with type 2 diabetes and may be caused by infection, increased glucose consumption, or a cerebrovascular accident. Clinical findings of NHHK include hyperosmolarity without ketosis. The elevated ketone bodies in the blood and urine rule out NHHK.

Chapter 20

Respiratory System

I **General Features (Figure 20-1).** The respiratory system is divided into a **conduction portion** and **respiratory portion**. The conduction portion **only conducts air into the lung**; no blood–air gas exchange occurs. Airflow through the conduction portion follows this route: **nasal cavities → nasopharynx → oropharynx → larynx → trachea → bronchi → bronchioles → terminal bronchioles**. The respiratory portion is where **blood–air gas exchange occurs**. Airflow through the respiratory portion follows this route: **respiratory bronchioles → alveolar ducts → alveoli**. The larger airways of the conduction portion (i.e., trachea and bronchi) are organized into a **mucosa (epithelium and lamina propria)**, **muscular layer**, **submucosa**, and **adventitia**. As the airways get progressively smaller down to the alveoli, the components of the wall change significantly and this organization is lost.

II **Trachea**

A. MUCOSA. The epithelium is a **respiratory epithelium** that is classically described as a **ciliated pseudostratified epithelium with goblet cells**, which contains the following cell types. **Ciliated cells** ($\cong$30%) beat toward the pharynx, thereby moving mucus and/or particulate matter to the mouth where it can be swallowed or expectorated. **Goblet cells** ($\cong$30%) secrete mucus. **Brush cells** contain microvilli and have been interpreted as either an intermediate stage in the differentiation to ciliated cells or as a sensory cell since it may be found in association with nerve terminals. **Endocrine cells (Kulchitsky cells)** secrete peptide hormones and catecholamines. **Basal cells** ($\cong$30%) have mitotic capacity and are thereby functioning as stem cells to regenerate the epithelium. The lamina propria consists of **collagen and elastic fibers**.

B. MUSCULAR LAYER. The muscular layer consists of smooth muscle that spans the dorsal ends of the cartilage rings called the **trachealis muscle**.

C. SUBMUCOSA. The submucosa consists of **seromucous glands** surrounded by **collagen and elastic fibers**.

D. ADVENTITIA. The adventitia consists of **C-shaped hyaline cartilage rings** surrounded by **collagen and elastic fibers**.

III **Bronchi**

A. MUCOSA. The epithelium is a **respiratory epithelium** as described previously. The lamina propria consists of **collagen and elastic fibers**.

B. MUSCULAR LAYER. The muscular layer consists of a **prominent circular layer of smooth muscle**.

C. SUBMUCOSA. The submucosa consists of **seromucous glands** surrounded by **collagen and elastic fibers**.

D. ADVENTITIA. The adventitia consists of **irregular hyaline cartilage plates** surrounded by **collagen and elastic fibers**.

IV Bronchioles

A. MUCOSA. The epithelium is a **simple ciliated columnar epithelium** with goblet cells and **Clara cells**. The lamina propria consists of **collagen and elastic fibers**. Clara cells **secrete a component of surfactant**; secrete Clara cell protein (CC16), which is used as a marker of pulmonary function in bronchopulmonary lavage fluid and serum; **metabolize airborne toxins** using cytochrome P_{450}; and **release Cl^- into the lumen** via a Cl^- ion channel regulated by the cyclic guanosine monophosphate (cGMP)-guanylate cyclase mechanism. Clara cells are nonciliated, have a dome-shaped protrusion extending into the lumen, and have the ultrastructural characteristics of a protein-secreting cell (rough endoplasmic reticulum [rER], Golgi, secretory granules).

B. MUSCULAR LAYER. The muscular layer consists of a **prominent circular layer of smooth muscle**.

V Terminal Bronchioles

A. MUCOSA. The epithelium is a **simple ciliated cuboidal epithelium** with Clara cells. The lamina propria consists of **collagen and elastic fibers**.

B. MUSCULAR LAYER. The muscular layer consists of a **reduced, incomplete circular layer of smooth muscle**.

VI Respiratory Bronchioles

A. MUCOSA. The epithelium is a **simple ciliated cuboidal epithelium** with numerous Clara cells. The lamina propria consists of **collagen and elastic fibers**.

B. MUSCULAR LAYER. The muscular layer consists of a **prominent, incomplete circular layer of smooth muscle**. Note that respiratory bronchioles are distinguished histologically by the presence of alveoli that open into its wall.

VII Alveolar Ducts

A. MUCOSA. The epithelium is a **simple squamous epithelium**. The lamina propria consists of **collagen and elastic fibers**.

B. MUSCULAR LAYER. The muscular layer consists of a **smooth muscle "knobs."**

VIII Alveoli contain the following:

A. TYPE I PNEUMOCYTES are a simple squamous epithelium joined by tight junctions (zonula occludens) that line alveoli and have no mitotic capacity.

B. TYPE II PNEUMOCYTES are cuboidal-shaped cells that are most commonly found at the junction of interalveolar septae and bulge into the air space. These cells secrete **surfactant** (which is stored as **lamellar bodies**) and have mitotic capacity, thereby functioning as stem cells to regenerate the epithelium. Hyperplasia of type II pneumocytes is an important marker of alveolar injury and repair of alveoli.

C. ALVEOLAR MACROPHAGES migrate over the surface of the alveoli and into the interalveolar septae to phagocytose inhaled dust, bacteria, and degraded surfactant.

D. ALVEOLAR PORES (PORES OF KOHN) are found within interalveolar septae and equalize pressure within alveoli. These pores play a significant role in obstructive lung disease by serving as a bypass to aerate alveoli distal to the blockage. The **interalveolar septae** of the alveoli contain **collagen and elastic fibers**.

	Mucosa	Muscular Layer	Submucosa	Adventitia	
	Epithelium and Lamina Propria	Smooth Muscle	Glands	Fibers	Cartilage
Trachea	Respiratory Collagen and elastic fibers	Spans dorsal end of cartilage rings (trachealis muscle)	Seromucous	Collagen and elastic fibers	C-shaped hyaline rings
Bronchi	Respiratory Collagen and elastic fibers	Prominent circular layer	Seromucous	Collagen and elastic fibers	Irregular hyaline plates
Bronchiole	Simple ciliated columnar and Clara cells Collagen and elastic fibers	Prominent circular layer	Absent	Absent	Absent
Terminal bronchiole	Simple ciliated cuboidal and Clara cells Collagen and elastic fibers	Reduced, incomplete circular layer	Absent	Absent	Absent
Respiratory bronchiole	Simple ciliated cuboidal and Clara cells Collagen and elastic fibers	Prominent, discontinuous ring	Absent	Absent	Absent
Alveolar duct	Simple squamous Collagen and elastic fibers	Smooth muscle "knobs"	Absent	Absent	Absent
Alveoli	Type I and type II pneumocytes, alveolar macrophages Collagen and elastic fibers	Absent	Absent	Absent	Absent

A

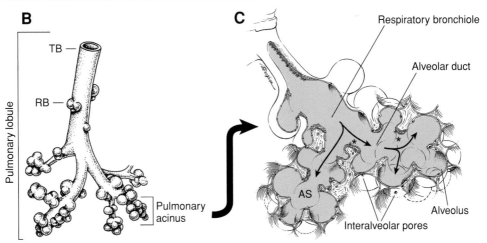

● **Figure 20-1 General features of the lung. A:** Table illustrating changes in the respiratory tree from the trachea to alveoli. In the trachea and bronchi, collagen and elastic fibers span the cartilage rings and plates, and also are found in the lamina propria beneath the epithelium. In the remaining portion of the respiratory tree, collagen and elastic fibers are found in the lamina propria where the elastic fibers are arranged in longitudinal bands. Collagen and elastic fibers (minor component) along with surfactant (major component) contribute to the elastance of the lung (i.e., the collapsing force that develops in the lung as the lung expands). Note that cilia extend farther down the respiratory tree than mucous glands and goblet cells. **B:** Diagram of a pulmonary lobule. A pulmonary lobule consists of a terminal bronchiole (TB), respiratory bronchioles (RB), alveolar ducts, and alveoli. **C:** Diagram of a pulmonary acinus. A pulmonary acinus consists of a respiratory bronchiole, alveolar ducts, and alveoli. Note the smooth muscle arranged in a circular layer in the respiratory bronchiole and as "knobs" (*) in the alveolar duct. The pulmonary lobule–respiratory acinus concept is important pathologically in classifying types of emphysema: (a) centriacinar emphysema involves widening of air spaces within the respiratory bronchioles only at the apex of an acinus, whereas (b) panacinar emphysema involves widening of air spaces distal to the terminal bronchiole involving the entire acinus.

IX **Surfactant** is composed of **cholesterol (50%)**, **dipalmitoylphosphatidylcholine (DPPC; 40%)**, and **surfactant proteins (10%) SP-A, SP-B, and SP-C**. SP-A and SP-B combine with DPPC in the lamellar bodies within type II pneumocytes. SP-B and SP-C stabilize the surfactant coat. Surfactant lines the alveoli and reduces surface tension (attraction), which prevents the collapse of small alveoli (atelectasis), cyanosis, and respiratory distress.

A. Surfactant (major component) contributes to the elastance of the lung. **Elastance** is the collapsing force that develops in the lung as the lung expands. Elastance is described by the **Laplace Law**.

$$E = \frac{2T}{r}$$

where

E = collapsing force (elastance)

T = surface tension

r = radius of the alveolus

B. The Laplace law indicates that:
1. **Large alveoli** have a low collapsing force (elastance) and are easy to keep open.
2. **Small alveoli** have a high collapsing force (elastance) and are difficult to keep open.

X **Blood-Air Barrier.** The components of the blood-air barrier include the **surfactant layer, type I pneumocyte, basement membrane,** and **capillary endothelial cell**. The rate of diffusion across the blood-air barrier is governed by the **Fick Law**. The Fick Law indicates that increases in the thickness of the blood-air barrier will decrease the rate of diffusion of O_2 and CO_2 across the blood-air barrier.

$$RD = \frac{A}{T} \times D \times (P_1 - P_2)$$

where

RD = rate of diffusion

A = surface area of the alveoli

T = thickness of the blood-air barrier

D = solubility of the gas

$P_1 - P_2$ = pressure difference across the blood-air barrier

Note that increases in the thickness of the blood-air barrier will decrease the rate of diffusion of O_2 and CO_2 across the blood-air barrier.

XI **Air Flow** through the lung from the bronchi to alveoli is inversely proportional to airway resistance.

A. AIRWAY RESISTANCE is described by **Poiseuille Law**. The Poiseuille Law indicates that if airway radius is reduced by a factor of 2, then airway resistance is increased by a factor of 16 (2^4). Therefore, air flow will be dramatically reduced.

$$R = \frac{8n\,l}{\pi r^4}$$

where

R = resistance

n = the viscosity of the inspired gas

l = length of the airway

r = radius of the airway

Note the strong relationship of r to R. If airway radius (r) is reduced by a factor of 2, then airway resistance (R) is increased by a factor of 16 (2^4). Therefore, airflow will be dramatically reduced.

B. The **medium-sized bronchi** are the **main site of airway resistance** through the contraction or relaxation of smooth muscle.

1. **Parasympathetic stimulation, leukotrienes (LTC$_4$, LTD$_4$), prostaglandin (PGF$_2\alpha$), and thromboxane (TXA$_2$)** constrict the airways (i.e., reduce r) and thereby increase airway resistance (R). These are bronchoconstrictors.

2. **Sympathetic stimulation, PGE$_2$, and β_2-adrenergic agonists (e.g., terbutaline, albuterol, metaproterenol, salmeterol)** dilate the airways (i.e., increase r) and thereby decrease airway resistance (R). These are bronchodilators.

XII   Clinical Considerations

A. INFANT RESPIRATORY DISTRESS SYNDROME (RDS) is caused by a deficiency of surfactant, which may be due to prolonged intrauterine asphyxia or premature birth or occur in infants of diabetic mothers. **Thyroxine and cortisol treatment** increase production of surfactant. Not only does RDS threaten the infant with immediate asphyxiation, but also repeated gasping inhalations can damage the alveolar lining, leading to **hyaline membrane disease.**

B. BRONCHOGENIC CARCINOMA begins as hyperplasia of respiratory epithelium that lines the bronchi. Types of bronchogenic carcinoma include:

1. **Adenocarcinoma (AD)** is the most common type (35%). The lesions are peripherally located within the lung as they arise from distal airways and alveoli. AD forms well-circumscribed gray-white masses with obvious glandular elements that contain **mucin**. AD is less closely associated with a smoking history than squamous cell carcinoma.

2. **Squamous cell carcinoma (SQ)** is the second most common type (25%). The lesions are centrally located as they arise from larger bronchi. SQ begins as a small, red, granular plaque and progresses to a large intrabronchial mass that may produce **keratin** and secrete **parathyroid hormone–related peptide (PTHrP)**, causing humoral hypercalcemia of malignancy. SQ is closely associated with a **smoking history.**

3. **Small cell carcinoma (SC)** is the least common type (15%). The lesions are centrally located as they arise from larger bronchi. SC forms large, soft, gray-white masses and contains small, oval-shaped cells ("**oat cells**") derived from **Kulchitsky cells** that may produce **adrenocorticotropic hormone (ACTH)** or **antidiuretic hormone (ADH)**, causing Cushing syndrome or syndrome of inappropriate secretion of ADH (SIADH), respectively. SC is associated with a smoking history.

C. CYSTIC FIBROSIS (CF) is an autosomal recessive genetic disorder caused by more than 1000 mutations (almost all are point mutations or small deletions [1 to 84 bp]) in the *CFTR* gene on **chromosome 7q31.2** for the **cystic fibrosis transmembrane conductance regulator**, which functions as a chloride ion (Cl⁻) channel. The Cl⁻ ion channel normally transports Cl⁻ out of the cell and H_2O follows by osmosis. The H_2O maintains the mucus in a wet and less viscous form. CF is most commonly ($\approx$70% of cases in the North American population) caused by a **three base deletion**, which codes for the amino acid **phenylalanine at position 508** (delta F508) such that phenylalanine is missing from CFTR. However, there are a large number of deletions that can cause CF, and parents of an affected child can carry different deletions of the *CFTR* gene. These mutations result in absent/near-absent CFTR synthesis, a block in CFTR regulation, or a destruction of Cl⁻ transport.

D. LUNG INFECTIONS
1. ***Staphylococcus aureus*** produces lung abscesses and is a common secondary infection in rubeola or influenza.
2. ***Chlamydia trachomatis*** produces pneumonia that is contracted as a newborn infant passes through the birth canal.
3. ***Candida albicans*** produces pneumonia that is associated with an indwelling catheter and immunodeficiency states.
4. ***Coxiella burnetii*** is a respiratory pathogen that is commonly found in individuals who have close association with cows, sheep, or goats.
5. ***Histoplasma capsulatum*** is a fungal infection characterized by multiple granulomas with calcification in the lung. It is acquired by inhalation of spores and is the most common systemic fungal in Midwest United States.
6. ***Aspergillus fumigatus*** is a fungal infection that resides in old tuberculous cavities.
7. ***Coccidioides immitis*** ("valley fever") is a fungal infection. It is acquired by inhalation of spores and is most common in the Southwest United States (San Joaquin Valley).
8. ***Pneumocystis carinii*** is an opportunistic fungal infection that is a common initial presentation of acquired immunodeficiency syndrome (AIDS).

E. ALLERGIES, SEASONAL HAYFEVER, RHINITIS, AND URTICARIA can be treated with the following drugs:
1. **Diphenhydramine (Benadryl), Dimenhydrinate (Dramamine), Chlorpheniramine (Chlor-Trimeton), and Meclizine (Antivert)** are first-generation H_1-receptor antagonists that block the effect of histamine released from mast cells on vascular permeability, vasodilation, and smooth muscle contraction of bronchi. The H_1 receptor is a G protein–linked receptor that increases inositol triphosphate (IP_3) and diacylglycerol (DAG) levels.
2. **Loratadine (Claritin), Desloratadine, and Fexofenadine** are second-generation H_1-receptor antagonists. These drugs do not cross the blood-brain barrier and therefore do not have a sedative effect like the first-generation drugs listed previously.

F. EMPHYSEMA
1. **General Features.** Patients are referred to as **"pink puffers"** with the following characteristics: a thin, barrel-shaped chest; increased breathing rate (tachypnea); a mildly decreased PaO_2 (mild hypoxemia); and a mildly decreased or normal $PaCO_2$ (hypocapnia or normocapnia).
2. **Pathology**
   a. **Panacinar emphysema** (related to α_1-antitrypsin deficiency). Pathologic findings include a widening of the air spaces distal to the terminal bronchioles due to destruction of the alveolar walls by enzymes.
   b. **Centriacinar emphysema** (related to **smoking**). Pathologic findings include a widening of the air spaces within the respiratory bronchioles only while the surrounding alveoli remain fairly well preserved.

G. CHRONIC BRONCHITIS (related to smoking)
1. **General Features.** Patients are referred to as **"blue bloaters"** with the following characteristics: a muscular, barrel-shaped chest; severely decreased PaO_2 (severe hypoxemia with cyanosis); increased $PaCO_2$ (hypercapnia), which leads to chronic respiratory acidosis; increased HCO_3^- reabsorption by kidney to buffer the acidemia; right ventricular failure; and systemic edema.

2. **Pathology.** Pathologic findings include an excessive mucus production leading to copious, purulent sputum production; bronchi demonstrating inflammatory cell infiltrates; and hypertrophy of mucous glands (increase in Reid index).

H. ASTHMA (FIGURE 20-2)

1. **General Features.** Asthma is associated with **smooth muscle hyperactivity within bronchi and bronchioles, increased mucus production, and edema of the bronchial wall.**

2. **Pathology.** Pathologic findings include inflammatory cell infiltrates containing numerous **eosinophils** within the bronchial wall, hyperplasia of bronchial smooth muscle cells, hyperplasia of mucous glands, **Curschmann spirals** (formed from shed epithelium), and **Charcot-Leyden crystals** (formed from eosinophil granules) within the mucous plugs.

3. **Pharmacology**

   a. **Terbutaline, Albuterol, Metaproterenol, and Salmeterol** are β_2-adrenergic receptor agonists (i.e., β_2 agonists) that promote bronchodilation. The β_2-adrenergic receptor is a G protein–linked receptor that increases cyclic adenosine monophosphate (cAMP) levels. **In asthma, the FEV_1 (the volume of air that can be expired in 1 second following a maximal inspiration) is reduced. After treatment with a β_2 agonist, the FEV_1 is increased.**

   b. **Atropine and Ipratropium** are muscarinic acetylcholine receptor (mAChR) antagonists that inhibit bronchoconstriction. The mAChR is a G protein–linked receptor that increases IP_3 and DAG levels.

   c. **Cromolyn (NasalCrom)** inhibits the release of histamine from mast cells.

   d. **Beclomethasone, Budesonide, and Triamcinolone** are corticosteroids that have an anti-inflammatory effect by reducing the synthesis of arachidonic acid by phospholipase A_2 and inhibiting the expression of cyclooxygenase II (COX II).

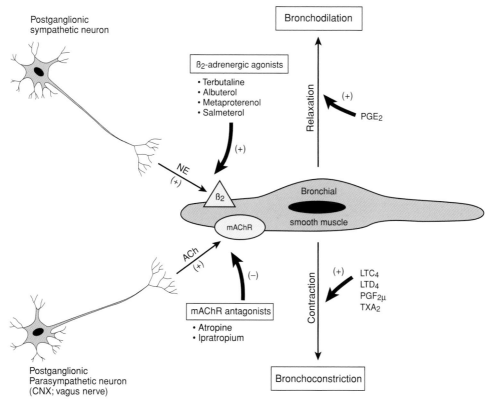

● **Figure 20-2 Control of bronchial smooth muscle.** This diagram shows the various factors that control bronchial smooth muscle relaxation and contraction.

XIII Selected Photomicrographs

A. BLOOD-AIR BARRIER AND TYPE II PNEUMOCYTE (FIGURE 20-3)

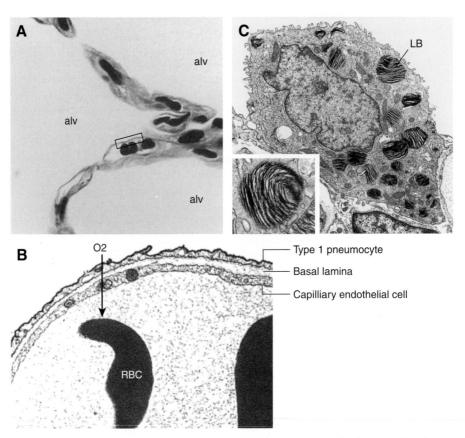

● **Figure 20-3 Blood-air barrier and type II pneumocyte. A:** Light micrograph of an interalveolar septum. The junction of three alveoli (alv) is shown. The area within the box demonstrates the blood-air barrier, which separates the blood (red blood cells within the capillary) and air within the alveolus. **B:** Electron micrograph (EM) of boxed area in A shows the components of the blood-air barrier. The type I pneumocyte borders the air interface, whereas the capillary endothelial cell borders the blood interface. The basal lamina lies between the type 1 pneumocyte and capillary endothelial cell. The surfactant layer covering the type 1 pneumocyte is not shown. Note the histologic layers that O_2 must traverse to get to the red blood cells (RBC). **C:** EM of a type II pneumocyte with lamellar bodies (LB; and *inset*) that contain surfactant.

B. HYALINE MEMBRANE DISEASE, SQUAMOUS CELL CARCINOMA, CYSTIC FIBROSIS (FIGURE 20-4)

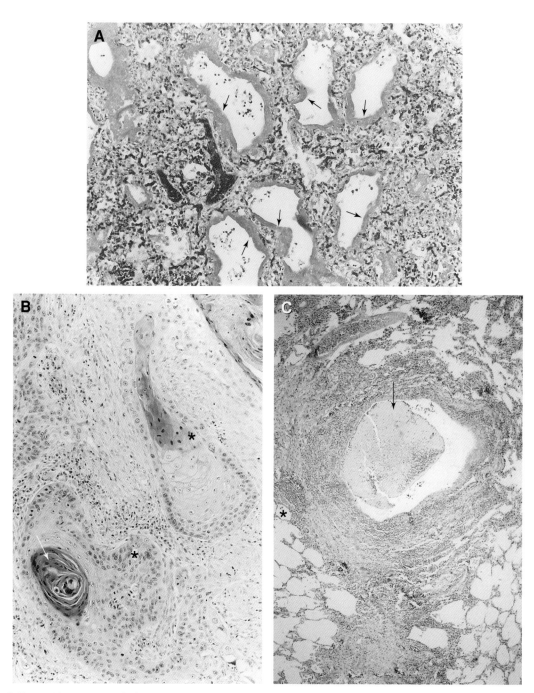

● **Figure 20-4 Lung pathology. A:** Light micrograph (LM) of hyaline membrane disease due to respiratory distress syndrome (i.e., deficiency of surfactant). Note the air-filled bronchioles and alveolar ducts that are widely dilated. They are lined by a homogenous hyaline material consisting of fibrin and necrotic cells. In addition, there is atelectasis and collapse of more distal alveoli is present. **B:** LM of squamous cell carcinoma. Note the irregular nests (*) of squamous cell carcinoma. In some nests, keratinization is present (*arrow*). **C:** LM of cystic fibrosis. A bronchus that is filled with thick mucus and inflammatory cells is shown (*arrow*). Smaller bronchi may be completely plugged by this material. In addition, surrounding the bronchus there is a heavy lymphocyte infiltration (*).

C. LUNG INFECTIONS (FIGURE 20-5)

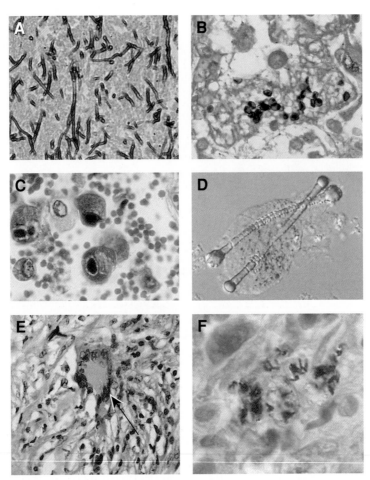

● **Figure 20-5 Lung infections. A:** Aspergillosis. Fungal hyphae are impregnated with silver and appear as branching strands. **B:** *Pneumocystis carinii.* The lung alveoli are filled with bubbly, protein-rich exudates. The cysts of *P. carinii* in the exudates are impregnated with silver and appear black. **C:** Cytomegalovirus (CMV). Desquamated alveolar cells infected with CMV are markedly enlarged with large purple intranuclear inclusions surrounded by a clear halo. **D:** Asbestosis. Asbestos bodies are beaded, dumbbell-shaped rods, which stain with Prussian blue iron stain. **E, F:** Tuberculosis. **E:** Tuberculosis is characterized by caseating granulomas containing giant Langerhans cells (*arrow*), which have a horseshoe-shaped pattern of nuclei. **F:** *Mycobacterium tuberculosis* organisms are identified as red rods ("red snappers") by acid-fast Ziehl-Neelsen stain.

Case Study 20-1

A mother brings her 4-year-old son to your office complaining that "he coughs constantly and spits up a green mucus." After some discussion, she informs you that her son also has pungent, fatty stools; has had several bouts of severe coughing and fever within the past few months; and had meconium ileus (obstruction of the bowel with a thick meconium) as a baby. Finally, she asks you this question: "Why is my son so small?" What is the most likely diagnosis?

Differentials

- Asthma, foreign body aspiration, pneumonia, selective immunoglobulin A (IgA) deficiency

Relevant Physical Examination Findings

- The boy is in the 10th percentile for height and 5th percentile for weight for children 4 years of age.
- Fever = 101°F, tachypnea = 40breaths/min, tachycardia = 155 bpm
- Auscultation of the lungs reveals diffuse, bilateral wheezing; rales; and coarse breath sounds.

Relevant Lab Findings

- Sweat test: Na^+ = high; Cl^- = high
- Stool sample showed steatorrhea.
- Pulmonary function test: residual volume:total lung volume = high; FEV_1:FVC (forced vital capacity) = low
- Sputum culture: *S. aureus* and *P. aeruginosa* positive
- Radiograph: hyperinflation of lungs, early signs of bronchiectasis

Diagnosis: Cystic Fibrosis

- **Cystic Fibrosis (CF).** CF is caused by production of abnormally thick mucus by epithelial cells lining the respiratory (and gastrointestinal) tract. This results in obstruction of airways and recurrent bacterial infections (e.g., *S. aureus, P. aeruginosa*). CF is the most common lethal genetic disorder among whites. The primary manifestation of CF occurs in the lungs and pancreas. In the lungs, the excessively viscous mucus leads to plugging of the lungs. In the pancreas, the release of pancreatic digestive enzymes is deficient, leading to malabsorption and steatorrhea. One of the earliest signs of CF is failure to thrive in early childhood.
- Asthmatic patients have a low FEV_1:FVC and hyperinflation (similar to CF), but asthma is characterized by the reversibility of attacks and predisposes the patient to infections.
- Foreign body aspiration is usually unilateral and occurs most often on the right side.
- This 4-year-old boy has pneumonia but it is secondary to CF and the sputum culture is classic for pneumonia secondary to CF.
- Selective IgA deficiency is a congenital disorder in which class switching in the heavy chain fails to occur and is the most common congenital B-cell defect. IgA is found in bodily secretions and plays an important role in preventing bacterial colonization of mucosal surfaces, which makes these patients susceptible to recurrent sinopulmonary infections.

Case Study 20-2

A 70-year-old man comes to your office complaining that "I'm starting to cough up blood. It's bright red and it scares me. I know I cough a lot because I'm a heavy smoker and when I get a cold in the winter it gets real bad. But, it's always been green mucus, never blood." He also tells you that "I'm short of breath and I've lost 15 pounds this past month because I have no appetite. I can't describe it, but this cough seems different." After some discussion, he informs you that he has smoked 3 packs of cigarettes a day for about 50 years and drinks a lot. "You know, Doc, when I smoke I like to drink and when I drink I like to smoke. It's a vicious cycle. But, like I tell my wife, I only have two bad habits in life. That's pretty good, isn't it?" What is the most likely diagnosis?

Differentials

- Bronchiectasis, Goodpasture syndrome, pneumonia, tuberculosis

Relevant Physical Examination Findings

- Tachypnea, positive end-expiratory wheezing, clubbing of the digits
- Lung auscultation: decreased breath sounds on the right side
- Patient appears frail

Relevant Lab Findings

- Blood chemistry: white blood cells (WBCs) = 8500/μL (normal); hematocrit (Hct) = 30% (low); mean corpuscular volume = 100 μm^3 (high); serum Ca^{2+} = 14.1 mg/dL (high)
- Sputum culture: normal respiratory flora; no acid-fast bacilli
- Urinalysis: ketones = none; leukocyte esterase = none; bacteria = none
- Chest radiograph: large mass in the lower right hilum; atelectasis in the right lower lobe
- Biopsy: keratin pearls and intercellular bridging are observed

Diagnosis: Squamous Cell Carcinoma

- **Squamous Cell Carcinoma (SQ).** SQ has a 35% incidence and is most closely associated with smoking history. SQ is centrally located as it arises from larger bronchi due to injury of the bronchial epithelium followed by regeneration from the basal layer in the form of squamous metaplasia. SQ begins as a small red granular plaque and progresses to a large intrabronchial mass. Cavitation of the lung may occur distal to the mass. SQ may secrete parathyroid hormone (PTH), causing hypercalcemia. SQ appears histologically as polygonal-shaped cells arranged in solid cell nests and bright eosinophilic aggregates of extracellular keratin ("pearls"). Intracellular keratinization may also be apparent such that the cytoplasm appears glassy and eosinophilic. In well-differentiated squamous cell carcinomas, intercellular bridges may be observed that are cytoplasmic extensions between adjacent cells. Another important histologic characteristic of squamous cell carcinoma is the in situ replacement of the bronchial epithelium. As a rule, neither adenocarcinoma nor small cell carcinoma replaces the bronchial epithelium, but instead, tends to grow beneath the epithelium.
- Bronchiectasis is the abnormal, permanent dilatation of bronchi due to chronic necrotizing infection (e.g., *Staphylococcus*, *Streptococcus*, *H. influenzae*), bronchial obstruction (e.g., foreign body, mucous plugs, or tumors), or congenital conditions (e.g., Kartagener syndrome, cystic fibrosis, immunodeficiency disorders). The lower lobes of the lung are predominately affected and the affected bronchi have a saccular appearance. Clinical findings of bronchiectasis include cough; fever; expectoration of large amounts of foul-smelling purulent sputum; crackles, rhonchi, and wheezing heard upon lung auscultation; and chest radiograph showing prominent cystic spaces.

- Antiglomerular basement membrane glomerulonephritis (ABMG; Goodpasture syndrome) is caused by deposition of IgG immune complexes (i.e., autoantibodies to a globular non-collagenous domain of type IV collagen) within the glomerular basement membrane. The autoantibodies generally cross-react with pulmonary basement membranes, and therefore, when both the lungs and kidneys are involved, the term Goodpasture syndrome is used. Pathologic findings of ABMG include glomerular crescents in greater than 50% of glomeruli, which are formed by an inflammatory exudate containing macrophages and fibrin filling the urinary space and a proliferation of the simple squamous epithelium lining the Bowman capsule; immunofluorescence localizing IgG in a linear fashion along the glomerular basement membrane (GBM); and electron microscopy showing focal breaks in the GBM but not immune dense deposits. Clinical findings of ABMG include patients presenting with a rapidly progressive renal failure; severe bloody cough (hemoptysis); dyspnea; hematuria; and nephritic syndrome.
- *Streptococcus pneumoniae* causes pneumococcal pneumonia. Pneumococcal pneumonia is the most common bacterial pneumonia in older adults (>65 years of age). Pneumococcal pneumonia is generally a consequence of altered immunity within the respiratory tract most frequently following a viral infection (e.g., influenza), which damages the mucociliary elevator, or chronic obstructive pulmonary disease (COPD) or alcoholism. Four stages of classic bacteria pneumonia are described: (a) The initial stage features acute congestion, intra-alveolar fluid containing many bacteria, and few neutrophils. (b) The early consolidation or "red hepatization" (2 to 4 days) stage features consolidation with infiltration of a large number of neutrophils and intra-alveolar hemorrhage. The lung is red due to extravasated RBCs, firm, and airless with a liverlike consistency. (c) The late consolidation or "gray hepatization" (4 to 8 days) stage features large amounts of fibrin within the alveoli, lysis of the neutrophils, and appearance of macrophages, which phagocytose the inflammatory debris. The lung has a gray-brown dry surface. (d) The resolution stage begins after 8 days. Clinical findings of pneumococcal pneumonia include acute onset with fever, chills, chest pain secondary to pleural involvement, and hemoptysis (rusty, blood-tinged sputum); the chest radiograph shows lobar lung infiltrate.
- *Mycobacterium tuberculosis* causes tuberculosis (TB), which is the classic mycobacterial disease. Aerosolized infectious particles travel to terminal airways where *M. tuberculosis* penetrates inactivated alveolar macrophages and inhibits acidification of endolysosomes so that alveolar macrophages cannot kill the bacteria. However, replicating intracellular *M. tuberculosis* stimulates $CD8^+$ cytotoxic T cells, which lyse infected cells, and $CD4^+$ helper T cells, which release interferon-γ and other cytokines that activate macrophages to phagocytose and kill the bacteria. The Ghon complex is the first lesion of primary TB and consists of a parenchymal granuloma (location is subpleural and in lower lobes of the lung) and prominent, infected mediastinal lymph nodes. Most cases of primary TB are asymptomatic and resolve spontaneously. The genus *Mycobacterium* are poorly gram-positive bacilli (rods), obligate aerobic, acid-fast (due to a waxy, hydrophobic, arabinogalactanmycolate cell wall), endospore-negative, nonmotile, intracellular pathogens. Clinical findings of TB include hemoptysis, weakness, night sweats, and weight loss; the chest radiograph shows localized consolidation, possibly with cavitation.

Chapter 21

Urinary System

I **General Features (Figure 21-1).** The kidneys are retroperitoneal organs that lie on the ventral surface of the quadratus lumborum muscle and lateral to the psoas muscle and vertebral column. They are covered by a fibrous capsule called the **renal capsule (or true capsule)**, which can be readily stripped from the surface of the kidney except in some pathologic conditions where it is strongly adherent due to scarring. A fresh kidney that is hemisected in the sagittal plane shows a distinct outer **cortex** (a reddish brown band 1 to 2 cm thick; its color is due to its high degree of vascularization), inner **medulla** (lighter in color than the cortex), and **collecting system**. The functions of the kidney include:

A. Regulation of the volume, osmolarity, mineral composition, and acidity (acid-base balance) of the body by excreting water and inorganic electrolytes (Na^+ Cl^-, K^+, Ca^{2+}, Mg^{2+}, SO_4^{2-}, PO_4^{2-}, H^+) in adequate amounts to achieve total-body balance and maintain their normal concentration in the extracellular fluid

B. Excretion of metabolic waste products (urea, uric acid, creatinine, end products of hemoglobin breakdown, metabolites of various hormones, etc.)

C. Excretion of many foreign chemicals (drugs, pesticides, food additives, etc.)

D. Gluconeogenesis (during prolonged fasting, the kidneys synthesize glucose from amino acids and release glucose into the blood)

E. Secretion of the hormone **erythropoietin** by peritubular interstitial fibroblasts in the kidney cortex, which acts on the bone marrow to stimulate red blood cell (RBC) formation (erythropoiesis)

F. Secretion of the enzyme **renin** by juxtaglomerular (JG) cells, which regulates blood pressure

G. 1-α-Hydroxylation of **25-(OH) vitamin D** to form 1,25-$(OH)_2$ vitamin D, which acts directly on osteoblasts to secrete interleukin-1 (IL-1), which stimulates osteoclasts to increase bone resorption and increases the absorption of Ca^{2+} from the intestinal lumen, thereby elevating blood Ca^{2+} levels

II **Internal Structure of the Kidney**

A. RENAL CAPSULE. The kidney surface is covered by a connective tissue capsule that consists of fibroblasts, collagen, and myofibroblasts (with a contractile function).

B. RENAL CORTEX. The renal cortex lies under the capsule and also extends between the renal pyramids as the **renal columns of Bertin**. The renal cortex may be divided into the **cortical labyrinth** and the **medullary rays of Ferrein** (which appear as striations perpendicular to the kidney surface that emanate from the renal medulla).

C. RENAL MEDULLA. The renal medulla is composed of **5 to 11 renal pyramids of Malpighi**, whose tips terminate as **5 to 11 renal papillae**. The base of a renal pyramid abuts the renal cortex, whereas the tip of a renal pyramid (i.e., the renal papillae) abuts a minor calyx.

D. RENAL LOBES. A renal lobe consists of a renal pyramid and its associated cortical tissue at its base and sides (half of each adjacent renal column). There are 5 to 11 renal lobes in the adult, which corresponds to the number of renal pyramids. The renal lobes are conspicuous in the fetal kidney as a number of convexities on the surface, but these typically disappear in the adult kidney.

E. RENAL LOBULE. A renal lobule consists of a central medullary ray and its surrounding cortical labyrinth. A renal lobule is basically composed of all the nephrons that drain into the single collecting duct located in the medullary ray.

F. COLLECTING SYSTEM. The collecting system of the kidney includes the following:
1. **Collecting Ducts.** The distal convoluted tubule is connected to the collecting ducts by **connecting tubules**. The collecting ducts located in the cortex are called **cortical collecting ducts**. As the cortical collecting ducts travel into the medulla, they are called **medullary collecting ducts**. As the medullary collecting ducts travel toward the renal papillae, they merge into larger collecting ducts called the **papillary ducts of Bellini**. The papillary ducts open onto the surface of the renal papillae at the **area cribrosa**. The collecting ducts are lined by a simple cuboidal epithelium that transitions into a simple columnar epithelium as the collecting ducts increase in size toward the renal papillae. The epithelium is composed of two cell types: **principal cells** and **intercalated cells (type A and type B)**.
2. **Five to 11 Minor Calyces.** The minor calyces are cup-shaped structures that abut the 5 to 11 renal papillae. The minor calyces consist of a transitional epithelium, a lamina propria rich in collagen and elastic fibers, and a smooth muscle layer, which undergoes rhythmic peristaltic movements.
3. **Two to Three Major Calyces.** The major calyces are continuous with the minor calyces. The major calyces consist of a transitional epithelium, a lamina propria rich in collagen and elastic fibers, and a smooth muscle layer, which undergoes rhythmic peristaltic movements.
4. **Renal Pelvis.** The renal pelvis is continuous with the major calyces. The renal pelvis consists of a transitional epithelium, a lamina propria rich in collagen and elastic fibers, and a smooth muscle layer, which undergoes rhythmic peristaltic movements.

G. RENAL (URINIFEROUS) TUBULES are classically considered the structural and functional units of the kidney and consist of the **nephron** and **collecting duct**.

III **Nephrons (Figure 21-1 and Table 21-1)** consist of the following components:

A. RENAL GLOMERULUS
1. A renal glomerulus is a capillary bed (or tuft) that consists of a single layer of endothelial cells surrounded by a glomerular basement membrane. The capillaries within the renal glomerulus are **continuous, fenestrated capillaries without diaphragms**.

2. A renal glomerulus receives blood from an **afferent arteriole** (a major site of autoregulation of renal blood flow) and is drained by an **efferent arteriole** (i.e., the **vascular pole**).

3. A renal glomerulus is surrounded by a **glomerular (Bowman) capsule.**

4. A renal glomerulus is associated with a **glomerular mesangium**, which lies between the capillaries and consists of a **mesangial matrix** and **glomerular mesangial cells.**

B. THE GLOMERULAR MESANGIUM

1. **The mesangial matrix** is an extracellular matrix of microfibrils and contains collagen (types III, IV, V, and VI), microfibrillar proteins (fibrillin, microfibril-associated glycoprotein [MAGP], MP78, MP340), and fibronectin.

2. The glomerular **mesangial cells** are irregular in shape, have many cell processes that extend toward the glomerular basement membrane, are attached to each other by desmosomes, and communicate with each other by gap junctions.

3. The functions of mesangial cells include the following:
   a. Synthesis of the mesangial matrix, which is frequently increased in glomerular disease
   b. Phagocytosis of colloids, macromolecules, protein aggregates, and immune complexes trapped by the glomerular basement membrane
   c. Contraction and relaxation in response to a number of vasoactive agents (e.g., angiotensin II and atrial natriuretic peptide [ANP])
   d. Production of cytokines and prostaglandins
   e. Serving as a target cell in many glomerular diseases and responding by repair and proliferation

C. GLOMERULAR (BOWMAN) CAPSULE

1. The glomerular capsule is a double-layered capsule that consists of an outer **parietal layer** and an inner **visceral layer**.

2. The parietal layer consists of a **simple squamous epithelium** that lines the outer wall of the glomerular capsule and becomes continuous with the simple cuboidal epithelium of the proximal convoluted tubule.

3. The visceral layer consists of **podocytes** that extend cell processes to the glomerular basement membrane surrounding the capillaries of the renal glomerulus and is reflected to become continuous with the parietal layer.

4. The space between the parietal and visceral layers of the glomerular capsule is called the **urinary (Bowman) space.**

5. The urinary space receives an ultrafiltrate of plasma produced by filtration through the glomerular filtration barrier and is continuous with the lumen of the proximal convoluted tubule (i.e., the **urinary pole**).

D. PROXIMAL CONVOLUTED TUBULE (PCT).
The PCT consists of simple cuboidal epithelial cells with a distinctly acidophilic cytoplasm, brush border (i.e., microvilli), intercellular zonula occludens (tight junctions), apical endocytic vesicles, lateral interdigitations, and basal infoldings with numerous mitochondria.

E. LOOP OF HENLE.
The loop of Henle consists of the following:

1. **Proximal Straight Tubule (PST).** The PST is similar in morphology to the PCT.

2. **Descending Thin Limb (DTL).** The DTL consists of simple squamous epithelial cells with deep intercellular zonula occludens (tight junctions), no lateral interdigitations, and a few microvilli.

3. **Ascending Thin Limb (ATL).** The ATL consists of simple squamous epithelial cells with shallow intercellular zonula occludens (tight junctions) and extensive lateral interdigitations.

4. **Distal Straight Tubule (DST).** The DST consists of simple cuboidal epithelial cells with intercellular zonula occludens (tight junctions), lateral interdigitations, and basal infoldings with numerous mitochondria. The DST has no conspicuous brush border (i.e., microvilli). In the region of the afferent and efferent arterioles, the DST contains specialized cells called **macula densa cells**. The DST synthesizes the **Tamm-Horsfall glycoprotein**, which is the most abundant constituent of renal tubule casts found in many diseases.

F. **DISTAL CONVOLUTED TUBULE (DCT).** The DCT consists of simple cuboidal epithelial cells with intercellular zonula occludens (tight junctions), lateral interdigitations, and basal infoldings with numerous mitochondria. The DCT has no conspicuous brush border (i.e., microvilli).

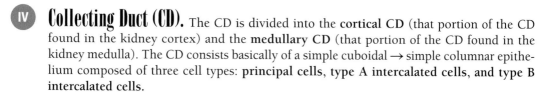

IV **Collecting Duct (CD).** The CD is divided into the **cortical CD** (that portion of the CD found in the kidney cortex) and the **medullary CD** (that portion of the CD found in the kidney medulla). The CD consists basically of a simple cuboidal → simple columnar epithelium composed of three cell types: **principal cells, type A intercalated cells, and type B intercalated cells.**

A. **PRINCIPAL CELLS**
   1. Principal cells are found in both cortical and medullary collecting ducts and change in size from simple cuboidal → simple columnar.
   2. Principal cells possess **antidiuretic hormone (ADH) receptors**.
   3. Principal cells reabsorb (tubular fluid → plasma) **5% of the filtered Na^+**, reabsorb **5% to 25% of the filtered H_2O** depending on the H_2O balance of the person, reabsorb **5% of the filtered Ca^{2+}**, reabsorb **10% of the filtered urea**, and secrete (plasma → tubular fluid) **plasma K^+** when a person is on a high/normal K^+ diet.

B. **TYPE A INTERCALATED CELLS**
   1. Type A intercalated cells are found predominately in the cortical collecting ducts and their number gradually decreases in the medullary collecting ducts until they are completely absent in the largest papillary ducts.
   2. Type A intercalated cells possess a **H^+ adenosine triphosphatase (ATPase)** on the <u>luminal</u> membrane.
   3. Type A intercalated cells reabsorb (tubular fluid → plasma) **10% of the filtered HCO_3^-**, reabsorb **filtered K^+** when a person is on a low K^+ diet (K^+ depleted), and secrete (plasma → tubular fluid) **H^+**.

C. **TYPE B INTERCALATED CELLS**
   1. Type B intercalated cells are found predominately in the cortical collecting ducts and their number gradually decreases in the medullary collecting ducts until they are completely absent in the largest papillary ducts.
   2. Type B intercalated cells possess a **H^+ ATPase** located on the <u>basolateral</u> membrane.
   3. Type B intercalated cells reabsorb (tubular fluid → plasma) **5% of the filtered Cl^-** and, **secrete HCO_3^-** during alkalosis.

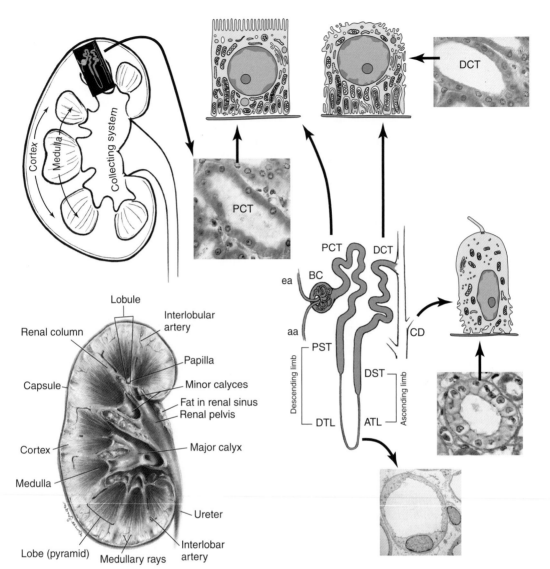

● **Figure 21-1 Diagram of the kidney and renal tubules.** The renal tubules consist of a nephron and collecting duct. The nephron (*shaded area*) consists of the renal glomerulus formed by the afferent arteriole (aa) and efferent arteriole (ea), Bowman capsule (BC), proximal convoluted tubule (PCT), proximal straight tubule (PST), descending thin limb (DTL), ascending thin limb (ATL), distal straight tubule (DST), and distal convoluted tubule (DCT). Note the histologic appearance of each of the tubules.

TABLE 21-1	**PHYSIOLOGIC FUNCTIONS OF RENAL TUBULES**

Tubules	Functions
PCT	**Reabsorption from tubular fluid → plasma:** 100% of organic nutrients (glucose, amino acids, water-soluble vitamins [B complex and C], lactate, acetate, ketones [β-hydroxybutyrate, acetoacetate], Krebs cycle intermediates) 100% of proteins and polypeptides and 50% of urea 65% of Na^+ 65% of Cl^- 65% of H_2O 55% of K^+ 80% of Ca^{2+} 85% of PO_4^{2-} 80% of HCO_3^- **Secretion from plasma → tubular fluid:** 100% of organic anions (para-aminohippuric acid, urate, bile salts, fatty acids, hydroxybenzoates, acetazolamide, chlorothiazide, penicillin, salicylates, sulfonamides) 100% of organic cations (acetylcholine, creatinine, dopamine, epinephrine, norepinephrine, histamine, serotonin, atropine, isoproterenol, cimetidine, morphine) H^+ and NH_4^+
Loop of Henle	
PST	**Reabsorption from tubular fluid → plasma:** 5% of H_2O (permeable to H_2O)
DTL	**Reabsorption from tubular fluid → plasma:** 5% of H_2O (permeable to H_2O)
ATL	**Reabsorption from tubular fluid → plasma:** 10% of Na^+, 10% of Cl^- (impermeable to H_2O)
DST	**Reabsorption from tubular fluid → plasma:** 15% of Na^+, 15% of Cl^-, 30% of K^+, 10% of Ca^{2+}, 10% of HCO_3^- (impermeable to H_sO) **Secretion from plasma → tubular fluid:** H^+
DCT	**Reabsorption from tubular fluid → plasma:** 5% of Na^+, 5% of Cl^-, K^+ (low K^+ diet), 5% of Ca^{2+} (impermeable to H_2O)
CD (Principal cells)	**Reabsorption from tubular fluid → plasma:** 5% of Na^+, 5% to 25% of H_2O (depending on water balance), 5% of Ca^{2+}, 10% of urea **Secretion from plasma → tubular fluid:** K^+ (high/normal diet)
CD (Type A cells)	**Reabsorption from tubular fluid → plasma:** 10% of HCO_3^-, K^+ (low K^+ diet) **Secretion from plasma → tubular fluid:** H^+
CD (Type B cells)	**Reabsorption from tubular fluid → plasma:** 5% of Cl^- **Secretion from plasma → tubular fluid:** HCO_3^- (during alkalosis)

PCT, proximal convoluted tubule; PST, proximal straight tubule; DTL, descending thin limb; ATL, ascending thin limb; DST, distal straight tubule; DCT, distal convoluted tubule; CD, collecting duct.

Renal Vasculature (Figure 21-2)

A. ARTERIAL SUPPLY. The **renal artery** branches into **five segmental arteries**. The segmental arteries branch into **5 to 11 interlobar arteries**. The interlobar arteries branch into the **arcuate arteries**, which travel along the base of the renal pyramids at the corticomedullary junction. The arcuate arteries branch into the **interlobular arteries**, which travel through the cortex toward the capsule and branch into numerous **afferent arterioles**. Each afferent arteriole forms a capillary bed (or tuft) called the **renal glomerulus**, which is drained by an **efferent arteriole**. The efferent arteriole has two fates:

1. **Formation of the Cortical Peritubular Capillary Bed.** The efferent arteriole of renal glomeruli from cortical and midcortical nephrons branches into a **cortical peritubular capillary bed** that is intimately associated with renal tubules in the cortex. Note that the renal glomerulus and cortical peritubular capillary bed are two capillary beds connected in series by the efferent arteriole.

2. **Formation of the Vasa Recta (Hairpin Loop).** The efferent arteriole of renal glomeruli from juxtamedullary nephrons branches into **12 to 25 descending vasa recta**, which are long, straight capillaries that run to varying depths of the medulla. The ends of the descending vasa recta give rise to a **medullary peritubular capillary bed** that is intimately associated with renal tubules in the medulla. The venous ends of the capillaries converge to form **ascending vasa recta**, which then complete the hairpin loop. The vasa recta are part of the **countercurrent exchanger system**, which maintains the hyperosmolarity gradient of the interstitial fluid in the medulla that is crucial for urine concentration. Note that the renal glomerulus and the vasa recta/medullary peritubular capillary bed are two capillary beds connected in series by the efferent arteriole.

B. VENOUS DRAINAGE

1. **Kidney Surface and Capsule.** The venous ends of a capillary bed near the kidney surface and capillaries of the kidney capsule drain into **stellate veins**. Stellate veins drain into **interlobular veins**. The interlobular veins drain into **arcuate veins**. The arcuate veins drain into **interlobar veins**, which anastomose and converge to form the **renal vein**.

2. **Cortical Venous Drainage.** The venous ends of the cortical peritubular capillary bed converge to drain into **interlobular veins**. The interlobular veins drain into **arcuate veins**. The arcuate veins drain into **interlobar veins**, which anastomose and converge to form the **renal vein**.

3. **Medullary Venous Drainage.** The venous ends of the medullary capillary bed converge to form **ascending vasa recta**, which complete the hairpin loop. The ascending vasa recta drain into both **the interlobular veins** and **arcuate veins**. The arcuate veins drain into **interlobar veins**, which anastomose and converge to form the **renal vein**.

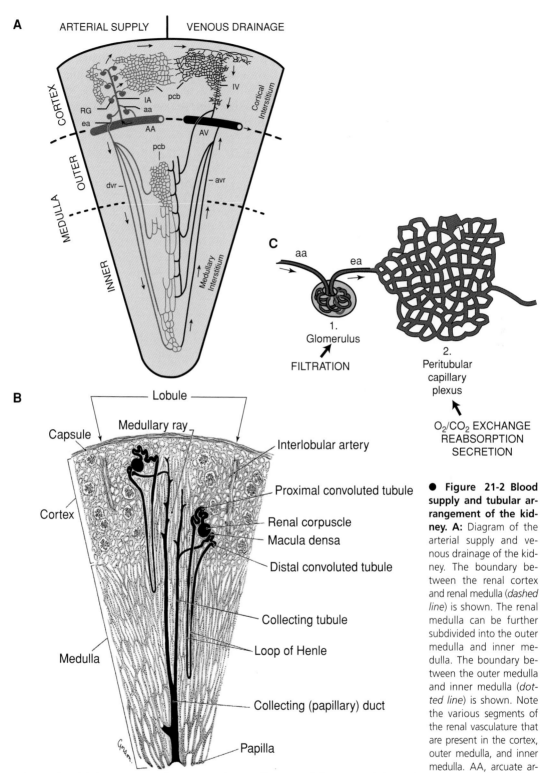

● **Figure 21-2 Blood supply and tubular arrangement of the kidney. A:** Diagram of the arterial supply and venous drainage of the kidney. The boundary between the renal cortex and renal medulla (*dashed line*) is shown. The renal medulla can be further subdivided into the outer medulla and inner medulla. The boundary between the outer medulla and inner medulla (*dotted line*) is shown. Note the various segments of the renal vasculature that are present in the cortex, outer medulla, and inner medulla. AA, arcuate arteries; IA, interlobular artery; aa, afferent arteriole; ea, efferent arteriole; RG, renal glomerulus; pcb, peritubular capillary bed; dvr, descending vasa recta; avr, ascending vasa recta; IV, interlobular vein; AV, arcuate vein. **B:** Diagram indicating the renal tubules (*black*) in the cortex and medulla of the kidney. The difficulty in understanding the histology of the kidney involves the superimposition of the renal vasculature network on the renal tubule system. Figure 21-1A and B will help the student in this superimposition. **C:** A diagram to indicate that in the kidney there are two capillary networks **arranged in series**. The afferent arteriole forms a capillary network called the renal glomerulus, which is involved in filtration of the blood. The efferent arteriole forms the peritubular capillary plexus, which is involved in O_2/CO_2 exchange for the renal tubules, reabsorption of substances from the tubular fluid into the blood (tubular fluid → plasma), and secretion of substances from the blood into the tubular fluid (plasma → tubular fluid).

Hormonal Control of the Kidney (Figure 21–3)

A. ANGIOTENSIN II. Angiotensin II is produced by the conversion of angiotensin I by **angiotensin-converting enzyme (ACE)** primarily by the endothelium of lung capillaries. Angiotensin II has many widespread actions, including actions on the kidney.

1. Angiotensin II acts on the **epithelial cells of the proximal convoluted tubule** and causes **increased Na^+ reabsorption** (tubular fluid → plasma) and therefore **decreased Na^+ excretion in the urine.**

2. Angiotensin II acts on the **smooth muscle cells of the afferent and efferent arterioles** and causes **vasoconstriction** of the afferent and efferent arterioles and therefore **decreases the glomerular filtration rate (GFR).**

3. Angiotensin II also plays a role in ADH and aldosterone secretion.

B. ADH. ADH is secreted by axon terminals within the **neurohypophysis** whose cell bodies are located in the **supraoptic nucleus** and **paraventricular nucleus** of the hypothalamus. The most important inputs to these neurons are from baroceptors and osmoreceptors. **Baroreceptors** in the walls of the common carotid arteries (carotid sinus), great veins, atria, and aortic arch respond to decreased blood pressure and stimulate ADH secretion. **Osmoreceptors** in the hypothalamus respond to increased plasma osmolarity and stimulate ADH secretion. **Angiotensin II** also stimulates ADH secretion.

1. ADH acts on the **principal cells of the cortical and medullary collecting ducts** and causes **increased H_2O reabsorption** (tubular fluid → plasma) and therefore **decreased H_2O excretion in the urine.**

2. **Clinical Consideration.** Syndrome of inappropriate ADH secretion (SIADH) is caused by pulmonary disorders (e.g., small cell carcinoma with ectopic secretion of ADH, tuberculosis), drugs (e.g., chlorpropamide, cyclophosphamide, morphine, carbamazepine, oxytocin), and central nervous system disorders (e.g., tumor, infection, hypopituitarism) and causes the loss of the inhibitory effect of cortisol on ADH. SIADH is characterized by **excessively increased H_2O reabsorption** (tubular fluid → plasma) and therefore **excessively decreased H_2O excretion** in the urine. This results in a dilutional hyponatremia (low serum Na^+) and a great increase in total body water. Eventually, the effective arterial blood volume is increased, leading to an inhibition of the renin-angiotensin system; hence, no aldosterone is secreted. This leads to decreased Na^+ reabsorption, increased loss of urea, and increased loss of uric acid. The triad of **hyponatremia, low serum blood urea nitrogen (BUN),** and **hypouricemia** is virtually pathognomonic for SIADH.

C. ALDOSTERONE (ALD). ALD is secreted by the **zona glomerulosa cells of the adrenal cortex.** The secretion of ALD is controlled by **angiotensin II** of the renin-angiotensin system.

1. ALD acts on the **principal cells of the cortical collecting duct** and causes **increased Na^+ reabsorption** (tubular fluid → plasma) and therefore **decreased Na^+ excretion in the urine.** ALD is the most important controller of Na^+ reabsorption.

2. ALD acts on the **principal cells of the cortical collecting duct** and causes **increased K^+ secretion** (plasma → tubular fluid) and thereby **increased K^+ excretion in the urine.**

3. ALD acts on the **type A intercalated cells of the cortical collecting duct** and causes **increased H^+ secretion** (plasma → tubular fluid).

D. A-TYPE NATRIURETIC PEPTIDE (ANP). ANP is secreted by **myocardial endocrine cells** located within the right and left atria of the heart. ANP is secreted in response to increased blood volume (pressure) or increased venous pressure with the atria of the heart. ANP binds to the natriuretic peptide receptor (NPR)-A and NPR-C. NPR-A is a G protein–linked receptor. NPR-C is believed to be a "decoy receptor," because it lacks an intracellular domain.

1. ANP acts on the **principal cells of the medullary collecting ducts** and causes **decreased Na$^+$ reabsorption** (tubular fluid $\rightarrow$ plasma) and therefore **increased Na$^+$ secretion in the urine.**

2. ANP acts on the **smooth muscle cells of the efferent arteriole** and causes vasoconstriction of the efferent arteriole and therefore **increases GFR.**

E. **B-TYPE NATRIURETIC PEPTIDE (BNP).** BNP is secreted by myocardial endocrine cells located within the right and left ventricles of the heart. BNP binds to NPR-A and NPR-C. BNP is secreted in congestive heart failure and has a diuretic effect on the kidney (similar to that of ANP). **Natrecor (nesiritide)** is a relatively new recombinant DNA human sequence of BNP and has been approved for short-term management of decompensated congestive heart failure.

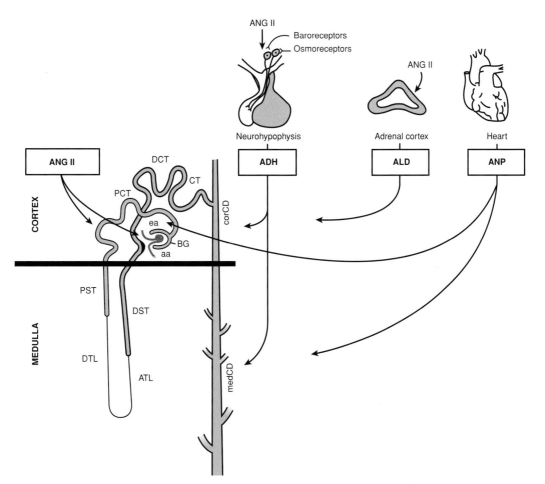

● **Figure 21-3 Diagram of hormonal control of the kidney.** BG, Bowman or glomerular capsule; PCT, proximal convoluted tubule; PST, proximal straight tubule of the loop of Henle; DTL, descending thin limb of the loop of Henle; ATL, ascending thin limb of the loop of Henle, DST, distal straight tubule of the loop of Henle; DCT, distal convoluted tubule; corCD, cortical collecting duct; medCD, medullary collecting duct; CT, connecting tubule; aa, afferent arteriole; ea, efferent arteriole; ANG II, angiotensin II; ADH, antidiuretic hormone; ALD, aldosterone; ANP, atrial natriuretic peptide.

VII **Glomerular Filtration Barrier (GFB) (Figure 21-4).** Urine formation begins with filtration, which occurs where the renal glomerulus and the glomerular (Bowman) capsule interact to form the GFB. Filtration is the bulk flow of fluid from the glomerular capillaries into the urinary (Bowman) space to form tubular fluid.

A. The components of the GFB include:

1. **Glomerular Capillary Endothelium.** The glomerular capillary endothelium is a **continuous, fenestrated (without diaphragms) endothelium**. The fenestrae are 70- to 90-nm-diameter pores that are not bridged by diaphragms as usually occurs in other capillaries. The endothelial cells possess **aquaporin H_2O channels** that allow fast movement of H_2O through the endothelium, **cell surface polyanionic glycoproteins** (e.g., podocalyxin) that impart a negative surface charge to the endothelial cells, and **integrins** that bind to fibronectin in the glomerular basement membrane.

2. **Glomerular Basement Membrane (GBM).** The GBM is a 300- to 350-nm-thick basement membrane that is synthesized jointly by the glomerular capillary endothelium and podocytes. The GBM consists of **type IV collagen (α_1 through α_6 chains); heparan sulfate proteoglycan**, which is important in imparting a negative charge to the GBM; **laminin (a glycoprotein)**; and **fibronectin (a glycoprotein**.

3. **Slit Diaphragms of Podocytes.** The podocytes have large cell bodies that bulge into the urinary space and make up the visceral layer of the glomerular (Bowman) capsule. The cell bodies give rise to **foot processes** that extend toward and make contact with the GBM. The foot processes from neighboring podocytes regularly interdigitate with one another, thereby forming elongated 25-nm-wide spaces called the **filtration slits**. The filtration slits are bridged by **slit diaphragms**. The podocytes possess **cell surface polyanionic glycoproteins** (e.g., podocalyxin) that impart a negative surface charge to the foot processes and slit diaphragms and **integrins** that bind to fibronectin in the glomerular basement membrane.

B. **THE FUNCTIONS OF THE GFB** include:

1. Prevents passage of red blood cells, leukocytes, and platelets

2. Restricts passage of proteins greater than 70,000 d ("**size filter**") and negatively charged substances ("**charge filter**"). The GFB provides no hindrance to molecules less than **7000 d** and almost total hindrance to plasma albumin (**70,000 d**). For molecules between **7000 d and 70,000 d**, the amount filtered becomes progressively smaller as the molecule becomes larger. For any given molecular size, negatively charged molecules are filtered to a lesser extent and positively charged molecules to a greater extent versus neutral molecules. The reason is that the GFB is negatively charged (due to heparan sulfate), which repels negatively charged molecules. Since almost all plasma proteins are negatively charged, the charge hindrance of the GFB plays an important role of enhancing the size hindrance. Note that the "charge filter" does not affect ions.

3. Permits passage of water, cations, anions, and other small molecules

4. Forms an ultrafiltrate of blood

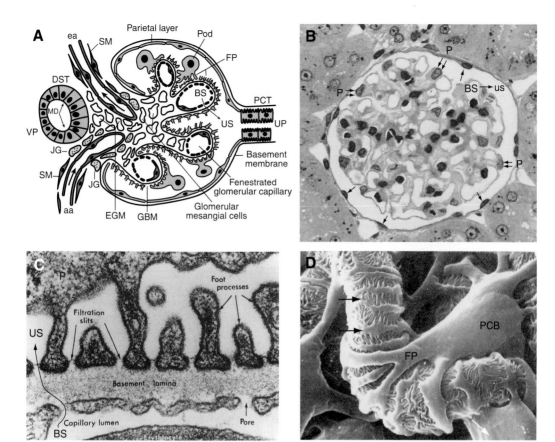

● **Figure 21-4 Histology of the glomerular filtration barrier. A:** Diagram of the renal glomerulus and the glomerular (Bowman) capsule. Note that the renal glomerulus is actually part of the renal vasculature, but there is an intimate histologic relationship between the glomerular capillaries and the glomerular capsule. Hence, the glomerular capillaries and the glomerular capsule are sometimes called the **renal corpuscle**. The glomerular capillaries are covered by podocytes and their foot processes are called the visceral layer of glomerular capsule. The podocytes reflect to become continuous with the simple squamous epithelium of the parietal layer of the glomerular capsule. The parietal layer of the glomerular capsule becomes continuous with the simple cuboidal epithelium of the proximal convoluted tubule at the urinary pole (UP). The renal glomerulus receives blood from the afferent arteriole (aa) and is drained by the efferent arteriole (ea) at the vascular pole (VP). JG, juxtaglomerular cells; MD, macula densa cells; DST, distal straight tubule; EGM, extraglomerular mesangial cells; SM, smooth muscle; Pod, podocyte; FP, foot process; PCT, proximal convoluted tubule; BS, blood space; US, urinary space; GBM, glomerular basement membrane. **B:** Light micrograph of the glomerulus and Bowman capsule. Podocytes (*double arrows*; P), which make up the visceral layer of Bowman capsule, are indicated. Simple squamous epithelium (*single arrows*), which makes up the parietal layer of Bowman capsule, is also indicated. Filtration from the blood space (BS) to the urinary space (US) is also indicated; see *arrow*. **C:** Electron micrograph of the glomerular filtration barrier. A podocyte (P) with its foot processes and filtration slits is adjacent to the basement lamina. The glomerular capillary consists of an endothelium that is fenestrated (pore) with no diaphragms. Filtration from the blood space (BS) to the urinary space (US) is indicated; see *arrow*. **D:** Scanning electron micrograph of the renal glomerulus. A podocyte cell body (PCB) and foot processes (FP; *arrows*) are shown covering a capillary.

VIII **Juxtaglomerular (JG) Complex.** The JG complex is a composite specialized structure located where the DST of the nephron makes contact with the vascular pole of the glomerulus (i.e., the afferent and efferent arterioles).

A. THE COMPONENTS OF THE JG COMPLEX include:

1. **Macula Densa (MD) Cells.** The MD cells are **modified epithelial cells of the DST** that are located where the DST makes contact with the vascular pole of the glomerulus. MD cells have the following characteristics: columnar shaped, crowded nuclei that appear to be superimposed on each other, microvilli, and connected by desmosomes. **MD cells monitor changes in Na^+ levels in the DST fluid and stimulate the release of renin from JG cells.**

2. **JG Cells.** The JG cells are **modified smooth muscle cells** that are located in clusters of four to five cells in the tunica media of the afferent arteriole and early portion of the efferent arteriole. JG cells have the following characteristics: have a spherical nucleus, have many cell processes, communicate with neighboring cells through gap junctions, and have distinct granules that contain **renin** (a proteolytic enzyme). **JG cells secrete renin, monitor changes in blood pressure** (i.e., act as intrarenal baroreceptors), and are **innervated by postganglionic sympathetic nerves.**

3. **Extraglomerular Mesangium.** The extraglomerular mesangium is located at the vascular pole of the renal glomerulus and is continuous with the glomerular mesangium. The extraglomerular mesangium consists of a **mesangial matrix** and **extraglomerular mesangial cells (also called Lacis cells or Goormaghtigh cells).** Although the function of the extraglomerular mesangial cells is not quite clear, it appears that extraglomerular **mesangial cells mediate signals received from MD cells for transmission to JG cells and glomerular mesangial cells.**

B. THE FUNCTION OF THE JG COMPLEX. The JG complex is one of the most important regulators of **arterial blood pressure.** In most people, the daily average mean arterial blood pressure is strictly regulated at about **100 mm Hg** with fluctuations of **± 20 mm Hg.** This strict regulation provides organs with a blood flow at a constant perfusion pressure and minimizes cardiac, vascular, and renal damage. There are two main mechanisms that regulate arterial blood pressure:

1. **Baroreceptor Mechanism** involves the **autonomic nervous system** and regulates blood pressure in a **fast, moment-to-moment, neurotransmitter fashion.** The baroreceptors are stretch receptors that monitor **changes in blood pressure** and are located in the walls of the common carotid arteries (i.e., **carotid sinus**), great veins, atria, and aortic arch.

2. **Renin-Angiotensin II Mechanism** involves the **JG complex** of the kidney and regulates blood pressure in a **slow, long-term, hormonal fashion.** The JG complex regulates blood pressure through **renin** release from JG cells.

IX **Pharmacology of Diuretics (Figure 21-5).** Diuretics cause an increase in the volume of urine. Many diuretics have been developed that elicit their action on a specific renal tubule. Most diuretics act on the luminal side of the renal tubule and therefore must be present in the tubular fluid for action to occur. Diuretics in conjunction with other drugs are frequently used in the management of congestive heart failure and hypertension.

A. ACETAZOLAMIDE (DIAMOX) inhibits **carbonic anhydrase** by acting primarily on the **PCT**, resulting in decreased reabsorption of Na^+ (H_2O) and HCO_3^-. It is used clinically to treat glaucoma and altitude sickness.

B. MANNITOL (OSMITROL) promotes osmotic diuresis by acting primarily on the **PCT, PST, and DTL of the loop of Henle.** Mannitol is filtered at the glomerulus but is poorly reabsorbed so that mannitol "holds" H_2O within the lumen by virtue of its osmotic effect. It is used clinically to treat cerebral edema, increased intracranial pressure, or increased intraocular pressure.

C. LOOP DIURETICS (SULFONAMIDE DERIVATIVES). Furosemide (Lasix; "lasts six" hours), Bumetanide (Bumex), and Torsemide (Demadex) are Na^+-K^+-$2Cl^-$ symporter inhibitors that act on the **DST of the loop of Henle** and cause a decreased NaCl reabsorption (tubular fluid $\rightarrow$ plasma). This results in **NaCl diuresis**, and **hypokalemic alkalosis** due to the delivery of large amounts of Na^+ to the cortical collecting duct causing K^+ secretion (plasma $\rightarrow$ tubular fluid; K^+ wasting) and H^+ secretion (plasma $\rightarrow$ tubular fluid). Clinical uses include edema associated with congestive heart failure, liver disease, renal disease, and pulmonary disease; and hypertension (due to decrease in blood volume).

D. THIAZIDES DIURETICS (SULFONAMIDE DERIVATIVES). Hydrochlorothiazide (HydroDIURIL), Chlorthalidone (Hygroton), Indapamide (Lozol), and Metolazone (Mykrox) are Na^+-Cl^- symporter inhibitors that act on the early **DCT** and cause a decreased NaCl reabsorption (tubular fluid $\rightarrow$ plasma). This results in **NaCl diuresis**, and **hypokalemic alkalosis** due to the delivery of large amounts of Na^+ to the cortical collecting duct causing K^+ secretion (plasma $\rightarrow$ tubular fluid; K^+ wasting) and H^+ secretion (plasma $\rightarrow$ tubular fluid). Clinical uses include edema associated with congestive heart failure, liver disease, renal disease, and corticosteroid therapy; and hypertension (due to decrease in blood volume).

E. K^+-SPARING DIURETICS

1. **Spironolactone (Aldactone) is an aldosterone antagonist** that acts by reducing gene expression of Na^+ ion channels and Na^+-K^+ ATPase in the cortical collecting ducts. This causes a decreased NaCl reabsorption (tubular fluid $\rightarrow$ plasma), decreased K^+ secretion (plasma $\rightarrow$ tubular fluid; **K^+ sparing**), and decreased H^+ secretion (plasma $\rightarrow$ tubular fluid). This results in **NaCl diuresis with K^+ sparing**. Clinical uses include hypertension, edematous states, and primary hyperaldosteronism (Conn syndrome).

2. **Amiloride (Midamor) and Triamterene (Dyrenium) are Na^+ ion channel antagonists** that block Na^+ ion channels in the late DCT and CDs. This causes a decreased NaCl reabsorption (tubular fluid $\rightarrow$ plasma), decreased K^+ secretion (plasma $\rightarrow$ **tubular fluid; K^+ sparing**), and decreased H^+ secretion (plasma $\rightarrow$ tubular fluid). This results in **NaCl diuresis with K^+ sparing**. Clinical uses include hypertension and edematous states.

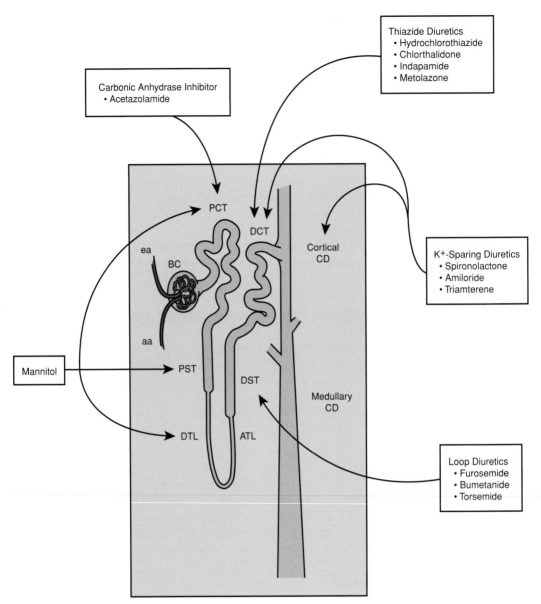

● **Figure 21-5 Pharmacologic site of action of diuretics.** ea, efferent arteriole; aa, afferent arteriole; PCT, proximal convoluted tubule; BC, Bowman capsule; PST, proximal straight tubule; DTL, descending thin limb of the loop of Henle; ATL, ascending thin limb of the loop of Henle; DCT, distal convoluted tubule; CD, collecting duct.

Clinical Considerations (Figure 21-6)

A. WILMS TUMOR (WT)

1. WT is a neoplasm associated with a loss-of-function mutation in the *WT1* **gene** on **chromosome 11p13** for the <u>W</u>ilms <u>t</u>umor <u>1</u> **protein**, which is a tumor suppressor protein. In addition, WT has been associated with mutations in the *WT2* **gene locus** on **chromosome 11p15.5**, which contains a cluster of imprinted genes. Imprinted genes are genes that demonstrate selective gene expression based on parental origin.

2. WT is the **most common renal malignancy of childhood**, which usually presents between 1 and 3 years of age.

3. WT presents as a large, solitary, well-circumscribed mass that on cut section is soft, homogeneous, and tan-gray in color. WT is interesting histologically in that this tumor tends to recapitulate different stages of embryologic formation of the kidney so that three classic histologic areas are described: a stromal area, a blastemal area of tightly packed embryonic cells, and a tubular area.

4. In 95% of the cases, the WT is sporadic and unilateral. In 5% of the cases, the WT arises in association with the **WAGR syndrome**, **Denys-Drash syndrome**, or **Beckwith-Wiedemann syndrome**.

B. AUTOSOMAL DOMINANT POLYCYSTIC KIDNEY DISEASE (ADPKD; ALSO CALLED ADULT POLYCYSTIC KIDNEY DISEASE)

1. **General Features.** ADPKD is an autosomal dominant genetic disorder caused (85% of cases) by mutations in the *PKD1* **gene** on **chromosome 16p13.3** for the protein **polycystin-1**, which is an integral membrane protein involved in cell-to-cell and cell-to-matrix interactions. The remaining cases of ADPKD are caused by mutations in the *PKD2* **gene** on **chromosome 4q21** for the protein **polycystin-2**, which is involved in calcium signaling.

2. **Pathologic Findings.** Pathologic findings include: bilaterally enlarged palpable kidneys; numerous cysts filled with a straw-colored fluid that distort the external contours of the kidney; cysts lined by simple cuboidal or columnar epithelium; and cysts arising from any point along the nephron; it is associated with cystic disease in other organs (especially the liver) and with berry aneurysms within the circle of Willis.

3. **Clinical Findings.** Clinical findings include: symptoms becoming apparent around 40 years of age, heaviness in the loins, bilateral flank and abdominal masses, hematuria, hypertension, azotemia, and uremia; it leads to end-stage renal disease.

C. AUTOSOMAL RECESSIVE POLYCYSTIC KIDNEY DISEASE (ARPKD; ALSO CALLED CHILDHOOD POLYCYSTIC KIDNEY DISEASE)

1. **General Features.** ARPKD is an autosomal recessive genetic disorder caused by mutations in the *PKHD1* **gene** on **chromosome 6p21.2** for the protein **fibrocystin** found in the cortical and medullary collecting duct of the kidney.

2. **Pathologic Findings.** Pathologic findings include: bilaterally enlarged spongy kidneys that may impede delivery of the infant, numerous cysts present but do not distort the external contours of the kidney, cysts arising from collecting ducts and tubules, and cysts arranged in a radial pattern perpendicular to the kidney surface; it is associated with congenital hepatic fibrosis.

3. **Clinical Findings.** Clinical findings include: that it leads to end-stage renal disease, where 75% of these infants die in the perinatal period.

D. GLOMERULONEPHRITIS (TABLE 21-2). Glomerulonephritis is a general term applied to kidney diseases where inflammation is prominent due to the deposition of immune complexes within the glomeruli, in situ formation of immune complexes, or antineutrophil cytoplasmic autoantibodies. The inflammation may cause proliferation of endothelial cells lining the glomerular capillaries, mesangial cells, or epithelial cells (both simple squamous epithelium lining Bowman capsule and podocytes). In severe cases, glomerular necrosis occurs. Glomerulonephritis causes **nephritic syndrome**, whose clinical findings include **hematuria (hallmark finding), proteinuria, edema, hypoalbuminemia**, and **hypertension**. The various types of glomerulonephritis are indicated here.

1. **Immunoglobulin A (IgA) Nephropathy (Berger Disease)**
   a. **General Features.** IgA nephropathy is caused by the deposition of IgA immune complexes within the mesangium whose etiology is unknown but usually follows infection of the respiratory or gastrointestinal tracts. IgA nephropathy is the most common type of glomerulonephritis.
   b. **Pathologic Findings.** Pathologic findings include: mesangial cell proliferation, immunofluorescence localizing IgA to the mesangium, and electron microscopy showing dense deposits within the mesangium.
   c. **Clinical Findings.** Clinical findings include: clinical presentation highly variable, ranging from asymptomatic microscopic hematuria → gross hematuria → end-stage renal disease; symptoms usually follow an episodic pattern exacerbated by respiratory and gastrointestinal infections.

2. **Acute Poststreptococcal Glomerulonephritis (APG)**
   a. **General Features.** APG is caused by the deposition of IgG immune complexes within the GBM and complement (C3) activation most commonly as a result of infection with **group A (β-hemolytic) streptococci** (e.g., poststreptococcal pharyngitis, "strep throat," impetigo).
   b. **Pathologic Findings.** Pathologic findings include: increased size of glomeruli; glomerular hypercellularity due to proliferation of endothelial cells, mesangial cells, neutrophils, and monocytes; immunofluorescence localizing IgG and C3 to "**lumpy-bumpy**" areas; and electron microscopy showing "lumpy-bumpy" subepithelial (beneath the podocytes) dense deposits.
   c. **Clinical Findings.** Clinical findings include: it most commonly being seen in children with a primary infection of the pharynx; diagnosis relying on a rise of antibody titers to streptococcal products; hematuria; oliguria; proteinuria; facial edema; hypertension; and a short-lived nephritic syndrome where most children recover spontaneously.

3. **Type I Membranoproliferative Glomerulonephritis (MPG)**
   a. **General Features.** Type I MPG is caused by the deposition of immune complexes within the mesangium and subendothelial (i.e., beneath the endothelium of the glomerular capillaries) as a result of persistent, indolent infections causing chronic antigenemia.
   b. **Pathologic Findings.** Pathologic findings include: increased size of glomeruli; capillary wall thickening; lobular distortion of glomeruli (hypersegmentation); mesangial cell proliferation; immunofluorescence localizing IgG and C3 to the mesangium and subendothelial areas; and electron microscopy showing a focal loss of podocytic foot processes and a "**train track**" GBM, which appears as two layers.
   c. **Clinical Findings.** Clinical findings include: it presenting as either a nephritic syndrome or nephrotic syndrome, or a combination of both.

4. **Type II Membranoproliferative Glomerulonephritis (MPG) or Dense Deposit Disease**
   a. **General Features.** Type II MPG is caused by deposition of complement within the GBM and mesangium, the basis of which is unknown. In most patients, **C3 nephritic factor** (a circulating IgG autoantibody that stabilizes the activated C3 convertase enzyme and causes increased C3 cleaving activity) is present.
   b. **Pathologic Findings.** Pathologic findings are similar to type I MPG with capillary wall thickening and include: lobular distortion of glomeruli (hypersegmentation), but mesangial cell proliferation may be reduced or absent; immunofluorescence localizes C3 within the GBM and mesangium, and electron microscopy shows **ribbonlike dense deposits** with the GBM.

    c.   **Clinical Findings.** Clinical findings include: presents as either a nephritic syndrome or nephrotic syndrome, or a combination of both.

5.   **Lupus Glomerulonephritis (LG)**

    a.   **General Features.** LG is caused by the deposition of immune complexes (IgG, IgM, IgA) within the mesangium, subendothelial (i.e., beneath the endothelium of the glomerular capillaries), and subepithelial (i.e., beneath the podocytes) and complement activation as a complication of **systemic lupus erythematosus (SLE)**. SLE is an autoimmune disease characterized by the hyperactivity of B lymphocytes with the production of a wide variety of autoantibodies including those against DNA (**anti ds-DNA**).

    b.   **Pathologic Findings.** Pathologic findings are highly variable and include the following: **class I**: SLE patient with no glomerular lesion, no immune complexes, and no glomerular dysfunction; **class II**: mesangial proliferation, immune complexes located in the mesangium, and mild hematuria and proteinuria; **class III**: focal proliferative (<50% of glomeruli affected), immune complexes located in the mesangium and subendothelial, and moderate nephritis (poor prognosis); **class IV**: diffuse proliferative (>50% of glomeruli affected), immune complexes located in the mesangium and subendothelial ("wire loop lesion"), and severe nephritis (worst prognosis); **class V**: membranous glomerulonephritis, immune complexes located subepithelial (i.e., beneath the podocytes), and nephrotic syndrome.

    c.   **Clinical Findings.** Clinical findings include: 70% of all SLE patients develop kidney disease, the clinical manifestations of which are varied as indicated by the different classes; renal biopsies of SLE patients are taken to evaluate the class, activity, and chronicity of the SLE rather than to diagnose LG. Currently, immunosuppressive therapy is only given in class III, IV, and V SLE nephritis (25% of class IV SLE patients reach end-stage renal disease within 5 years).

6.   **Antiglomerular Basement Membrane Glomerulonephritis (ABMG; Goodpasture Syndrome)**

    a.   **General Features.** ABMG is caused by deposition of IgG immune complexes (i.e., autoantibodies to a globular noncollagenous domain of type IV collagen) within the GBM. The autoantibodies generally cross-react with pulmonary basement membranes, and therefore when both the lungs and kidneys are involved, the term **Goodpasture syndrome** is used.

    b.   **Pathologic Findings.** Pathologic findings include: **glomerular crescents** in greater than 50% of glomeruli, which are formed by an inflammatory exudate containing macrophages and fibrin filling the urinary space and a proliferation of the simple squamous epithelium lining Bowman capsule; immunofluorescence localizing IgG in a linear fashion along the GBM; and electron microscopy showing focal breaks in the GBM but not immune dense deposits.

    c.   **Clinical Findings.** Clinical findings include: patients present with a rapidly progressive renal failure, and nephritic syndrome.

7.   **Antineutrophil Cytoplasmic Autoantibody Glomerulonephritis (ANCAG)**

    a.   **General Features.** ANCAG is not caused by immune complexes within the GBM, but instead is an aggressive, neutrophil-mediated disease causing glomerular necrosis and crescents. However, 90% of ANCAG patients have circulating **antineutrophil cytoplasmic autoantibodies (ANCAs)** directed against myeloperoxidase and proteinase 3. ANCAG may also affect the lungs, and therefore when both the lungs and kidney are involved, the term **Wegener granulomatosis** is used.

    b.   **Pathologic Findings.** Pathologic findings include: focal glomerular necrosis and glomerular crescents in greater than 50% of glomeruli, which are formed by an inflammatory exudate containing macrophages and fibrin filling the urinary space and a proliferation of the simple squamous epithelium lining Bowman capsule; immunofluorescence does not localize immune complexes along the GBM, and electron microscopy shows no immune dense deposits.

  c. **Clinical Findings.** Clinical findings include: patients present with a rapidly progressive renal failure, and nephritic syndrome; 75% of ANCAG patients have systemic small vessel vasculitis, and 80% of ANCAG patients develop end-stage renal disease within 5 years.

8. **Hereditary Nephritis (Alport Syndrome)**
  a. **General Features.** Hereditary nephritis is caused by an X-linked mutation in the COL4A5 gene that encodes for the α_5 chain of **type IV collagen,** which is a key component of the GBM and leads to a leaky GBM. Hereditary nephritis is a proliferative and sclerosing glomerular disease that is accompanied by defects of the ears and eyes.
  b. **Pathologic Findings.** Pathologic findings include: mild mesangial matrix expansion; mesangial hypercellularity; focal and diffuse glomerular sclerosis; and interstitial foam cells; immunofluorescence does not localize the α_5 chain of type IV collagen to the GBM, and electron microscopy shows an **irregularly thickened GBM with interlacing lamellae** surrounding electron lucent areas.
  c. **Clinical Findings.** Clinical findings include: disease being more severe in males; hematuria; proteinuria; hypertension; and progressive renal failure; nearly all males and 20% of females develop end-stage renal disease by 40 to 50 years of age.

E. **GLOMERULOPATHY (TABLE 21-3).** Glomerulopathy is a general term applied to kidney diseases where glomerular pathology can be observed but no inflammation is present. Glomerulopathy causes **nephrotic syndrome,** whose clinical findings include **proteinuria greater than 3.5 g of protein/day (hallmark finding), edema, hypoalbuminemia,** and **hyperlipidemia.** The various types of glomerulopathy are indicated here.

1. **Membranous Glomerulopathy**
  a. **General Features.** Membranous glomerulopathy is caused by the deposition of IgG and C3 immune complexes in a subepithelial (beneath the podocytes) location within the glomerulus whose etiology is unknown but may be secondary to SLE, hepatitis B, cancer, or penicillamine. Membranous glomerulopathy is the most common primary renal cause of nephrotic syndrome in young adults.
  b. **Pathologic Findings.** Pathologic findings include: slightly increased size of glomeruli; no hypercellularity of glomeruli; silver staining showing spikes of basement membrane; glomerular sclerosis in advanced stages; immunofluorescence localizing IgG and C3 to subepithelial domes that lie between the spikes of basement membrane; and electron microscopy showing spikes of basement membrane and domelike subepithelial dense deposits ("**spike and dome**" appearance).
  c. **Clinical Findings.** Clinical findings include: a clinical course that is highly variable; 25% of patients shows spontaneous remission, 50% of patients have persistent proteinuria and only partial loss of kidney function, and 25% of patients develop end-stage renal disease.

2. **Minimal Change Disease (Lipoid Nephrosis)**
  a. **General Features.** Minimal change disease is caused by immune system irregularities whose etiology is unknown. Minimal change disease is the most common cause of nephrotic syndrome in children under 5 years of age.
  b. **Pathologic Findings.** Pathologic findings include: glomeruli appearing normal or "minimally changed" and lipid droplets found in the renal cortex (i.e., lipoid nephrosis); immunofluorescence does not localize immune complexes, and electron microscopy shows fusion of podocyte foot processes, which leads to a disruption of the negative charge of the glomerular filtration barrier.

    c.   **Clinical Findings.** Clinical findings include: proteinuria due to large amounts of albumin in the urine (although this is not diagnostic); 90% of the patients show complete remission within 8 weeks of the start of corticosteroid therapy.

3. Focal Segmental Glomerulosclerosis

    a.   **General Features.** Focal segmental glomerulosclerosis is caused by many factors both idiopathic (primary) or secondary to obesity, renal mass reduction, sickle cell disease, cyanotic heart disease, acquired immunodeficiency syndrome (AIDS), and intravenous drug abuse.

    b.   **Pathologic Findings.** Pathologic findings include: a variable number of glomeruli (focal) and only a portion of the glomerulus (segmental) showing scarring (sclerosis) of the capillary loops; scarring involving collagen deposition along with lipid and proteinaceous material (e.g., plasma proteins; hyalinosis) accumulation; the remainder of the glomeruli appearing normal; immunofluorescence localizing IgM and C3; and electron microscopy showing fusion and focal detachment of podocyte foot processes along with dense deposits within the sclerotic areas, which correspond to the hyalinosis seen in light microscopy.

    c.   **Clinical Findings.** Clinical findings include: insidious onset with asymptomatic proteinuria; it frequently progressing to nephrotic syndrome; and progressive decline in renal function, leading to end-stage renal disease in 5 to 20 years.

4. Diabetic Glomerulosclerosis

    a.   **General Features.** Diabetic glomerulosclerosis is caused by type 1 or type 2 diabetes.

    b.   **Pathologic Findings.** Pathologic findings include: glomerular basement membrane (GBM) thickening; diffuse mesangial matrix expansion or focal, segmental, sclerotic lesions called **Kimmelstiel-Wilson nodules**; immunofluorescence localizing IgG, albumin, fibrinogen, and other plasma proteins, which represents nonimmunologic adsorption of these proteins to the GBM; and electron microscopy showing thickening of the lamina densa of the GBM and dense deposits containing lipid debris corresponding to the Kimmelstiel-Wilson nodules.

    c.   **Clinical Findings.** It is the leading cause of end-stage renal disease; the earliest sign is microalbuminuria; overt proteinuria occurs 10 to 15 years after the onset of diabetes and causes nephrotic syndrome; and it always progresses to end-stage renal disease.

5. Renal Amyloidosis

    a.   **General Features.** Renal amyloidosis is caused by complications of **amyloidosis**, which is a group of diseases that have in common the deposition of **amyloid** protein in the intercellular space of various organs. Renal amyloidosis is associated with **AL amyloid protein** and **AA amyloid protein**. AL amyloid is derived from lambda immunoglobulin light chains and is associated with AL amyloidosis, multiple myeloma, light chain deposition disease, and light chain cast nephropathy. AA amyloid is derived from an inflammatory serum protein called SAA and is associated with rheumatoid arthritis, chronic tuberculosis, and familial Mediterranean fever.

    b.   **Pathologic Findings.** Pathologic findings include: amyloid appearing as an amorphous, eosinophilic material, which can be specifically stained with Congo red or thioflavine T; early deposition of amyloid occurring in the mesangium that eventually spreads to obliterate capillary lumens; increased size of glomeruli due to amyloid deposition; and electron microscopy showing 10-nm nonbranching amyloid fibrils within the mesangium that are oriented perpendicular to the GBM along with the loss of podocyte foot processes.

    c.   **Clinical Findings.** Clinical findings include: proteinuria, nephrotic syndrome, and end-stage renal disease.

F. MALIGNANT NEPHROSCLEROSIS
1. **General Features.** Malignant nephrosclerosis is caused by malignant hypertension (i.e., >125 mm Hg diastolic pressure, retinal blood vessel changes, papilledema, and renal functional impairment) whereby the endothelium is damaged, leading to thrombosis (a type of thrombotic microangiopathy).
2. **Pathologic Findings.** Pathologic findings include: the following: size of kidney varies from small to enlarged; cut surface of kidney has a red/yellow mottled appearance with small cortical infarcts; kidney exhibits a microscopic background similar to benign nephrosclerosis; glomeruli show fibrinoid necrosis and consolidation; large arteries show edematous tunica intima expansion; afferent and efferent arterioles show fibrinoid necrosis; and vascular thrombosis is present.
3. **Clinical Findings.** Clinical findings include: headache, dizziness, visual disturbances, hematuria, and proteinuria; it occurs more frequently in men, and aggressive antihypertensive medication controls this disease very well.

G. PYELONEPHRITIS ("PYELO" = RENAL PELVIS). Pyelonephritis is a type of infectious tubulointerstitial nephritis caused by bacterial infection with involvement of the renal parenchyma, calyces, and pelvis. The various types of pyelonephritis are indicated here.
1. **Acute Pyelonephritis (APY)**
   a. **General Features.** APY is caused by bacterial infection either by the ascending route or hematogenous route. APY is a clinical syndrome. APY is characterized by an acute suppurative (purulent; pus-forming) inflammation of the kidney.
   b. **Pathologic Findings.** Pathological findings include: patchy suppurative inflammation of the renal interstitium and renal tubular necrosis (glomeruli are generally spared); suppuration causing discrete focal abscesses involving one or both kidneys or large, wedge-shaped areas where the suppuration has coalesced; infiltration with predominately neutrophils within the renal interstitium and renal tubules; renal papillary necrosis where the distal portion of the renal pyramids show gray-white to yellow necrosis that resembles infarction; pyonephrosis where the suppurative exudate fills the renal calyces, pelvis, and ureter; perinephric abscess where the suppurative inflammation breaks through the renal capsule into the perinephric tissue; and pyelonephritic scar that is associated with fibrosis and deformation of the underlying renal calyx and pelvis.
   c. **Clinical Findings.** Clinical findings include: flank pain; costovertebral angle tenderness; fever; chills; nausea and vomiting; diarrhea; bacteriuria; pyuria; and leukocyte casts (pus casts) within the urine, which indicate renal involvement. Urine and blood cultures are performed to determine infection; uncomplicated acute pyelonephritis follows a benign course and symptoms disappear within a few days after antibiotic treatment.
2. **Chronic Pyelonephritis (CPY)**
   a. **General Features.** CPY is caused by recurrent or persistent bacterial infection secondary to either vesicoureteral reflux or urinary tract obstruction. CPY is a radiologic diagnosis. CPY is characterized by a chronic tubulointerstitial nephritis (inflammation) along with a blunting deformity and dilatation of renal calyces with overlying corticomedullary scarring of kidney parenchyma, resulting in marked parenchymal loss. Of all the causes of tubulointerstitial nephritis, only CPY and analgesic nephropathy produce a deformity and dilatation of renal calyces with overlying corticomedullary scarring of kidney parenchyma.
   b. **Pathologic Findings.** Pathologic findings include: kidney scarring irregular and asymmetric; deformed (blunted) and dilated renal calyces with coarse,

discrete, overlying corticomedullary scarring; renal tubule atrophy, hypertrophy, and dilatation; dilated renal tubules containing colloidal casts that resemble thyroid follicles (called thyroidization); infiltration with neutrophils, lymphocytes, and plasma cells within the renal interstitium.

    c. **Clinical Findings.** Clinical findings are usually nonspecific. Some patients have recurrent acute symptomatic exacerbations of renal infection, some patients have no clear-cut symptoms despite persistent bacteriuria, and some patients complain of vague flank pain, abdominal pain, or intermittent low-grade fever.

    d. **Forms of CPY:** There are two main forms of CPY:

        i. **Chronic Reflux-associated Pyelonephritis (CRPY; Reflux Nephropathy).** CRPY is caused by recurrent or persistent bacterial infection secondary to vesicoureteral reflux and is the most common type of CPY. CRPY lacks an abrupt onset and is usually completely silent and diagnosed only during the investigation of acute urinary tract infections (UTIs), hypertension, or chronic renal failure especially in adult men, who are seen for treatment of UTIs less often than women. Generally, renal involvement in CRPY occurs early in childhood as a result of congenital vesicoureteral reflux, which may be unilateral or bilateral. The scars associated with CRPY occur in the upper and lower poles of the kidney where the renal papillae are concave shaped instead of convex shaped, which occurs in the rest of the kidney.

        ii. **Chronic Obstructive Pyelonephritis (COPY).** COPY is caused by recurrent or persistent bacterial infection secondary to urinary tract obstruction (e.g., calculi; "kidney stones"). COPY may be insidious in onset and present with many of the clinical findings of acute pyelonephritis. The scars associated with COPY occur in all renal papillae.

H. RENAL CELL CARCINOMA (RCC)

    1. **General Features.** RCC is a malignant neoplasm involving the epithelium lining the renal tubules and ducts and is the most common cancer of the kidney. In 95% of the cases, RCC is sporadic and unilateral. In 5% of the cases, RCC is hereditary and arises in association with von Hippel-Lindau (vHL) disease, hereditary (autosomal dominant) clear cell carcinoma, or hereditary (autosomal dominant) papillary carcinoma and is multifocal and bilateral.

    2. **Clinical Findings.** Clinical findings include: more frequent in men; risk factors that include tobacco use and obesity; incidence peaking at about 60 years of age; hematuria being the most common presenting sign; the classic triad of hematuria, flank pain, and a palpable abdominal mass observed in only 10% of patients; fever; weakness; malaise; weight loss; and production of ectopic hormones (e.g., parathyroidlike hormone) leading to a number of paraneoplastic syndromes (e.g., hypercalcemia, polycythemia, hypertension, feminization or masculinization, or Cushing syndrome; one of the great mimics in medicine); RCC tends to metastasize (to lungs and bones) before giving any clinical signs.

    3. The most common RCC is the **clear cell carcinoma** (70% frequency). The clear cell carcinoma tumor is solid and yellow-orange in color due to the presence of cytoplasmic lipid and glycogen, with cream-colored necrotic areas. A clear cell carcinoma shows spherical collections of neoplastic cells with a clear or granular cytoplasm that resemble proximal tubule cells. If the clear cell carcinoma is sporadic or hereditary, a deletion or an unbalanced chromosomal translocation (3;6, 3;8, 3;11) is present, resulting in a **deletion of the chromosome 3p12-p2G region.** This region contains the *VHL* gene. The VHL gene is an antioncogene (tumor suppressor gene) that encodes a protein that suppresses the cell cycle.

TABLE 21-2	VARIOUS TYPES OF GLOMERULONEPHRITIS	
Disease	General Features	Pathologic and Clinical Findings
IgA nephropathy	Deposition of IgA. Most common type of glomerulonephritis	Mesangial cell proliferation; IgA localized to mesangium; dense deposits within mesangium; asymptomatic to gross hematuria; follows a respiratory or GI infection
Acute poststreptococcal glomerulonephritis	Deposition of IgG	Glomerular hypercellularity; "lumpy-bumpy" deposits of IgG; short-lived nephritic syndrome; spontaneous recovery; follows a group A (β-hemolytic) streptococcal infection
Type I membranoproliferative glomerulonephritis	Deposition of immune complexes	Hypersegmentation of glomeruli; mesangial cell proliferation; IgG localized to mesangium and subendothelial areas; "train track" GBM; nephritic syndrome; nephrotic syndrome; combination of both syndromes
Type II membranoproliferative glomerulonephritis	Deposition of C3. C3 nephritic factor is present	Hypersegmentation of glomeruli; no mesangial cell proliferation; C3 localized to GBM and mesangium; ribbonlike GBM; nephritic syndrome; nephrotic syndrome; combination of both syndromes
Lupus glomerulonephritis	Deposition of IgG, IgM, and IgA. Complication of SLE	Class I; class II; class III; class IV: diffuse proliferative, immune complexes localized to the mesangium and subendothelial ("wire loop" lesion); severe nephritis (worst prognosis); class V; 70% of all SLE patients develop kidney disease; 25% of class IV patients reach end-stage renal disease within 5 y
Antiglomerular basement membrane glomerulonephritis (Goodpasture syndrome)	Deposition of IgG autoantibodies to type IV collagen; called Goodpasture syndrome when both lungs and kidney are involved	Glomerular crescents; IgG autoantibodies localized linearly along the GBM; focal breaks in the GBM; rapidly progressive renal failure; nephritic syndrome
Antineutrophil cytoplasmic autoantibody glomerulonephritis (Wegener granulomatosis)	No deposition of immune complexes; neutrophil-mediated disease; circulating antineutrophil cytoplasmic autoantibodies are present; called Wegener granulomatosis when both lungs and kidney are involved	Glomerular crescents; no IgG autoantibodies localized; no immune dense deposits along the GBM; rapidly progressive renal failure; nephritic syndrome; vasculitis; end-stage renal disease within 5 y
Hereditary nephritis (Alport syndrome)	X-linked mutation of the α_5 chain of type IV collagen	Mesangial matrix expansion; mesangial hypercellularity; focal and diffuse glomerular sclerosis; interstitial foam cells; irregularly thickened GBM with interlacing lamellae; disease is more severe in males; progressive renal failure; end-stage renal disease by 40–50 y of age

Nephritic syndrome: hematuria (hallmark finding), proteinuria, edema, hypoalbuminemia, and hypertension.

Ig, immunoglobulin; GI, gastrointestinal; GBM, glomerular basement membrane; C3, complement; SLE, systemic lupus erythematosus.

TABLE 21-3	VARIOUS TYPES OF GLOMERULOPATHY	
Disease	General Features	Pathologic and Clinical Findings
Membranous glomerulopathy	Deposition of IgG and C3 Unknown etiology Secondary to SLE, hepatitis B, cancer, or penicillamine Most common cause of nephrotic syndrome in young adults	No hypercellularity of glomeruli; basement membrane spikes; IgG and C3 localized to subepithelial domes; "spike and dome" GBM; highly variable clinical course; 25% of patients develop end-stage renal disease
Minimal change disease (lipoid nephrosis)	Immune system irregularities Unknown etiology Most common cause of nephrotic syndrome in children under 5 y of age	Minimally changed glomeruli; lipid droplets found in cortex; no immune complexes localized; fusion of podocyte foot processes; 90% of patients show complete remission after corticosteroid therapy
Focal segmental glomerulosclerosis	Idiopathic Secondary to obesity, renal mass reduction, sickle cell disease, cyanotic heart disease, AIDS, intravenous drug use	A variable number (focal) and only a portion of the glomerulus (segmental) show scarring (sclerosis); IgM and C3 localized; fusion and focal detachment of podocyte foot processes; insidious onset with asymptomatic proteinuria; end-stage renal disease in 5–20 y
Diabetic glomerulosclerosis	Caused by type 1 or type 2 diabetes	Diffuse mesangial matrix expansion; Kimmelstiel-Wilson nodules; IgG, albumin, fibrinogen, and plasma proteins localized to the GBM; thickened GBM; earliest sign is microalbuminemia; always progresses to end-stage renal disease
Renal amyloidosis	Caused by complication of amyloidosis Associated with AL amyloid and AA amyloid	Amorphous, eosinophilic material; specifically stained with Congo red or thioflavin T; 10-nm nonbranching amyloid fibrils within the mesangium; proteinuria; nephrotic syndrome; end-stage renal disease

Nephrotic syndrome: proteinuria >3.5–4.0 g of protein/day (hallmark finding), edema, hypoalbuminemia, and hyperlipidemia

Ig, immunoglobulin; C3, complement; SLE, systemic lupus erythematosus; GBM, glomerular basement membrane.

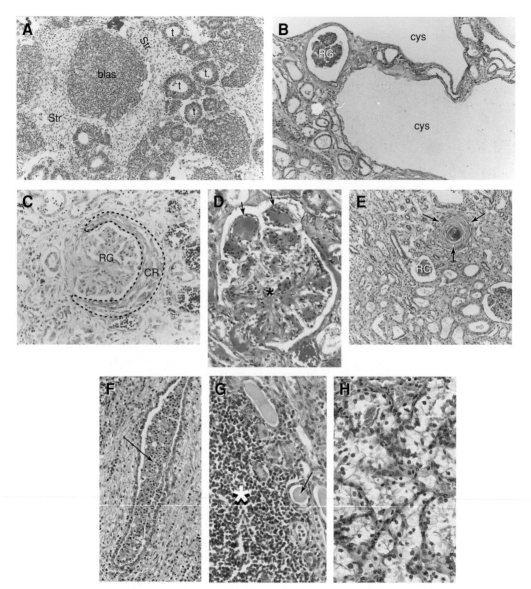

● **Figure 21-6 A:** Wilms tumor. Light micrograph (LM) shows the following three components: (a) metanephric blastema elements (blas) consisting of clumps of small, tightly packed embryonic cells; (b) stromal elements (str); and (c) epithelial elements generally in the form of abortive attempts at forming tubules (t) or glomeruli. **B:** Autosomal dominant polycystic kidney disease (ADPKD; also called adult polycystic kidney disease). LM shows large, fluid cysts (cys), which are found throughout the substance of the kidney. In between the cysts, some functioning nephrons can be found. ADPKD is associated in about 10% to 30% of the patients with a **Berry aneurysm** and subarachnoid hemorrhage. RG, renal glomerulus. **C:** Antiglomerular basement membrane glomerulonephritis (Goodpasture syndrome). LM shows the accumulation of cells in the urinary space (Bowman space) in the form of **"crescents"** (CR; *dotted lines*). The crescents are formed by an inflammatory exudate containing macrophages and fibrin filling the urinary space and the proliferation of simple squamous epithelium lining Bowman capsule. These crescents eventually obliterate the urinary space and compress the renal glomerulus (RG). **D:** Diabetic glomerulosclerosis. LM shows glomerular basement membrane thickening, a diffuse mesangial matrix expansion (*), and Kimmelstiel-Wilson nodules (*arrows*), which are hyaline masses situated at the periphery of the glomerulus. **E:** Malignant nephrosclerosis. Malignant nephrosclerosis is associated with the malignant phase of **hypertension.** Interlobular arteries and arterioles within the kidney show a tunica intima thickening due to a proliferation of smooth muscle cells and a concentric layering of collagen. This is called "onion skinning" or hyperplastic arteriolitis (*arrows*). RG, renal glomerulus **F:** Acute polynephritis. LM shows neutrophilic exudates within the collecting duct (*arrow*) and within the parenchyma. **G:** Chronic polynephritis. LM shows that interstitial spaces are wide and contain lymphocytes, macrophages, plasma cells, and neutrophils (*). The renal tubules become atrophic and contain hyaline casts in their lumen (*arrow*). The entire kidney parenchyma may histologically resemble the thyroid gland (thyroidization). **H:** Renal cell carcinoma (clear cell carcinoma). LM shows renal tubular epithelium consisting of clear, cuboidal cells arranged in tubules.

Case Study 21-1

A 30-year-old woman comes to your office complaining that "I feel like my body is swelling up. This has been going on for about 6 weeks now." She also tells you that "I'm feeling very tired and weak lately. I don't even feel like going out to the bars with my girl-friends." After some discussion, she informs you that she is an alcoholic who started abusing alcohol when she was 14 years old and "I'm not going to quit and go into any recovery program, so you can just forget about that. It's not going to happen." What is the most likely diagnosis?

Differentials

- Alcoholic cirrhosis, hypothyroidism, nephritic syndrome

Relevant Physical Examination Findings

- Tachypnea and tachycardia
- Blood pressure = 100/70 mm Hg
- Generalized 2+ pitting edema
- No enlargement of liver or spleen
- No ascites

Relevant Lab Findings

- Blood chemistry: aspartate aminotransferase (AST) = 15 U/L (normal); alanine amino-transferase (ALT) = 12 U/L (normal); albumin = 1.2g/L (low); thyroid-stimulating hormone (TSH) = 3.5 uIU/mL (normal)
- Urinalysis: protein = 5.1 g/24 hours (high)
- Kidney biopsy: sliver staining shows spikes of basement membrane.

Diagnosis: Membranous Glomerulopathy

- **Membranous Glomerulopathy (MG).** MG is caused by the deposition of IgG and C3 immune complexes in a subepithelial (beneath the podocytes) location within the glomerulus whose etiology is unknown but may be secondary to SLE, hepatitis B, cancer, or penicillamine. Membranous glomerulopathy is the most common primary renal cause of nephrotic syndrome in young adults. Pathologic findings of MG include slightly increased size of glomeruli; no hypercellularity of glomeruli; silver staining showing spikes of basement membrane; glomerular sclerosis in advanced stages; immunofluorescence localizing IgG and C3 to subepithelial domes that lie between the spikes of basement membrane; and electron microscopy showing spikes of basement membrane and domelike subepithelial dense deposits ("spike and dome" appearance). Clinical findings of MG include the clinical course being highly variable: 25% of patients shows spontaneous remission, 50% of patients have persistent proteinuria and only partial loss of kidney function, and 25% of patients develop end-stage renal disease.
- Cirrhosis is the end stage of chronic liver disease. Cirrhosis is defined as the destruction of normal hepatic architecture by fibrous septae that encompass regenerative nodules of hepatocyte parenchyma. Cirrhosis can progress to liver failure and present with jaundice (due to hyperbilirubinemia) and edema (due to hypalbuminemia). The spectrum of alcoholic liver disease involves three major morphologic and clinical conditions: fatty liver, alcoholic hepatitis, and alcoholic cirrhosis. Alcoholic cirrhosis is differentiated from other types of cirrhosis by the elevation of both AST and ALT, with AST twice that of ALT. The most common cause of cirrhosis is alcohol related.

- Severe hypothyroidism is called myxedema in adults or cretinism in children. Clinical findings of myxedema include cold intolerance; weight gain; mental and physical slowness; nonpitting edema; hair loss; and a dry, waxy swelling of the skin. The most common cause of myxedema is hyperthyroid therapy (surgery, radiation, or drugs).
- Glomerulonephritis is a general term applied to kidney diseases where inflammation is prominent due to the deposition of immune complexes within the glomeruli, in situ formation of immune complexes, or antineutrophil cytoplasmic autoantibodies. The inflammation may cause proliferation of endothelial cells lining the glomerular capillaries, mesangial cells, or epithelial cells (both simple squamous epithelium lining Bowman capsule and podocytes). In severe cases, glomerular necrosis occurs. Glomerulonephritis causes nephritic syndrome, whose clinical findings include hematuria (hallmark finding), proteinuria, edema, hypoalbuminemia, and hypertension.

Chapter 22

Hypophysis

The Adenohypophysis (Figure 22-1) has three subdivisions, called the **pars distalis**, **pars tuberalis**, and **pars intermedia**.

A. PARS DISTALIS contains the following endocrine cells:

1. **Somatotrophs (Acidophils)** secrete **growth hormone (GH)** under the control of the hypothalamic factors **growth hormone–releasing factor (GHRF)** and **growth hormone–inhibiting factor (somatostatin)**. GH binds to the GH receptor, which is a **receptor tyrosine kinase.** The functions of GH include the following.
   a. **In muscle,** GH decreases glucose uptake and increases protein synthesis.
   b. **In adipose tissue,** GH decreases glucose uptake and increases lipolysis.
   c. **In hepatocytes,** GH increases gluconeogenesis, increases glycogen degradation, and stimulates release of insulinlike growth factor 1 (IGF-1; somatomedin C).
   d. **IGF-1 (somatomedin C)** increases protein synthesis in chondrocytes at the epiphyseal growth plate and therefore causes **linear bone growth (pubertal growth spurt).**
   e. **Hyposecretion** of GH causes dwarfism.
   f. **Hypersecretion** of GH causes giantism or acromegaly.

2. **Mammotrophs (Acidophils)** secrete **prolactin (PRL)** under the control of the hypothalamic factors **thyrotropin-releasing factor (TRF)** and **prolactin-inhibiting factor (dopamine).** PRL binds to the PRL receptor, which is a **receptor tyrosine kinase.** The functions of PRL include the following:
   a. Promotes milk secretion in lactating women
   b. Promotes growth of mammary gland during pregnancy
   c. Inhibits release of gonadotropin-releasing factor (GnRF) and thereby prevents ovulation (in women) or spermatogenesis (in men).

3. **Thyrotrophs (Basophils)** secrete **thyroid-stimulating hormone (TSH)** under the control of the hypothalamic factor **TRF.** TSH binds to the TSH receptor, which is a **G protein–linked receptor.** The function of TSH is to stimulate triiodothyronine (T_3) and thyroxine (T_4) secretion from thyroid follicular cells.

4. **Corticotrophs (Basophils)** secrete **adrenocorticotropic hormone (ACTH)** under the control of the hypothalamic factor **corticotropin-releasing factor (CRF).** ACTH binds to the ACTH receptor, which is a **G protein–linked receptor.** ACTH is derived from a large precursor protein called **pro-opiomelanocortin (POMC).** POMC is cleaved into ACTH and **β-lipotrophic hormone (β-LPH).** β-LPH is further cleaved into γ-LPH and **β-endorphin.** γ-LPH may give rise to **β-melanocyte–simulating hormone (β-MSH),** which explains the hyperpigmentation observed in Addison disease. The functions of ACTH include the following:
   a. Stimulates the enzyme desmolase that converts cholesterol → pregnenolone, a key step in the synthesis of all steroids
   b. Stimulates the zona fasciculata and zona reticularis to secrete cortisol, androstenedione, and dehydroepiandrosterone (DHEA)

5. **Gonadotrophs (Basophils)** secrete follicle-stimulating hormone (FSH) and leuteinizing hormone (LH) under the control of the hypothalamic factor **GnRF.** FSH and LH bind to the FSH receptor and LH receptor, respectively, both of which are **G protein–linked receptors.** The functions of FSH and LH are as follows:

   a. **FSH.** In women, FSH promotes the growth of secondary follicles → Graafian follicles. In men, FSH maintains spermatogenesis and stimulates synthesis of androgen-binding protein (ABP) in Sertoli cells.

   b. **LH.** In women, LH promotes ovulation (LH surge), formation of corpus luteum (luteinization), and progesterone secretion. In men, LH stimulates testosterone secretion from Leydig cells.

B. **PARS TUBERALIS.** The pars tuberalis surrounds the median eminence and infundibular stem of the neurohypophysis. The par tuberalis contains the portal venules of the hypophyseal portal system.

C. **PARS INTERMEDIA.** The pars intermedia (rudimentary in humans) contains numerous colloid-filled cysts (**Rathke cysts**).

II. Hormonal Secretion from the adenohypophysis is controlled by hypothalamic neurons and the hypophyseal portal system.

A. **HYPOTHALAMIC NEURONS.** Neuronal cell bodies are located in the **arcuate nucleus, medial preoptic nucleus,** and **paraventricular nucleus** of the hypothalamus. The cell bodies synthesize **releasing factors (RFs)** and **inhibiting factors (IFs).** Axons project to the **median eminence,** where axon terminals secrete RFs and IFs into the primary capillaries of the hypophyseal portal system. RFs and IFs control hormone secretion from the adenohypophysis and include the following: **GHRF, growth hormone–inhibiting factor (somatostatin), prolactin-inhibiting factor (dopamine), TRF, CRF,** and **GnRF.**

B. **THE HYPOPHYSEAL PORTAL SYSTEM** has three components.

   1. **Primary capillaries** (fenestrated) are formed by the superior hypophyseal artery. They are located in the median eminence and are the site where RFs and IFs are secreted into the bloodstream.

   2. **Portal venules** are located in the pars tuberalis. They transport RFs and IFs to the pars distalis.

   3. **Secondary capillaries** (fenestrated) are located in the pars distalis. They are the site where RFs and IFs leave the bloodstream to stimulate or inhibit endocrine cells of the adenohypophysis.

III. The Neurohypophysis (Figure 22-1) receives axonal projections from neurons that have cell bodies located in the **supraoptic nucleus** and **paraventricular nucleus** of the hypothalamus.

A. The cell bodies synthesize **oxytocin,** which causes **milk ejection** (by stimulating myoepithelial cells in the mammary gland to contract) and **uterine contraction during childbirth** (by stimulating smooth muscle cells of the myometrium).

B. The cell bodies also synthesize **antidiuretic hormone (ADH),** which increases water reabsorption from tubular fluid to blood by the medullary collecting ducts of the kidneys.

C. As axons project to the neurohypophysis, large aggregations of neurosecretory vesicles (called **Herring bodies**) containing oxytocin or ADH (plus a carrier protein called **neurophysin**) can be observed.

D. Axon terminals secrete oxytocin and ADH into a capillary network formed by the inferior hypophyseal artery.

E. **PITUICYTES** also are found within the neurohypophysis and may function as glial-type cells.

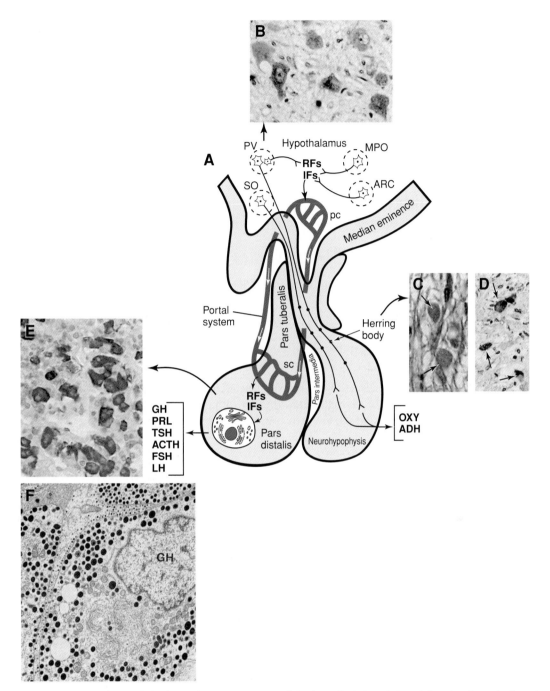

● **Figure 22-1 Histology of the hypophysis. A:** Diagram of the hypophysis (consisting of the adenohypophysis and neurohypophysis) and hypothalamus. Releasing factors (RFs) or inhibitory factors (IFs) from the arcuate nucleus (ARC), medial preoptic nucleus (MPO), and paraventricular nucleus (PV) of the hypothalamus enter the primary capillaries (pc) of the portal system. RFs and IFs travel to the secondary capillaries (sc), where they either stimulate or inhibit endocrine cells of the pars distalis. Oxytocin (OXY) and antidiuretic hormone (ADH) from the supraoptic nucleus (SO) and PV nucleus of the hypothalamus travel down axons to the neurohypophysis, where they are secreted at axon terminals into the blood. ACTH, adrenocorticotropin; ADH, antidiuretic hormone; FSH, follicle-stimulating hormone; GH, growth hormone; LH, luteinizing hormone; OXY, oxytocin; PRL, prolactin; TSH, thyroid-stimulating hormone. **B:** Light micrograph (LM) of neuronal cell bodies immunocytochemically stained for ADH within the PV nucleus of the hypothalamus. **C:** LM of Herring bodies (*arrows*) that characterize axons of the neurohypophysis (hematoxylin and eosin stain). **D:** LM of Herring bodies (*arrows*) immunocytochemically stained for ADH. **E:** LM of somatotrophs of the adenohypophysis immunocytochemically stained for GH. **F:** Electron micrograph of a somatotroph of the adenohypophysis. Note the abundant secretory granules, which contain GH.

Chapter 23

Thyroid

I **Thyroid Follicles** are bounded by **follicular cells** and **parafollicular cells**. They are filled with a colloid that consists of **iodinated thyroglobulin**.

II **Follicular Cells (Figure 23-1).** These cells:

A. Contain **thyroid-stimulating hormone (TSH) receptors**, which are G protein–linked receptors

B. Synthesize **thyroglobulin** and secrete thyroglobulin into the follicular lumen

C. Take up iodide (I^-) from the blood using a Na^+-I^- **cotransporter** and transport it to the follicular lumen

D. Oxidize iodide ($2I^- + H_2O_2 \rightarrow I_2$) using the enzyme **thyroid peroxidase** and **iodinate tyrosine residues in thyroglobulin**, thereby forming monoiodotyrosine (MIT) and di-iodotyrosine (DIT), which are then coupled to form triiodothyronine (T_3) and thyroxine (T_4)

E. Are stimulated by **TSH** to begin endocytosis of iodinated thyroglobulin. TSH is secreted from the adenohypophysis and is under the control of **thyrotropin-releasing factor (TRF)** released from hypothalamic neurons.

F. Break down iodinated thyroglobulin into MIT, DIT, T_3, and T_4 through **lysosomal degradation**

G. Deiodinate MIT and DIT using the enzyme **deiodinase** to recycle iodide (I^-), and secrete T_3 and T_4 into the bloodstream, which then circulate bound to **thyroid-binding globulin (TBG)**

H. T_3 (more potent) accounts for 10% of the thyroid output and has a half-life of 1 day. T_4 (less potent) accounts for 90% of the thyroid output and has a half-life of 8 days.

I. T_3 and T_4 function like **steroid hormones** in that they use a cytoplasmic receptor that belongs to the steroid-hormone receptor superfamily.

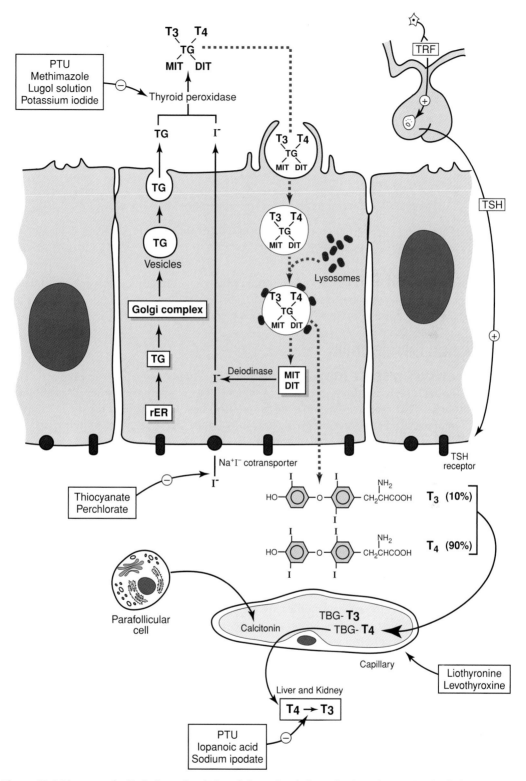

● **Figure 23-1 Diagram of triiodothyronine (T₃) and thyroxine (T₄) synthesis and secretion by follicular cells.**
The secretion of calcitonin by parafollicular cells also is shown. Note the location of drug action. DIT, diiodotyrosine; MIT, monoiodotyrosine; TBG, thyroid-binding globulin; TG, thyroglobulin; TSH, thyroid-stimulating hormone; TRF, thyroid-releasing factor; rER, rough endoplasmic reticulum; PTU, propylthiouracil.

III Functions of T_3 and T_4 include the following:

A. Increase basal metabolic rate (BMR; i.e., rate of oxygen consumption and heat production)

B. Increase cardiac output, increase systolic blood pressure, and decrease diastolic blood pressure

C. Increase gluconeogenesis, increase glycogen degradation, increase glucose oxidation, and increase lipolysis

D. Increase eating and glucose absorption

E. Stimulate cartilage growth

F. Stimulate endochondral ossification and linear growth of bone

G. Play a crucial role in central nervous system (CNS) development (a deficiency of T_3 and T_4 results in permanent brain damage)

IV Parafollicular Cells secrete **calcitonin**, which acts directly on osteoclasts to decrease bone resorption, thereby lowering blood Ca^{2+} levels. Calcitonin binds to the calcitonin receptor, which is a G protein–linked receptor.

V Clinical Considerations

A. **GRAVES DISEASE (GD)** is hyperthyroidism caused by a diffuse, hyperplastic (toxic) goiter. GD is relatively common in women. GD is an autoimmune disease that produces **TSH receptor–stimulating autoantibodies.** Clinical features include: ophthalmopathy (lid stare, eye bulging), heat intolerance, nervousness, irritability, and weight loss in the presence of a good appetite.

B. **SECONDARY HYPERTHYROIDISM** is relatively uncommon and may be caused by a TSH adenoma in the adenohypophysis.

C. **HASHIMOTO THYROIDITIS (HT)** is the most common cause of goitrous hypothyroidism. HT is relatively common in middle-aged women. HT is an autoimmune disease that produces **thyroid peroxidase autoantibodies.** Clinical features include: goiter and hypothyroidism. In some variants of Hashimoto thyroiditis, only hypothyroidism, and no goiter, exists.

D. **PRIMARY HYPOTHYROIDISM (PH)** is most commonly idiopathic, whereby **TSH receptor–blocking autoantibodies** are present. Clinical features include: low blood pressure, low heart rate, low respiratory rate, reduced body temperature, and myxedema (peripheral nonpitting edema).

E. **SECONDARY HYPOTHYROIDISM** is relatively uncommon and caused by a deficiency in the adenohypophysis (low TSH secretion) or hypothalamus (low thyrotropin-releasing factor [TRF] secretion).

F. **ESTROGEN EFFECT.** The use of oral contraceptive pills or the use of diethylstilbestrol for treatment of prostatic cancer increases synthesis of TBG.

G. **DIFFUSE NONTOXIC (SIMPLE) GOITER** is an enlargement of the entire thyroid gland in a diffuse manner without producing nodules. A simple goiter occurs most commonly in particular geographic areas (called **endemic goiter**), most often caused by deficiency of iodine in the diet. Wherever endemic goiter is prevalent, endemic **cretinism** occurs. A severe iodine deficiency during fetal development results in growth retardation and severe mental retardation.

H. DIAGNOSIS. Table 23-1 shows the laboratory findings used for diagnosis.

TABLE 23-1	LABORATORY FINDINGS USED FOR DIAGNOSIS OF THYROID DISORDERS					
Disorder	Mechanisms	Total T_4[a]	T_3RU (TBG)[b]	FTI[c]	TSH	I^{131} Uptake
Graves disease	Production of TSH receptor-stimulating autoantibodies	High	High (low)	High	Undetectable	High
Secondary hyperthyroidism	TSH adenoma	High	High (low)	High	High	High
Factitious thyrotoxicosis	Excessive exogenous thyroid hormone intake	High	High (low)	High	Low	Low
Thyroiditis	Inflammation of bacterial or viral origin	High	High (low)	High	Low	Low
Hashimoto thyroiditis	Production of thyroid peroxidase autoantibodies	Low	Low (high)	Low	High	Low
Primary hypothyroidism	Production of TSH receptor–blocking antibodies	Low	Low (high)	Low	Very high	Low
Secondary hypothyroidism	Low TSH secretion by adenohypophysis or low TRF secretion by the hypothalamus	Low	Low (high)	Low	Low	Low
Increased TBG (increased estrogen)	Oral contraceptives, DES therapy for prostate cancer	High	Low (high)	Normal	Normal	Normal
Decreased TBG (increased androgens)	Steroid abuse	Low	High (low)	Normal	Normal	Normal

T_4, thyroxine; T_3RU, triiodothyronine resin uptake test; TBG, thyroid-binding globulin; FTI, free thyroxine index; TSH, thyroid-stimulating hormone; I^{131}, radioactive iodine I^{131} uptake; TRF, thyrotropin-releasing factor; DES, diethylstilbestrol.
[a]Total T_4 measures both bound and free T_4.
[b]The T_3RU test is not a measure of serum T_3 levels; rather, it measures the percentage of free T_4. This test evaluates TBG levels via a competition assay between a resin and TBG for radioactive T_3. If TBG levels are low, then more radioactive T_3 will bind to the resin. TBG has an inverse relationship to T_3RU.
[c]The FTI is a measure of free T_4. It is calculated by multiplying the total $T_4 \times T_3RU$. The FTI is rapidly becoming obsolete as major medical centers are using assays that directly measure free T_4.

VI Pharmacology of the Thyroid

A. PROPYLTHIOURACIL (PTU) inhibits thyroid peroxidase and the peripheral conversion of $T_4 \rightarrow T_3$. It is used clinically to treat hyperthyroidism (e.g., Graves disease) and thyrotoxicosis in pregnant women since it crosses the placenta to a lesser degree than methimazole.

B. METHIMAZOLE (TAPAZOLE) inhibits thyroid peroxidase. It is used clinically to treat hyperthyroidism (e.g., Graves disease) but not thyrotoxicosis in pregnant women since it crosses the placenta to a greater degree than PTU.

C. LUGOL SOLUTION AND POTASSIUM IODIDE (THYRO-BLOCK, PIMA) inhibit the secretion of T_3 and T_4 and inhibit the iodination of thyroglobulin (Wolff-Chaikoff effect). They are used clinically to treat hyperthyroidism (e.g., Graves disease).

D. LIOTHYRONINE SODIUM (CYTOMEL, TRIOSTAT) is T_3. It is used clinically to treat myxedema coma, which is a medical emergency caused by long-standing hypothyroidism.

E. LEVOTHYROXINE SODIUM (SYNTHROID, LEVOTHROID) is T_4. It is used clinically as hormone replacement therapy to treat hypothyroidism or to prevent cretinism in newborns.

VII Selected Photomicrographs

A. Normal thyroid, Hashimoto thyroiditis, and Graves disease (Figure 23-2)

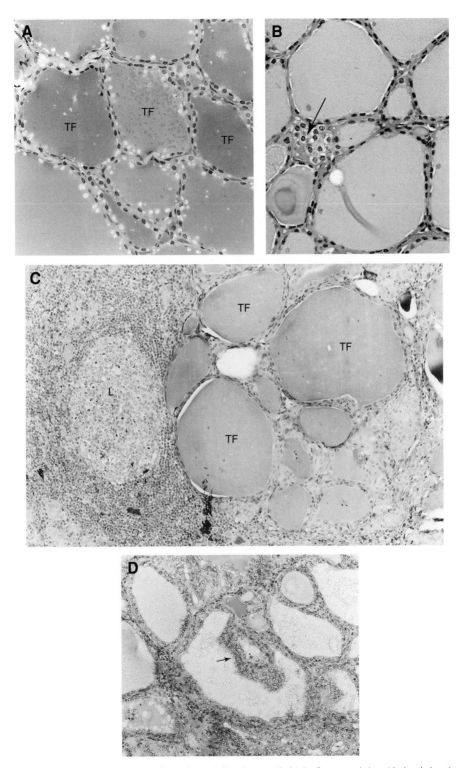

● **Figure 23-2 Normal and pathologic thyroid. A:** Light micrograph (LM) of a normal thyroid gland showing numerous thyroid follicles (TF) containing colloidal material. The follicles are lined by follicular cells arranged as a simple cuboidal epithelium. **B:** LM of a normal thyroid gland showing a cluster of parafollicular cells, which secrete calcitonin. **C:** LM of Hashimoto thyroiditis (HT). HT is characterized by a high lymphocytic infiltration that may form lymphoid follicles with germinal centers (L). Normal thyroid follicles (TF) also are observed. **D:** LM of Graves disease (GD). Graves disease is caused by a diffuse, hyperplastic goiter. The follicular cells are increased in number (hyperplasia) and arranged as a simple tall columnar epithelium. In addition, the follicular cells can form buds that encroach into the colloidal material (*arrow*).

B.   Papillary carcinoma and medullary carcinoma (Figure 23-3)

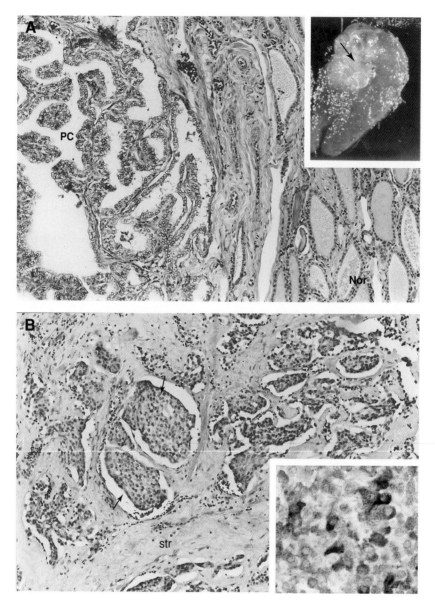

● **Figure 23-3 Thyroid carcinomas. A:** LM of papillary carcinoma (PC). Normal thyroid parenchyma can be observed (Nor). PC infiltrates normal thyroid parenchyma and forms elaborate branching papillae that are lined by single to multiple layers of follicular cells. The nuclei of follicular cells do not contain nucleoli ("Orphan Annie eyes"). Psammoma bodies sometimes surrounded by calcific lamellations are generally found within the core of the papillae. *Inset:* Gross photograph of a papillary carcinoma showing a yellow-white infiltrative mass (*arrow*) with some fibrous strands. **B:** LM of medullary carcinoma (MC). MC is an endocrine neoplasm of the parafollicular cells that secrete calcitonin. The parafollicular cells are usually arranged in cell nests (*arrow*) surrounded by bands of stroma (str) containing amyloid. *Inset:* LM of medullary carcinoma cells immunocytochemically stained for calcitonin.

Case Study 23-1

A 40-year-old woman comes to your office complaining that "About 4 weeks ago, I started feeling very nervous for no good reason. And, sometimes my heart starts to pump so fast it feels like it is going to jump out of my chest." She also tells you that "I have a real good appetite and have been eating a lot lately, but I still lost 15 pounds." After some discussion, she informs you that she can't stand this hot weather, has not had a period in 3 months, and frequently has diarrhea. What is the most likely diagnosis?

Differentials

- Hashimoto thyroiditis, menopause, pheochromocytoma

Relevant Physical Examination Findings

- Tachycardia
- Moist, warm skin
- Mild exophthalmos
- Goiter
- Resting tremor of the hands

Relevant Lab Findings

- Blood chemistry: total T_4 = 17.2 μg/mL (high); free thyroxine index (FTI) = 5.8 (high); TSH = undetectable
- Urinalysis: catecholamine = normal
- Thyroid scan: high I^{131} uptake
- Thyroid biopsy: follicular cells are increased in number (hyperplasia) and arranged as simple tall columnar epithelium; follicular cells form buds that encroach into the colloid material.

Diagnosis: Graves Disease

- **Graves Disease (GD).** GD is hyperthyroidism caused by a diffuse, hyperplastic (toxic) goiter. GD is the most common form of hyperthyroidism. GD is an autoimmune disease that produces TSH receptor–stimulating autoantibodies. These autoantibodies mimic TSH and cause increased secretion of T_3 and T_4. The normal negative feedback loop does not inhibit the autoantibodies so that the thyroid gland is constantly stimulated. Clinical findings of hyperthyroidism include restlessness, irritability, and fatigue; resting tremor in the hands; heat intolerance; sweating with warm, moist skin; tachycardia with palpitations; fat and muscle loss despite increased caloric intake; thinning of hair; diarrhea; and amenorrhea.
- Hashimoto thyroiditis (HT) is the most common cause of goitrous hypothyroidism. In some variants of Hashimoto thyroiditis, only hypothyroidism, and no goiter, exists. HT is relatively common in middle-aged women. HT is an autoimmune disease that produces thyroid peroxidase autoantibodies and destroys the thyroid gland. HT progresses from a euthyroid state → transient hyperthyroidism → hypothyroidism. Clinical findings of hypothyroidism include myxedema; cold intolerance; weight gain; low pitch of voice; mental slowing; increased menstrual bleeding; constipation; edema of face, eyelids, and hands; and brittle and dry hair that falls out.
- Menopause is the stoppage of the menstrual cycle in women around 50 years of age. Clinical findings of menopause include hot flashes, sweating, depression, and insomnia. It should be considered that menopause and GD may run concurrently.
- Pheochromocytoma is a relatively rare (usually not malignant) catecholamine-producing tumor (both epinephrine and norepinephrine) of the adrenal medulla. A pheochromocytoma occurs mainly in adults and is generally found in the region of the adrenal gland but also is found in extra-adrenal sites. It occurs within families as part of the multiple endocrine neoplasia type 2 (MEN 2) syndrome. Clinical findings of pheochromocytoma include persistent or paroxysmal hypertension, anxiety, tremor, profuse sweating, pallor, chest pain, abdominal pain, increased urine vanillylmandelic acid (VMA) and metanephrine levels, inability to suppress catecholamines with clonidine, and hyperglycemia.

Chapter 24

Parathyroid

I   **Chief Cells** secrete **parathyroid hormone (PTH)**. PTH binds to the PTH receptor, which is a G protein–linked receptor.

II   **Oxyphil Cells** are distinctly eosinophilic because of the numerous mitochondria within the cytoplasm, but they have no known function.

III   **Calcium Homeostasis (Figure 24-1).** The body regulates blood Ca^{2+} levels closely because hypocalcemia results in tetanic convulsions and death. The substances most important for elevating blood Ca^{2+} levels are the following:

A. PTH

1. PTH increases kidney reabsorption of Ca^{2+} from the tubular fluid $\rightarrow$ plasma by the distal convoluted tubule (DCT) and collecting duct (CD), thereby elevating blood Ca^{2+} levels.

2. PTH acts directly on osteoblasts to secrete **macrophage colony-stimulating factor (M-CSF)** and expression of a cell surface protein called **RANKL**.

   a. M-CSF stimulates monocytes to differentiate into macrophages and express a cell surface receptor called **RANK**.

   b. RANKL (on the osteoblast) and RANK (on the macrophage) interact and cause the differentiation of macrophages into **osteoclasts**.

   c. Osteoclasts increase bone resorption, thereby elevating blood Ca^{2+} levels.

3. PTH increases the synthesis of 1α-hydroxylase in the kidney by the proximal convoluted tubule (PCT), thereby elevating blood 1,25-hydroxyvitamin D [1,25-$(OH)_2$ vitamin D] levels.

B. 1,25-$(OH)_2$ VITAMIN D

1. 1,25-$(OH)_2$ vitamin D mainly stimulates absorption of Ca^{2+} and PO^{2-} ions from the intestinal lumen into the blood, thereby elevating blood Ca^{2+} and PO^{2-} levels.

2. 1,25-$(OH)_2$ vitamin D also acts directly on osteoblasts to secrete interleukin 1 (IL-1), which stimulates osteoclasts to increase bone resorption, thereby elevating blood Ca^{2+} levels.

C. CALCITONIN is secreted by parafollicular cells found with the thyroid gland. Calcitonin acts directly on osteoclasts to decrease bone resorption, thereby lowering blood Ca^{2+} levels.

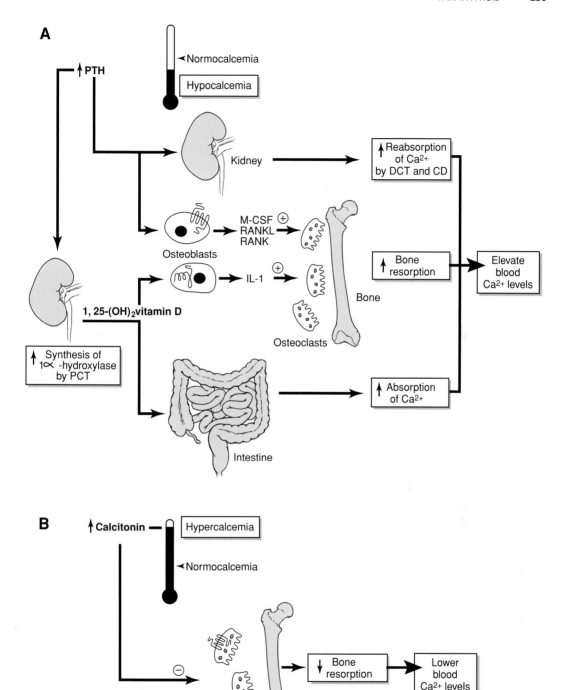

● **Figure 24-1 Calcium homeostasis. A:** Blood calcium levels can be depicted on a thermometer such that when blood calcium levels are too low, parathyroid hormone (PTH) is released. PTH and 1,25-(OH$_2$) vitamin D regulate blood calcium levels by acting on the kidney, bone, and intestine to elevate blood calcium levels. **B:** Blood calcium levels can be depicted on a thermometer such that when blood calcium levels are too high, calcitonin is released. Calcitonin regulates blood calcium levels by acting on bone to lower blood calcium levels. M-CSF, macrophage colony-stimulating factor; RANK, receptor for activation of nuclear factor-κB; RANKL, RANK ligand.

IV **Clinical Considerations**

A. **PRIMARY HYPOPARATHYROIDISM** (e.g., accidental surgical removal, DiGeorge syndrome, autoimmune destruction) is characterized by the absence of PTH, leading to **hypocalcemia**. Chronic renal failure and vitamin D deficiency also lead to hypocalcemia. Clinical findings include carpopedal spasm, laryngospasm, **Chvostek sign** (tapping facial nerve elicits spasm of facial muscles), **Trousseau phenomenon** (inflated blood pressure cuff on arm elicits carpal tunnel spasm), calcification of basal ganglia, cataracts, and tetany. Seizures and cardiac arrest may occur in severe cases.

B. **PSEUDOHYPOPARATHYROIDISM** is a rare condition characterized by abnormal PTH receptors, leading to **hypocalcemia**, although there are high PTH levels.

C. **PRIMARY HYPERPARATHYROIDISM** (e.g., adenoma, hyperplasia, associated with multiple endocrine neoplasia [MEN] syndromes) is characterized by excessive secretion of PTH, leading to **hypercalcemia**. Clinical findings include osteitis fibrosa cystica (bone softening and painful fractures), urinary calculi, abdominal pain (due to constipation, pancreatitis, or biliary stones), depression/lethargy, and cardiac arrhythmias. Think "painful bones, kidney stones, belly groans, mental moans."

D. **MALIGNANT TUMORS** (e.g., lung, breast, or ovarian carcinomas) may secrete **parathyroid hormone–related protein (PTH-rP)**, leading to **humoral hypercalcemia of malignancy**.

E. **DIAGNOSIS.** Table 24-1 shows laboratory findings used for diagnosis.

TABLE 24-1	LABORATORY FINDINGS USED FOR DIAGNOSIS OF PARATHYROID DISORDERS		
Disorder	**Calcium**	**Phosphorus**	**Parathyroid Hormone**
Hypocalcemia			
Primary hypoparathyroidism	Low	High	Low
Pseudohypoparathyroidism	Low	High	Normal → high
Secondary hypoparathyroidism (malabsorption)	Low	Low	High
Secondary hypoparathyroidism (renal failure)	Low	High	High
Hypoalbuminemia	Low (normal ionized calcium)	Normal	Normal
Alkalosis	Normal (decreased ionized calcium)	Normal	High
Hypercalcemia			
Primary hyperparathyroidism	High	Low	High
Malignant tumors	High	Low	Low

Ⓥ Pharmacology of Calcium Homeostasis

A. CALCIUM CARBONATE (TUMS), CALCIUM CHLORIDE, CALCIUM GLUCEPTATE, AND CALCIUM GLUCONATE are calcium salt preparations. They are used to treat hypocalcemia.

B. CALCIFEDIOL, CALCITRIOL, DIHYDROTACHYSTEROL, AND ERGOCALCIFEROL are vitamin D preparations. They are used to treat hypocalcemia.

C. ETIDRONATE (DIDRONEL) AND PAMIDRONATE (AREDIA) are bisphosphonates that inhibit osteoclast activity. They are used to treat hypercalcemia.

D. HUMAN CALCITONIN (CIBACALCIN) AND SALMON CALCITONIN (CALCIMAR) are the 32-amino-acid peptide secreted by the parafollicular cells of the thyroid gland that acts directly on osteoclasts to decrease bone resorption. They are used to treat hypercalcemia.

Ⓥ Selected Photomicrographs (Figure 24-2)

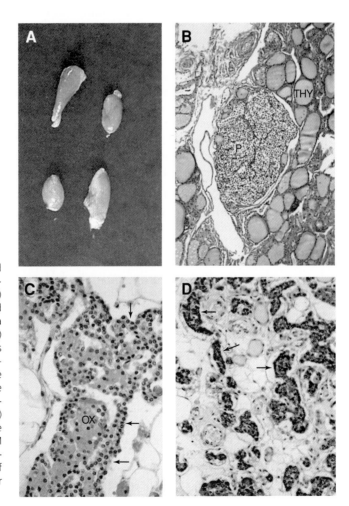

● **Figure 24-2 A:** Four normal parathyroid glands dissected at autopsy of a 53-year-old man. **B:** A normal parathyroid gland (P) embedded entirely within the thyroid gland (THY). **C:** Light micrograph (LM) of a parathyroid gland. The chief cells (*arrows*) are arranged in sheets or cords. Chief cells contain lipid droplets, glycogen, and lysosomes. Chief cells synthesize and secrete parathyroid hormone (PTH) and therefore contain a distinct Golgi and rough endoplasmic reticulum (rER). Oxyphil cells (Ox) have a distinctly eosinophilic cytoplasm due to a large number of mitochondria. **D:** LM of a parathyroid gland immunocytochemically stained for PTH. Note the staining of chief cells (*arrows*) arranged in sheets or cords.

Chapter 25

Adrenal

I **Cortex.** Cortical cells of the adrenal gland synthesize and secrete steroid hormones. They have abundant smooth endoplasmic reticulum (sER), mitochondria with tubular cristae, and lipid droplets, which are characteristic of all steroid-secreting cells.

A. ZONA GLOMERULOSA (ZG). This region constitutes **15%** of the cortical volume. ZG cells are arranged in a **glomerularlike fashion**. ZG cells synthesize and secrete **aldosterone**. The secretion of aldosterone is controlled by the **renin-angiotensin system**. Aldosterone has a **half-life of 20 minutes** as it is metabolized by the liver and excreted as a glucuronide. Urine levels of **aldosterone 3-glucuronide** are used for diagnostic purposes. The functions of aldosterone include the following:

1. **Increases Na^+ reabsorption** from tubular fluid $\rightarrow$ plasma (water follows) by the cortical collecting ducts of the kidneys

2. **Increases K^+ secretion** from plasma $\rightarrow$ tubular fluid by the cortical collecting ducts of the kidneys

3. **Increases H^+ secretion** from plasma $\rightarrow$ tubular fluid by the cortical collecting ducts of the kidneys

4. **Increases Na^+ absorption** by enterocytes of the large intestine

5. **Increases Na^+ reabsorption** from excretory ducts of eccrine sweat glands

B. ZONA FASCICULATA (ZF). This region constitutes **78%** of the cortical volume. ZF cells are arranged in **vertical cords**. ZF cells synthesize and secrete **cortisol**. The secretion of cortisol is controlled by **corticotropin-releasing factor (CRF)** and **adrenocorticotropic hormone (ACTH)** from the hypothalamus and adenohypophysis, respectively. Abnormally high levels of ACTH (e.g., adenoma of adenohypophysis) cause hypertrophy of the ZF. Abnormally low levels of ACTH (e.g., hypophysectomy) cause atrophy of the ZF. Cortisol has a **half-life of 70 minutes** as it is metabolized by the liver and excreted in the urine as a glucuronide. Urine levels of **17-hydroxycorticoids** are used for diagnostic purposes. The functions of cortisol include the following:

1. Inhibits glucose uptake and decreases insulin sensitivity in adipose tissue and muscle

2. Stimulates lipolysis in adipose tissue, which forms glycerol, used by the liver as substrate for gluconeogenesis, and fatty acids, which are metabolized by the liver for energy

3. Stimulates protein catabolism in muscle, which forms amino acids that are used by the liver as substrate for gluconeogenesis

4. Stimulates gluconeogenesis. Overall, the most important metabolic effect of cortisol is to provide glycerol (from fat lipolysis) and amino acids (from muscle catabolism) to the liver as gluconeogenic substrates.

5. Inhibits bone formation, causing osteoporosis by reducing the synthesis of type I collagen and decreasing the absorption of Ca^{2+} by the intestinal tract by blocking the action of 1,25-$(OH)_2$ vitamin D

6. Produces an anti-inflammatory response at high concentrations by inhibition of **phospholipase A_2**, which releases arachidonic acid (a precursor for many immune mediators); **interleukin-2 (IL-2) production**, thereby preventing proliferation of T lymphocytes; and **histamine and serotonin release** from mast cells

7. Stimulates surfactant production in the fetus

C. **ZONA RETICULARIS (ZR).** This region constitutes 7% of the cortical volume. ZR cells are arranged in an **anastomosing network of cords** and contain large amounts of **lipofuscin pigment**. ZR cells synthesize and secrete **dehydroepiandrosterone (DHEA)** and **androstenedione**. The secretion of DHEA and androstenedione is controlled by CRF and ACTH from the hypothalamus and adenohypophysis, respectively. Although DHEA and androstenedione are weak androgens, they are converted to testosterone by peripheral tissues. DHEA and androstenedione are metabolized by the liver to 17-ketosteroids. Urine levels of **17-ketosteroids** are used for diagnostic purposes. The functions of DHEA and androstenedione include the following.

1. In women, DHEA and androstenedione conversion to testosterone is a main source of testosterone. During puberty, DHEA and androstenedione also may serve as substrates for conversion to estrogen.

2. In men, DHEA and androstenedione conversion to testosterone is of little biologic significance because the testes produce most of the testosterone.

D. **SYNTHESIS OF ADRENOCORTICAL HORMONES USES CHOLESTEROL AS A PRECURSOR (FIGURE 25-1).**

E. **CLINICAL CONSIDERATIONS**

1. **Primary hyperaldosteronism**

a. **Cause.** Elevated levels of aldosterone (i.e., hyperaldosteronism) are commonly caused by an aldosterone-secreting adenoma **(Conn syndrome)** within the ZG.

b. **Symptoms.** Primary hyperaldosteronism is characterized clinically by hypertension, hypernatremia due to increased Na^+ reabsorption, weight gain due to water retention, and hypokalemia due to increased K^+ secretion.

c. **Treatment.** It is treated by **surgery and/or spironolactone**, which is an aldosterone receptor antagonist and therefore an effective antihypertensive and diuretic agent.

2. **Cushing syndrome**

a. **Cause.** Cushing syndrome is most commonly caused by administration of **large doses of steroids** for treatment of primary disease. If not iatrogenic, elevated levels of cortisol (i.e., hypercortisolism) are caused by an **ACTH-secreting adenoma** within the adenohypophysis (75% of the cases; strictly termed **Cushing disease**) or **adrenal cortical adenoma** (25% of the cases).

b. **Symptoms.** Cushing syndrome is characterized clinically by mild hypertension, impaired glucose tolerance, acne, hirsutism, oligomenorrhea, impotence and loss of libido in men, osteoporosis with back pain and buffalo hump, central obesity, moon facies, and purple skin striae (bruise easily).

c. **Treatment.** Surgery is an option. **Aminoglutethimide, metyrapone, and ketoconazole** are used in the treatment of Cushing syndrome.

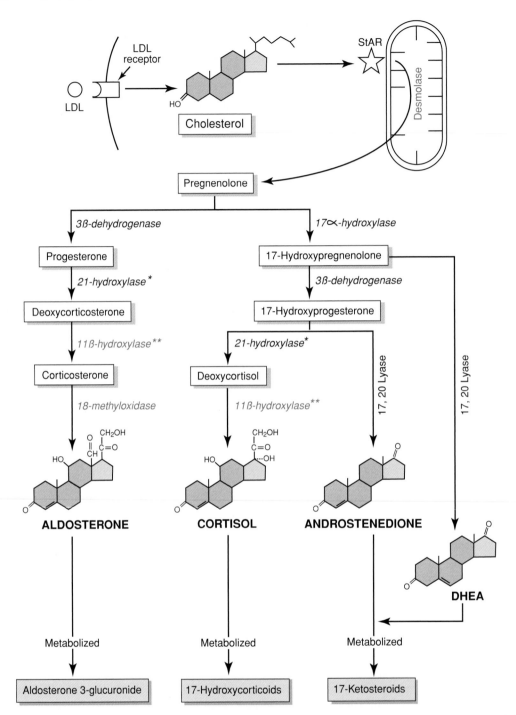

● **Figure 25-1 Synthesis and metabolism of adrenocortical steroid hormones. Cholesterol** is the precursor of all steroid hormones. Most of the cholesterol is derived from **low-density lipoprotein (LDL),** which binds to the **LDL receptor** and enters the cell by **receptor-mediated endocytosis.** Cholesterol is then transported into the mitochondria by **steroidogenic acute regulatory protein StAR (StAR).** Within the mitochondria, cholesterol is metabolized to pregnenolone by the enzyme desmolase. Pregnenolone is then transported to the cytoplasm. In general, enzymes for steroid biosynthesis are located either in the mitochondria or smooth endoplasmic reticulum (sER) such that substrate intermediates are shuttled back and forth from mitochondria to the sER. Enzymes located in the mitochondria are shaded. All other enzymes are located in the sER. The metabolic urine breakdown products (in *shaded boxes*) are used for diagnostic purposes. 21-Hydroxylase (*asterisk*) and 11β-hydroxylase (*double asterisk*) are enzymes involved in congenital adrenal hyperplasia.

3. **Congenital adrenal hyperplasia**
   a. **Cause.** Congenital adrenal hyperplasia is caused most commonly by mutations in genes for enzymes involved in adrenocortical steroid biosynthesis (e.g., **21-hydroxylase deficiency, 11β-hydroxylase deficiency**). In 21-hydroxylase deficiency (90% of all cases), there is virtually no synthesis of the aldosterone or cortisol, so that intermediates are funneled into androgen biosynthesis, thereby elevating androgen levels.
   b. **Symptoms.** The elevated levels of androgens lead to virilization of a female fetus ranging from mild clitoral enlargement to complete labioscrotal fusion with a phalloid organ (female pseudohermaphroditism). In the male fetus, macrogenitosomia occurs. Because cortisol cannot be synthesized, negative feedback to the adenohypophysis does not occur, so ACTH continues to stimulate the adrenal cortex, resulting in adrenal hyperplasia.
   c. **Treatment.** Depending on the severity, treatment may include surgical reconstruction and steroid replacement.
4. **Primary adrenal insufficiency (Addison disease)**
   a. **Cause.** Addison disease is commonly caused by autoimmune destruction of the adrenal cortex.
   b. **Symptoms.** It is characterized clinically by fatigue, anorexia, nausea, weight loss, hypotension, skin hyperpigmentation due to increased melanocyte-stimulating hormone (MSH) caused by an increase in ACTH secretion, hyponatremia, and hyperkalemia (may lead to fatal cardiac arrhythmias).
   c. **Treatment.** This condition is managed by steroid replacement therapy.
5. **Secondary adrenal insufficiency**
   a. **Cause.** Secondary adrenal insufficiency is caused by a disorder of the hypothalamus or adenohypophysis that reduces the secretion of ACTH.
   b. **Symptoms.** It is clinically very similar to Addison disease except there is no hyperpigmentation of the skin.

F. **PHARMACOLOGY OF ADRENAL GLAND**
1. **Aldosterone and Fludrocortisone (Florinef)** are mineralocorticoids. They are used clinically in steroid replacement therapy (e.g., Addison disease).
2. **Spironolactone** is an aldosterone receptor antagonist. It is used clinically to treat primary hyperaldosteronism (e.g., Conn syndrome).
3. **Cortisol, Cortisone, and Corticosteroid** are glucocorticoids. They are used clinically in steroid replacement therapy (e.g., Addison disease).
4. **Methylprednisolone (Medrol) and Prednisone (Deltasone)** are glucocorticoids. They are used clinically as anti-inflammatory agents, as immunosuppressive agents, and in chemotherapy (prednisone is part of the MOPP regimen).
5. **Dexamethasone (Decadron)** is a glucocorticoid. It is used clinically as an anti-inflammatory agent, as an immunosuppressive agent to suppress ACTH secretion, and in the diagnosis of Cushing disease (dexamethasone suppression test).
6. **Aminoglutethimide (Cytadren)** inhibits desmolase, thereby preventing synthesis of cortisol. It is used clinically to treat breast cancer and Cushing syndrome.
7. **Metyrapone (Metopirone)** inhibits 11β-hydroxylase, thereby preventing synthesis of cortisol. It is used clinically to treat Cushing syndrome.
8. **Ketoconazole** inhibits the cytochrome P_{450} enzymes, thereby preventing steroid biosynthesis in general. It is used clinically to treat Cushing syndrome.
9. **Mitotane (Lysodren)** destroys the cells of the zona fasciculata and zona reticularis. It is used clinically to treat adrenocortical carcinoma.

G. **DIAGNOSIS.** Table 25-1 shows the laboratory findings used for diagnosis.

| TABLE 25-1 | LABORATORY FINDINGS USED FOR DIAGNOSIS OF ADRENAL DISORDERS |

Clinical Condition	Dex^a	ALD	Cortisol	Androgens	ACTH	Other
Primary hyperaldosteronism (Conn syndrome)		High				
Cushing syndrome						
Normal patient	+		Normal		Normal	
ACTH adenoma	+		High		High	
Adrenal adenoma	−		High		Low	
Congenital adrenal hyperplasia						
21-Hydroxylase deficiency	Low	Low	High	High		Salt loss with volume depletion
11β-Hydroxylase deficiency	Low	Low	High	High		Salt retention with hypertension
Addison disease (primary adrenal insufficiency)	Low	Low	Low	High		
Secondary adrenal insufficiency	Normal	Low	Low	Low		

Dex, high-dose dexamethasone suppression test; ALD, aldosterone; ACTH, adrenocorticotropin.
^aThe Dex test is based on the ability of dexamethasone (a synthetic glucocorticoid) to inhibit ACTH and cortisol secretion. If the adenohypophysis–adrenal cortex axis is normal, dexamethasone will suppress ACTH and cortisol secretion and the test is considered positive (i.e., suppression occurred).

II The Medulla contains chromaffin cells, which are modified postganglionic sympathetic neurons.

Preganglionic sympathetic axons (via splanchnic nerves) synapse on chromaffin cells, and upon stimulation cause chromaffin cells to secrete catecholamines: epinephrine and norepinephrine. There are two types of chromaffin cells:

A. EPINEPHRINE-CONTAINING CELLS make up a majority of the chromaffin cells in the medulla and contain small, homogeneous, light-staining granules. All of the circulating epinephrine in the blood is derived from the adrenal medulla. Epinephrine binds to α- and β-adrenergic receptors, which are G protein–linked receptors. Epinephrine has a **half-life of 1 to 3 minutes** as it is metabolized by the liver and excreted in the urine as **free epinephrine** or **metanephrine**. Urinary levels of free epinephrine are used for diagnostic purposes in problems of adrenal medulla function.

B. NOREPINEPHRINE-CONTAINING CELLS make up a minority of the chromaffin cells in the medulla and contain large, electron-dense core granules. The majority of circulating norepinephrine in the blood is derived from the postganglionic sympathetic neurons and brain, with the secretion from the adrenal medulla contributing only a minor portion. Norepinephrine binds to α- and β-adrenergic receptors, which are G protein–linked receptors. Norepinephrine has a **half-life of 1 to 3 minutes** as it is metabolized by the liver and excreted in the urine as **free norepinephrine, normetanephrine, vanillylmandelic acid (VMA), or 3-methoxy-4-hydroxyphenyglycol (MOPEG)**. Urinary levels of VMA and MOPEG are used for diagnostic purposes in problems of the sympathetic nervous system.

C. FUNCTIONS OF EPINEPHRINE AND NOREPINEPHRINE basically include all the functions of the sympathetic nervous system as they elicit their effect via α- and β-adrenergic receptors. These functions include the following: contract dilator pupillae muscle, causing dilation of the pupil (mydriasis); contract arrector pili muscle in skin; contract vascular smooth muscle in skin and visceral vessels; relax vascular smooth muscle in skeletal muscle vessels; relax bronchial smooth muscle in lung (bronchodilation); relax gastrointestinal (GI) tract smooth muscle (decreases motility); contract

GI tract smooth muscle sphincters; relax smooth muscle in urinary bladder; contract smooth muscle in urinary tract sphincter; contract smooth muscle in ductus deferens, causing ejaculation; relax smooth muscle of uterus; accelerate the sinoatrial (SA) node (increases heart rate); increase conduction velocity at atrioventricular (AV) node; increase contractility of cardiac muscle; increases viscous secretion from salivary glands; increase eccrine sweat gland secretion (thermoregulation); increase apocrine sweat gland secretion; stimulate seminal vesicle and prostrate secretion during ejaculation; stimulate gluconeogenesis and glycogenolysis in hepatocytes; cause lipolysis in adipocytes; cause renin release from juxtaglomerular cells in kidney (increases blood pressure); and inhibit insulin secretion from pancreatic β cells.

D. BLOOD SUPPLY OF THE ADRENAL

1. **The superior and middle adrenal arteries** give rise to capillaries that supply the adrenal cortex and end in **medullary venous sinuses** within the adrenal medulla. This means that aldosterone, cortisol, androstenedione, and DHEA leave the adrenal cortex by first percolating through the adrenal medulla. This blood flow is significant because activation of **phenylethanolamine-N-methyltransferase (PNMT)**, a key enzyme in the synthesis of epinephrine by chromaffin cells within the adrenal medulla, is dependent on high levels of cortisol.

2. The **inferior adrenal artery** gives rise to **medullary arterioles** that supply only the adrenal medulla (i.e., bypass the adrenal cortex) and end in **medullary venous sinuses**.

3. Medullary venous sinuses drain into the **central vein** by which aldosterone, cortisol, androstenedione, DHEA, epinephrine, and norepinephrine leave the adrenal gland.

E. SYNTHESIS OF CATECHOLAMINES uses tyrosine as a precursor (**Figure 25-2**).

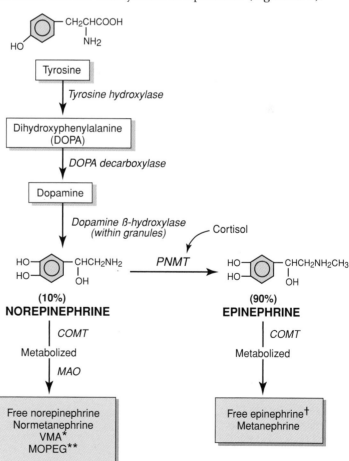

● **Figure 25-2 Synthesis and metabolism of adrenomedullary catecholamines.** Synthesis begins with tyrosine as a precursor. The metabolic urine breakdown products (in *shaded boxes*) are used for diagnostic purposes. Urinary levels of vanillylmandelic acid (VMA; *asterisk*) and 3-methoxy-4-hydroxyphenyglycol (MOPEG; *double asterisk*) are diagnostic of sympathetic nervous system function. Urinary levels of free epinephrine (*dagger*) are diagnostic of adrenal medulla function. The enzymes catecholamine O-methyltransferase (COMT) and monoamine oxidase (MAO) are key enzymes in the metabolism of catecholamines. When the adrenal medulla is stimulated, the secretion product is 90% epinephrine and 10% norepinephrine. All of the enzymes involved in catecholamine synthesis are found in the cytoplasm except dopamine β-hydroxylase, which is located within secretion granules. PNMT, phenylethanolamine-N-methyltransferase.

F. CLINICAL CONSIDERATIONS

1. **Pheochromocytoma** is a relatively rare (usually not malignant) catecholamine-producing tumor (both epinephrine and norepinephrine) of the adrenal medulla.

   a. **Characteristics.** Pheochromocytoma occurs mainly in adults and is generally found in the region of the adrenal gland but also is found in extra-adrenal sites. It occurs within families as part of the multiple endocrine neoplasia (MEN) type 2 syndrome.

   b. **Symptoms.** It is associated with persistent or paroxysmal hypertension, anxiety, tremor, profuse sweating, pallor, chest pain, and abdominal pain.

   c. **Diagnosis.** Increased urine VMA and metanephrine levels, inability to suppress catecholamines with clonidine, and hyperglycemia are common laboratory findings.

   d. **Treatment.** Pheochromocytoma is treated by surgery or phenoxybenzamine (an α-adrenergic antagonist).

2. **Neuroblastoma** is a common extracranial neoplasm containing primitive neuroblasts of neural crest origin.

   a. **Characteristics.** Neuroblastomas occur mainly in children. They are found in extra-adrenal sites usually along the sympathetic chain ganglia (60%) or within the adrenal medulla (40%). They metastasize widely.

   b. **Symptoms.** Neuroblastoma is associated with opsoclonus (rapid, irregular movements of the eye in horizontal and vertical directions; "dancing eyes").

   c. **Diagnosis.** A neuroblastoma contains small cells arranged in Homer-Wright pseudorosettes. Increased urine VMA and metanephrine levels are found.

   d. **Treatment** includes surgical excision, radiation, and chemotherapy.

Ⅲ   Selected Photomicrographs

A. Gross photograph and histology of a normal adrenal gland (Figure 25-3)

● **Figure 25-3 General features of the adrenal gland. A:** Gross photograph of a sliced normal adrenal gland. The zona glomerulosa and zona fasciculata appear as a light area (yellow color in fresh gross specimens) due to the large amount of lipid of these cells, whereas the zona reticularis appears as a dark area (dark brown color in fresh gross specimens) due to the eosinophilia and lipofuscin pigment of these cells. The medulla (M) appears as a gray area where dilated venules are observed (*arrows*). The *boxed area* is shown at higher magnification in B. **B:** Light micrograph (LM) of a normal adrenal gland. A capsule is present on the exterior of the gland. The three zones of the adrenal cortex and the adrenal medulla are clearly apparent. ZG, zona glomerulosa; ZF, zona fasciculata; ZR, zona reticularis; M, medulla. **C:** LM of the ZG. The ZG is a narrow, inconstant band (15% of the cortical volume) of cortex situated immediately below the capsule (cap). The cells of the ZG have distinct cell membranes and are arranged in glomerularlike clusters surrounded by small amounts of connective tissue. The ZG cell clusters may merge into short, hairpin-shaped trabeculae. The ZG cells have a round nucleus and a faintly eosinophilic, vacuolated cytoplasm. **D:** LM of the ZF. The ZF is a broad band of cortex (78% of the cortical volume). The ZF lies between the ZG and the ZR. The cells of the ZF have distinct cell membranes and are arranged as two-cell-wide vertical cords that run perpendicular to the capsule and are separated by parallel-running capillaries. The cells of the ZF have a round nucleus and a lipid-filled cytoplasm, which gives the ZF a vacuolated, clear appearance. The high lipid content of the ZF cells gives this zone a yellow color observed in fresh gross specimens. **E:** LM of the ZR. The ZR is a band of cortex (7% of cortical volume). The ZR lies deep to the ZF and in the head and body of the adrenal gland abuts on the medulla. The cells of the ZR have a distinct cell membrane and are arranged as one-cell-wide anastomosing rows of cells separated by capillaries. The cells of the ZR have a round nucleus and a lipid-sparse, distinctly eosinophilic cytoplasm. The deepest-located cells next to the medulla usually contain a yellow-brown lipofuscin pigment. The eosinophilia and lipofuscin pigment of the ZR cells gives this zone a dark brown color in fresh gross specimens. **F, G:** LM of the medulla. The medulla is located deep to the ZR in the head and body of the adrenal. The medulla is usually absent in the tail of the adrenal. The boundary between the cortex and medulla is quite distinct. At low magnification (F), venules (*) and nerve fibers (*arrows*) can be observed coursing through the medulla. At higher magnification (G), chromaffin cells have an indistinct cell membrane and are arranged in tight clusters. The chromaffin cells have variable-shaped nuclei and generally a finely granular basophilic cytoplasm, although some cells appear vacuolated, which gives the medulla a mottled appearance.

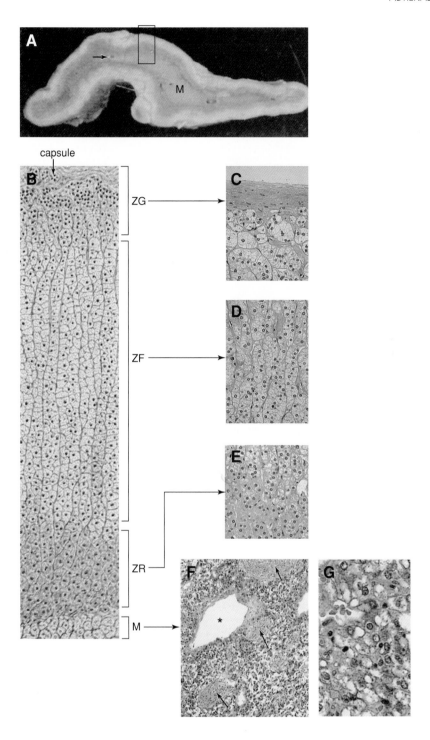

capsule

B. Hyperadrenalism (Cushing syndrome), normal adrenal gland, hypoadrenalism (Addison disease) (Figure 25-4)

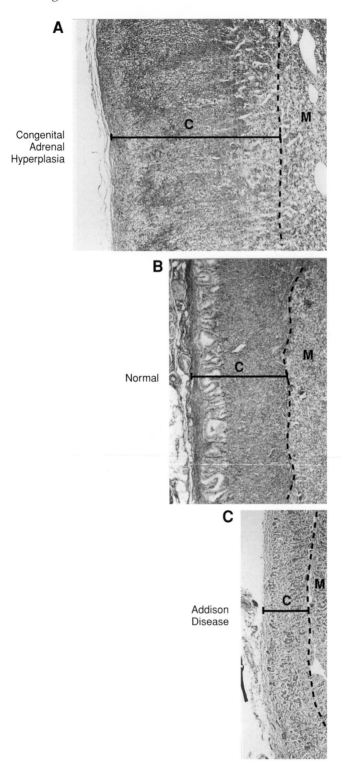

● **Figure 25-4 Normal and pathologic adrenal gland. A:** Hyperplasia of the adrenal cortex as might be found in congenital adrenal hyperplasia. **B:** Normal adrenal gland showing the normal thickness of the adrenal cortex. **C:** Hypoplasia of the adrenal cortex as might be found in Addison disease. All photomicrographs are taken at the same magnification so that the normal and pathologic changes may be compared. C, adrenal cortex; M, adrenal medulla.

C. Normal adrenal medulla, pheochromocytoma, neuroblastoma (Figure 25-5)

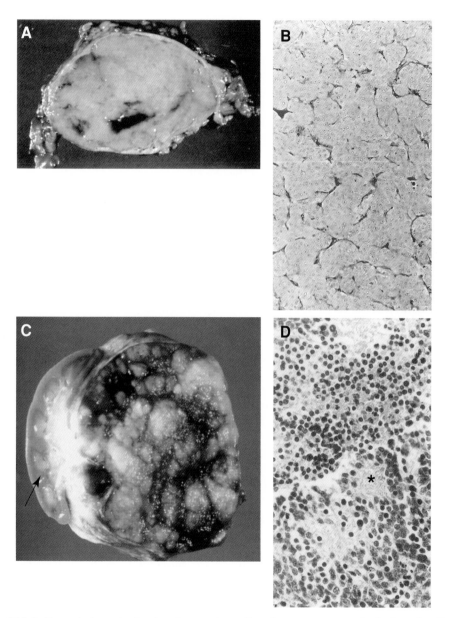

● **Figure 25-5 A:** Gross photograph of a pheochromocytoma. Pheochromocytomas vary in size from 3 to 5 cm in diameter. They are gray-white to pink-tan in color. Exposure of the cut surface often results in darkening of the surface due to formation of yellow-brown adrenochrome pigment. **B:** Light micrograph (LM) of a pheochromocytoma. A pheochromocytoma generally appears as a diffuse or nodular hyperplasia. The neoplastic cells are abundant cytoplasm with small centrally located nuclei. The neoplastic cells are separated into clusters by a slender stroma and numerous capillaries. **C:** Gross photograph of a neuroblastoma. Neuroblastomas vary in size from 1 cm to filling the entire abdomen. They are generally soft and white to gray-pink in color. As the size increases, the tumors become hemorrhagic and undergo calcification and cyst formation. Note the nodular appearance of this tumor with the kidney apparent on the left border (*arrow*). **D:** LM of a neuroblastoma, which is commonly composed of small, primitive-looking cells with dark nuclei and scant cytoplasm. The cells generally are arranged as solid sheets, and some cells arrange around a central fibrillar area, forming Homer-Wright pseudorosettes (*asterisk*).

Case Study 25-1

A 40-year-old woman comes to your office complaining that "I always feel nauseated and I get tired real fast even when I'm at home just puttering around. This has been going on for about 3 months." She also tells you that "I've been vomiting quite a bit and I don't have an appetite. The only good thing about all this is that I've lost 15 pounds." After some discussion, she informs you that she has been married for 10 years and denies any extramarital affairs. However, before she got married she admits that "I was pretty wild and would pick up the cutest guy in the bar and take him home for the night. I took megadoses of antibiotics to prevent sexually transmitted diseases and I loved to use amyl and butyl nitrite to heighten my orgasm." The woman does not seem to be very concerned about her condition as she says, "Doc, just give me something for this nausea and vomiting and I'll be good to go. I want to lose another 15 pounds." What is the most likely diagnosis?

Differentials

- Acquired immunodeficiency syndrome (AIDS), hemochromatosis, pituitary hypofunction

Relevant Physical Examination Findings

- Blood pressure = 100/70 mm Hg reclined; 80/60 mm Hg standing (orthostatic hypotension)
- Increased pigmentation on her knuckles, knees, and elbows
- Areolae are bluish-black
- Axillary and pubic hair is sparse
- No lymphadenopathy

Relevant Lab Findings

- Blood chemistry: hemoglobin (Hgb) = 16 g/dL (high); hematocrit (Hct) = 53% (high); Na^+ = 105 mEq/L (low); K^+ = 6.5 mEq/L (high); HCO_3^- = 19 mEq/L (low); blood urea nitrogen (BUN) = 26 mg/dL (high); fasting glucose = 45 mg/dL (low); serum ferritin = 200 ng/mL (normal); morning plasma cortisol = 3 mg/dL (low); morning plasma ACTH = 200 pg/mL (high)
- Human immunodeficiency virus (HIV) test: negative
- Purified protein derivative (PPD) test: negative
- Computed tomography (CT) scan: small, noncalcified adrenal glands

Diagnosis: Addison Disease (Primary Adrenocortical Insufficiency)

- Addison disease (AD) is commonly caused by the autoimmune destruction of the adrenal cortex resulting in a deficiency of cortisol, aldosterone, and dehydroepiandrosterone. Skin hyperpigmentation is seen as a result of increased MSH, which is a byproduct of ACTH synthesis in the adenohypophysis. The deficiency of cortisol results in the following: contributes to orthostatic hypotension; mild pressor effect on the heart and vasculature; hypoglycemia because cortisol plays a role in gluconeogenesis; nausea; vomiting; anorexia; weight loss; and an increase in ACTH levels because cortisol controls ACTH secretion by a negative feedback loop. The deficiency of aldosterone results in the following: hyponatremia, hypovolemia, decreased cardiac output, decreased renal blood flow, azotemia, and hyperkalemia (which can lead to cardiac dysrhythmia). Aldosterone acts on the principal cells of the cortical collecting ducts in the kidney and causes increased Na^+ reabsorption (tubular fluid → plasma). Aldosterone also acts on the principal cells of the cortical collecting ducts in the kidney and causes increased K^+ secretion (plasma → tubular fluid). A definitive diagnosis of AD is indicated by low cortisol levels, low aldosterone levels, low dehydroepiandrosterone levels, and high ACTH levels.

- Some AIDS patients (≈20%) present with cortisol resistance and adrenal insufficiency. The HIV test rules out AIDS in this case. Some believe that megadoses of antibiotics, amyl and butyl nitrites, and multiple blood transfusions may destroy $CD4^+$ lymphocytes and lead to AIDS.
- Hemosiderin is a golden brown hemoglobin-derived pigment consisting of iron. Iron is absorbed mainly by surface absorptive cells within the duodenum, transported in the plasma by a protein called transferrin, and normally stored in cells as ferritin, which is a protein–iron complex. During iron overload, intracellular ferritin undergoes lysosomal degradation, in which the ferritin protein is degraded and the iron aggregates within the cell as hemosiderin in a condition called hemosiderosis. The more extreme accumulation of iron is called hemochromatosis, which is associated with liver and pancreas damage. Hemochromatosis can be observed in patients with increased absorption of dietary iron, impaired utilization of iron, hemolytic anemias, and blood transfusions. Clinical findings of hemochromatosis include cirrhosis of the liver, diabetes, and increased skin pigmentation (bronze diabetes).
- Pituitary hypofunction (secondary adrenocortical insufficiency) presents with many of the same symptoms as AD because the adrenal cortex is under control of the adenohypophysis. A definitive diagnosis of pituitary hypofunction is indicated by low cortisol levels, normal aldosterone levels (because the zona glomerulosa of the adrenal cortex is controlled by the renin-angiotensin system), low dehydroepiandrosterone levels, and low ACTH levels. Since ACTH levels are low, MSH will not be increased so that no increased skin pigmentation would be observed.

Case Study 25-2

A 30-year-old woman comes to your office complaining that "I'm getting fat, I have pimples like when I was a teenager, and I have a beard and mustache. What the hell is going on?" After some discussion, she informs that she has not had a menstrual period in 4 months, she bruises easily, and she screams at her children over little things that never bothered her before. The woman is in an obvious high state of anxiety about her condition and begins to cry as she says, "Doc, I look like a circus freak! My husband won't even look at me. You've got to do something." What is the most likely diagnosis?

Differentials
- Adrenal adenoma or hyperplasia, alcoholism, small cell carcinoma of the lung

Relevant Physical Examination Findings
- Blood pressure = 175/115 mm Hg (high)
- Muscle weakness
- Central obesity; thin limbs
- Moon facies
- Purple striae

Relevant Lab Findings
- Blood chemistry: fasting blood glucose = 145 mg/dL (high); morning plasma cortisol = 55 μg/dL (high); plasma ACTH = 15 pg/mL (high)
- Urinalysis: 24-hour free cortisol = 375 μg (high); glucosuria = +1
- High-dose dexamethasone suppression test: positive
- Magnetic resonance imaging (MRI) of head: small pituitary adenoma
- Chest radiograph: negative

Diagnosis: Cushing Disease

- Cushing disease refers to high levels of cortisol caused by an ACTH-secreting adenoma within the adenohypophysis. Cushing syndrome refers to the constellation of clinical findings that appear secondary to high levels of cortisol. Clinical findings of Cushing syndrome include mild hypertension, impaired glucose tolerance, acne, hirsutism, oligomenorrhea, impotence and loss of libido in men, osteoporosis with back pain and buffalo hump, central obesity, moon facies, and purple skin striae (bruise easily). Cushing syndrome is caused by administration of large doses of steroids for treatment of primary disease (i.e., iatrogenic; most common cause), an ACTH-secreting adenoma within the adenohypophysis, an adrenal adenoma, or adrenal hyperplasia. A definitive diagnosis of Cushing disease is indicated by a positive dexamethasone suppression test, high cortisol levels, high levels of ACTH, and MRI indication of a pituitary adenoma.

- An adrenal adenoma will also cause Cushing syndrome. A definitive diagnosis of an adrenal adenoma is indicated by a negative dexamethasone suppression test, high cortisol levels, low levels of ACTH, and computed tomography (CT) scan indication of an adrenal adenoma. An adrenal adenoma usually occurs unilaterally, whereas adrenal hyperplasia occurs bilaterally. In adrenal hyperplasia, both adrenal glands are enlarged while maintaining their normal anatomic shapes. Note that in adrenal hyperplasia, except for the increased size, the adrenal glands appear normal, which may confound the diagnosis. In some cases of adrenal hyperplasia, the adrenal glands may demonstrate bilateral nodularity.

- Chronic alcoholics can develop signs of Cushing syndrome due to high levels of cortisol. However, this is associated with a negative dexamethasone suppression test. The ascites associated with chronic alcoholism is centrally located but is composed of fluid located in the peritoneal cavity, not fat.

- A small cell carcinoma of the lung can produce ACTH, which leads to high levels of cortisol and Cushing syndrome. However, the chest radiograph is negative in this case and there is no history of smoking.

Chapter 26

Female Reproductive System

I   Ovary (Figure 26-1). The ovaries are almond-shaped structures located posterior to the broad ligament. The ovaries are covered by a surface epithelium (simple cuboidal) called the **germinal epithelium** with a subjacent connective tissue layer called the **tunica albuginea**. The ovaries are divided into a **cortex** and **medulla**.

A. CORTEX. The cortex contains follicles in various stages of development, including the **primordial follicle, primary follicle, secondary follicle**, and **Graafian follicle**. Follicles are composed of an oocyte, follicular cells, and thecal cells.

B. MEDULLA. The medulla lies deep to the cortex and contains connective tissue, occasional smooth muscle cells, and numerous tortuous arteries (and veins) from which small branches radiate to the cortex.

C. CLINICAL CONSIDERATIONS

1. **Ovarian Cysts.** Functional cysts in the ovary are so common as to be virtually physiologic and resolve spontaneously. Functional cysts are physiologically and hormonally active cysts that have not yet involuted. They originate from either unruptured Graafian follicles or in Graafian follicles that have ruptured and immediately sealed. Ovarian cysts are nonneoplastic, fluid-filled cavities that may by solitary or multiple (up to 2 cm in diameter). There are three main types of cysts.

    a. **Follicular cysts** are generally large cysts (>2 cm) that may be diagnosed by palpation or ultrasound. Histologically, granulosa lutein cells can be identified if the pressure is not too great and theca lutein cells may be conspicuous.

    b. **Corpus luteum cysts** are lined by a conspicuous rim of granulosa lutein cells.

    c. **Theca lutein cysts** are caused by elevated levels of β**-human chorionic gonadotropin (β-hCG)** produced by the placenta during pregnancy. This causes a proliferation of theca lutein cells, which forms small nodules in the ovary.

2. **Polycystic Ovary Syndrome** is characterized biochemically by increased levels of androgens and leuteinizing hormone (LH), but decreased levels of follicle-stimulating hormone (FSH). This results in bilateral ovarian enlargement, cortical fibrosis, and multiple follicular cysts. Clinical features include: chronic anovulation with menstrual irregularities such as oligomenorrhea or amenorrhea; oily skin and acne; hirsutism; and obesity.

3. **Ovarian Tumors** originate from four cell types (germinal epithelium, oocyte, follicular cells, or stromal cells).
   a. **Germinal epithelium tumors** are the most common type. These tumors are cystic and may be filled with either a serous fluid or mucus. **Serous tumors** are generally malignant and bilateral with a poor prognosis.
   b. Oocyte tumors (or germ cell tumors)
   c. Follicular cell tumors (or sex cord cell tumors)
   d. Stromal cell tumors

II   Corpus Luteum is a temporary endocrine gland whose formation is **LH dependent**. After ovulation, the wall of the follicle collapses and becomes extensively infolded. Blood vessels and stromal cells invade the previously avascular granulosa cells. The granulosa and theca interna cells hypertrophy, develop smooth endoplasmic reticulum (sER), and accumulate lipid droplets (a process called **luteinization**), thereby becoming lutein cells.

A. **CELLULAR COMPOSITION.** There are two kinds of lutein cells:
   1. **Granulosa Lutein Cells**
      a. The granulosa lutein cells secrete **progesterone** and **estradiol** in response to FSH and LH stimulation.
      b. The granulosa lutein cells lack the steroidogenic enzymes required for the complete synthesis of estradiol. Consequently, theca lutein cells cooperate with the granulosa lutein cells by providing androstenedione, which is then converted into estradiol within the granulosa lutein cells.
      c. Progesterone maintains the endometrium of the uterus in the secretory (luteal) phase so that implantation and nutritional support of the blastocyst may occur.
      d. **Mifepristone (RU-486)** is a drug that binds to progesterone receptors and blocks progesterone action. RU-486 used in combination with **misoprostol (a prostaglandin E_1 [PGE_1] analogue)** is an effective and safe abortifacient.
   2. **Theca lutein cells** secrete **androstenedione** and **progesterone** in response to LH stimulation.

B. **EFFECT OF FERTILIZATION.** If fertilization occurs, the corpus luteum enlarges and becomes the predominant source of steroids needed to sustain pregnancy for approximately **8 weeks**. Thereafter, the placenta becomes the major source of the steroids required. If fertilization does not occur, the corpus luteum regresses and forms a **corpus albicans**.

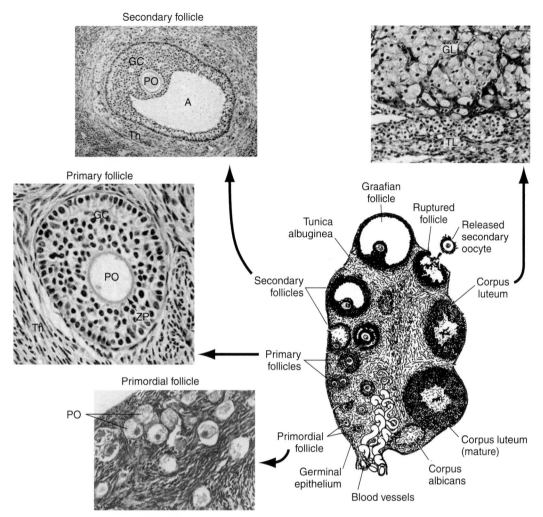

● Figure 26-1 Development of the ovarian follicles. The table shows the stages of follicle development along with the changes in the oocyte, follicular cells, and thecal cells. Diagram of the entire ovary shows the cycle of ovarian follicle maturation, luteinization, and residual scarring. *Curved arrows* point to light micrographs of primordial follicles, a primary follicle, a secondary follicle, and corpus luteum. PO, primary oocyte; GC, granulosa cells; Th, theca; A, antrum; ZP, zona pellucida; GL, granulosa lutein cells; TL, theca lutein cells.

Uterine Tubes (fallopian tubes; oviducts) (Figure 26-2) are tubular structures that provide a channel for the transport of the preimplantation embryo to the uterus and the site of fertilization.

A. REGIONS OF THE UTERINE TUBES

   1. **Infundibulum** is the flared open end of the uterine tube next to the ovary. Fimbriae are delicate, fingerlike projections that extend from the infundibulum toward the ovary.
   2. **Ampulla** is the longest segment of the uterine tube and has the largest diameter. This region is where **fertilization** occurs.
   3. **Isthmus** is the narrow segment of the uterine tube between the ampulla and uterus.
   4. **Intramural segment** is the portion of the uterine tube contained within the wall of the uterus.

B. HISTOLOGIC LAYERS

   1. **Mucosa.** The mucosa consists of an epithelium and lamina propria, but no muscularis mucosa. The **mucosal epithelium** consists of:
       a. **Secretory cells** (nonciliated) that secrete a nutrient-rich medium for the nourishment of the sperm and preimplantation embryo
       b. **Ciliated cells** whose cilia beat toward the uterus. The rate of ciliary beat is influenced by progesterone and estrogen and assists in transport of the preimplantation embryo to the uterus.
   2. **Muscularis layer** consists of smooth muscle oriented in an inner circular layer and an outer longitudinal layer. Peristaltic contractions may help to move the preimplantation embryo toward the uterus.
   3. **Serosa** consists of simple squamous epithelium (visceral peritoneum).

C. CLINICAL CONSIDERATIONS

   1. **Acute and Chronic Salpingitis** is a bacterial infection (most commonly *Neisseria gonorrhea* or *Chlamydia trachomatis*) of the uterine tube with acute inflammation (neutrophil infiltration) or chronic inflammation, which may lead to scarring of the uterine tube, predisposing to **ectopic tubal pregnancy.**
   2. **Ectopic tubal pregnancy** most often occurs in the **ampulla** of the uterine tube. Risk factors include salpingitis, pelvic inflammatory disease, pelvic surgery, or exposure to diethylstilbestrol (DES). Clinical features include: sudden onset of abdominal pain, which may be confused with appendicitis in a young woman; last menses 60 days ago; positive hCG test; and culdocentesis showing intraperitoneal blood. Ectopic tubal pregnancy is a medical emergency and should always be considered when a cycling female (no matter how young) presents with abdominal pain.

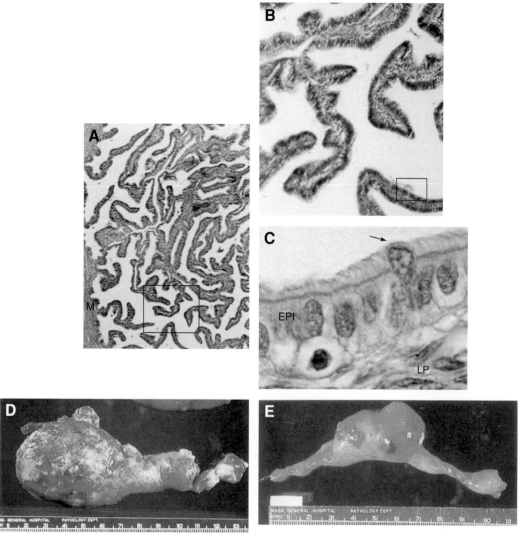

● **Figure 26-2 Normal and pathological uterine tubes. A:** Light micrograph (LM; low magnification) of the ampulla of the uterine tube. Note the long slender mucosal folds that project into the lumen. The muscularis layer (M) is also shown. The *boxed area* is shown at higher magnification in B. **B:** LM of the mucosal folds shows the epithelial lining and connective tissue of the lamina propria. The *boxed area* is shown at higher magnification in C. **C:** LM of the mucosal folds shows the epithelial lining (EPI) consisting of secretory nonciliated cells (peg cells; *arrow*) and ciliated cells along with the lamina propria (LP). **D:** Gross photograph of acute and chronic salpingitis. The uterine tube is markedly distended, the fimbriated end is closed, and there is hemorrhage on the serosal surface. **E:** Gross photograph of an ectopic tubal pregnancy.

Ⅳ Uterus

A. REGIONS OF THE UTERUS

1. The **body** is the expanded part of the uterus below the entrance of the uterine tubes.
2. The **fundus** is the rounded superior part of the uterus above the entrance of the uterine tubes.
3. The **cervix** is the most inferior part of the uterus that projects into the vagina.

B. **HISTOLOGIC LAYERS.** The uterine wall consists of:

1. **Endometrium** consists of simple columnar epithelium, which invaginates into the endometrial stroma to form **endometrial glands**. The endometrium can be divided into two layers.

    a. **Basal Layer** regenerates the functional layer each month during the menstrual cycle. The basal layer is NEVER sloughed off.

    b. **Functional Layer** undergoes alterations during the menstrual cycle. The functional layer is sloughed off each month during menses.

2. **Myometrium** consists of smooth muscle cells that are connected by gap junctions and contract upon stimulation by **oxytocin** and **prostaglandins** (PGE_2 and $PGE_{2\alpha}$) at parturition. During pregnancy, the myometrial smooth muscle cells hypertrophy and increase in number. The myometrium contains the **stratum vasculare**, which is highly vascular and is the source of the endometrial blood supply.

3. **Perimetrium** consists of connective tissue covered by peritoneal mesothelium.

Ⓥ The Menstrual Cycle (Figure 26-3) is a series of phases that repeats ideally every 28 days.

A. **THE MENSTRUAL PHASE (DAYS 1 TO 4)** is characterized by the **necrosis and shedding** of the functional layer of the endometrium. Spiral arterioles constrict episodically for a few days and finally constrict permanently, resulting in ischemia that leads to necrosis of endometrial glands and stroma. The spiral arterioles subsequently dilate and rupture, resulting in hemorrhage that sheds the necrotic endometrial glands and stroma.

B. **THE PROLIFERATIVE (FOLLICULAR) PHASE (DAYS 4 TO 15)** is characterized by the **regeneration** of the functional layer of the endometrium from the devastating effects of the menstrual phase. This phase is controlled by **estrogen** secreted by the granulosa cells of the secondary and Graafian follicle. Epithelial cells and fibroblasts of the basal layer of the endometrium regenerate to form **straight endometrial glands** and stroma, respectively.

C. **THE OVULATORY PHASE (DAYS 14 TO 16)** is characterized by **ovulation** of the secondary oocyte arrested in metaphase of meiosis II that coincides with **peak levels of LH (LH surge)**.

D. **THE SECRETORY (LUTEAL) PHASE (DAYS 15 TO 25)** is characterized by the **secretory activity** of the endometrial glands. This phase is controlled by **progesterone** secreted by the granulosa lutein cells of the corpus luteum. The endometrial glands become modified to **convoluted endometrial glands with secretion product** within their lumen.

E. **THE PREMENSTRUAL PHASE (DAYS 25 TO 28)** is characterized by **ischemia** due to reduced blood flow to the endometrium. This phase is controlled by the **reduction in progesterone and estrogen** as the corpus luteum involutes. As the endometrial glands begin to shrink, the spiral arterioles are compressed, thereby reducing blood flow and causing ischemic damage.

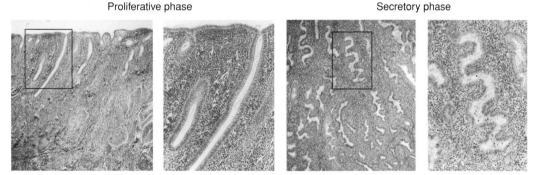

● **Figure 26-3 Hormonal control of the menstrual cycle.** The hypothalamus secretes gonadotropin-releasing factor (GnRF). In response to GnRH, the adenohypophysis secretes follicle-stimulating hormone (FSH) and luteinizing hormone (LH). In response to FSH, the development of a secondary follicle to a Graafian follicle is stimulated in the ovary. The granulosa cells within the secondary follicle and Graafian follicle secrete estrogen (E). In response to estrogen, the endometrium of the uterus enters the proliferative phase. In response to LH (LH surge), ovulation occurs. After ovulation, the granulosa lutein cells of the corpus luteum secrete progesterone (P). In response to progesterone, the endometrium of the uterus enters the secretory phase. Light micrograph (LM) of the proliferative phase of the endometrium showing straight endometrial glands. The *boxed area* is shown at higher magnification. LM of the secretory phase of the endometrium showing convoluted endometrium glands with secretion product within the lumen. The *boxed area* is shown at higher magnification. LM of the menstrual phase of the endometrium showing endometrial glands undergoing necrosis and shedding. Conditions that impair the secretion of GnRH from the hypothalamus will prevent the secretion of FSH that is necessary for follicle development and will result in infertility. **Female infertility** is usually treated with **clomiphene (Clomid, Serophene).** Clomiphene is an estrogen receptor partial agonist that imparts antiestrogen activity by competitive inhibition. This prevents feedback inhibition and increases FSH and LH secretion so that ovulation occurs. In **polycystic ovary syndrome**, increased LH secretion from the adenohypophysis stimulates excessive production of androgens by the theca interna cell of secondary and Graafian follicles, resulting in numerous atretic and/or cystic follicles.

F. CLINICAL CONSIDERATIONS

1. **Endometriosis** is the appearance of foci of endometrial tissue in abnormal locations outside the uterus (e.g., ovary, uterine ligaments, pelvic peritoneum). The ectopic endometrial tissue shows cyclic changes synchronous with the endometrium of the uterus. Endometriosis results in infertility, dysmenorrhea, and pelvic pain (most pronounced at the time of menstruation). The serosal surfaces of pelvic organs are sprinkled with red, bluish, or yellow punctate lesions. Bluish lesions are called "**gunpowder mark" lesions.** The ectopic endometrial tissue consists of a hemorrhagic endometrial stroma and glands. Blood-filled cysts ("**chocolate cysts**") up to 3 to 5 cm in diameter may be found on the ovaries.

2. **Leiomyomas (fibroids)** are very common benign tumors derived from smooth muscle within the myometrium of the uterus. They may be classified as subserosal, intramural, or submucosal. Subserosal and submucosal tumors may be pedunculated and therefore protrude from the uterine surface or protrude into the uterine cavity, respectively.

3. **Primary amenorrhea** is the complete absence of menstruation in a woman from puberty.

4. **Secondary amenorrhea** is the absence of menstruation for at least 3 months in a woman who previously had normal menstruation.

    a. **Causes.** The most common cause of secondary amenorrhea is pregnancy, which can be determined by assaying urine *β*-hCG. Other pathologic causes of secondary amenorrhea include hypothalamic/pituitary malfunction (e.g., **anorexia nervosa**), ovarian disorders (e.g., **ovariectomy**), and end-organ disease (e.g., **Asherman syndrome,** in which the basal layer of the endometrium has been removed by repeated curettages).

    b. **Diagnosis.** These causes are evaluated clinically by assaying serum FSH and LH levels along with a progesterone challenge. Bleeding after a **progesterone withdrawal test** indicates that the endometrium was primed by estrogen, thereby indicating that the hypothalamic/pituitary axis and the ovaries are functioning normally. The results of such clinical evaluations are indicated in Table 26-1.

TABLE 26-1	RESULTS OF CLINICAL EVALUATIONS FOR SECONDARY AMENORRHEA		
	Serum FSH	Serum LH	Bleeding after Progesterone Withdrawal Test[a]
Anorexia nervosa	Low	Low	No
Ovariectomy	High	High	No
Asherman syndrome	Normal	Normal	No

FSH, follicle-stimulating hormone; LH, leuteinizing hormone.
[a]10 mg of medroxyprogesterone is given daily for 5 days. Withdrawal bleeding suggests that sufficient estrogen production is present for uterine proliferation.

5. **Menorrhagia** is excessive bleeding at menstruation in either the amount of blood or number of days. It is usually associated with a leiomyoma (fibroids).

6. **Dysmenorrhea** is excessive pain during menstruation. It is commonly associated with endometriosis and an increased level of prostaglandin F in the menstrual fluid.

7. **Metrorrhagia** is bleeding that occurs at irregular intervals. It is commonly associated with cervical carcinoma or cervical polyps.

8. **Prepubertal bleeding** is bleeding that occurs before menarche. It is commonly associated with vaginitis, infection, sexual abuse, or embryonal rhabdomyosarcoma.

9. **Postmenopausal bleeding** occurs approximately 1 year after the cessation of the menstrual cycle. It is commonly associated with malignant tumors of the uterus.

VI **Cervix.** The cervix is the lower part of the uterus that measures about 2.5 to 3.0 cm in length. The cervix is divided into a **supravaginal portion** (lying above the vaginal vault) and a **vaginal portion (portio vaginalis)**, which protrudes into the vagina. The junction between the cervix and uterus is at the **internal os**. Histologically, the cervical wall consists of:

A. A **simple columnar epithelium**, which invaginates into the cervical stroma to form mucus-secreting cervical glands. This epithelium and cervical glands do not slough off during the menstrual cycle and are relatively unaffected by the menstrual cycle. The cervical mucus produced during the proliferative phase is **watery** and the cervical mucus produced during the proliferative phase is **viscous**.

B. The wall of the cervix is predominately **connective tissue** with very little smooth muscle (very different compared to the uterine wall, which is predominately smooth muscle). During pregnancy, the cervix undergoes little or no expansion. However, during childbirth, the connective tissue becomes pliable (called "**cervical softening**") due to the action of **relaxin**.

VII **Ectocervix (Figure 26-4).** The outer epithelial surface of the vaginal portion of the cervix (portio vaginalis) is called the **ectocervix**. The epithelial surface lining the lumen of the **endocervical canal** is called the **endocervix**.

A. During prepuberty, the ectocervix is covered by a **nonkeratinized, stratified squamous epithelium** that is continuous with the vaginal epithelium.

B. The **endocervical canal** connects the uterine cavity with the vaginal cavity and extends from the internal os to the **external os**. The endocervical canal is lined by **simple columnar epithelium**, which invaginates into the cervical stroma to form **mucus-secreting cervical glands**.

C. At puberty, the simple columnar epithelium of the endocervical canal extends onto the ectocervix. However, exposure of the simple columnar epithelium to the acidic (pH = 3) environment of the vagina induces a transformation from columnar to squamous epithelium (i.e., **squamous metaplasia**) and the formation of a **transformation zone**.

D. The transformation zone is the site of **Nabothian cysts**, which develop as stratified squamous epithelium grows over the mucus-secreting simple columnar epithelium and entraps large amounts of mucus.

E. The transformation zone is the most common site of **squamous cell carcinoma of the cervix**, which is usually preceded by epithelial changes called **cervical intraepithelial neoplasia (CIN)** diagnosed by a Pap smear. **Human papillomavirus (HPV)** has also been linked as an important factor in cervical oncogenesis and is often tested for.

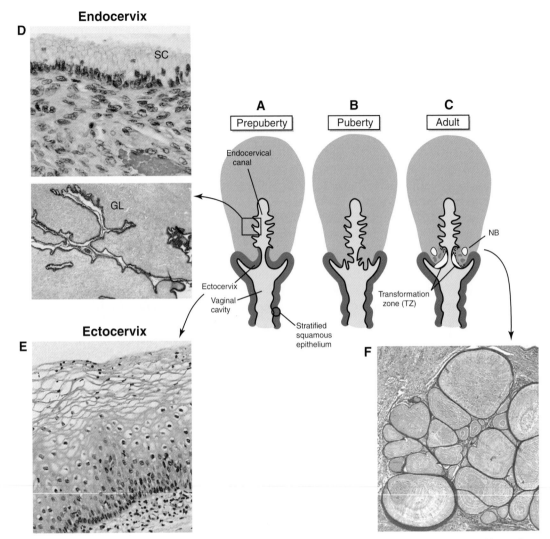

● **Figure 26-4 Diagram of the cervical–vaginal junction. A:** During prepuberty, the ectocervix is covered by nonkeratinized stratified squamous epithelium that is continuous with vaginal epithelium (*black area*). **B:** At puberty, the simple columnar epithelium and cervical glands extend onto the ectocervix. **C:** In the adult, exposure of the simple columnar epithelium to the acidic (pH = 3) environment of the vagina induces a squamous metaplasia, forming the transformation zone (*clear area*). Nabothian cysts (NB) may form in the transformation zone. TZ, transformation zone. **D:** Light micrograph (LM) of the endocervix shows a simple columnar epithelium (SC) and prominent mucus-secreting cervical glands (GL). **E:** LM of the ectocervix shows a nonkeratinized stratified squamous epithelium. Note the luminal cells have a clear cytoplasm indicative of large amounts of glycogen storage. **F:** LM of the transformation zone in the adult shows Nabothian cysts or tunnel clusters, which form as stratified squamous epithelium grows over mucus-secreting simple columnar epithelium and entraps large amounts of mucus.

VIII **Vagina (Figure 26-5).** The vagina is a fibromuscular tube that is kept moist by mucus produced by cervical glands that drain down through the cervical canal and additional mucus produced by the greater vestibular glands (of Bartholin) and lesser vestibular glands. Histologically, the vaginal wall consists of a mucosa (epithelium and lamina propria), muscularis layer, and adventitia.

A. EPITHELIUM. The vagina is lined by **nonkeratinized stratified squamous epithelium**.
  1. The most superficial layer of cells is continuously exfoliated during the menstrual cycle, but exfoliation increases during the late secretory phase and menstrual phase.
  2. Under the influence of estrogen, the epithelial cells accumulate large amounts of glycogen and undergo cell proliferation in the basal and parabasal layers.

3. The exfoliated cells contain **glycogen**, which is metabolized by commensal lacto-bacilli to lactic acid, which forms an **acidic (pH = 3) environment**. The acidic environment deters the invasion of bacterial pathogens and fungi (e.g., *Candida albicans*, which causes vaginal thrush).

4. A vaginal smear (stained with Schorr trichrome and Harris hematoxylin) may be used clinically to evaluate the hormonal status of a woman (**Table 26-2**). A vaginal smear contains three basic cell types.

    a. **Superficial squamous cells** (40 to 65 μm diameter) are flat with an irregular border and a light orange cytoplasm. These cells form under the influence of estrogen.

    b. **Intermediate squamous cells** (20 to 40 μm diameter) are flat with an irregular border and a blue cytoplasm. These cells form under the influence of progesterone.

    c. **Parabasal cells** (12 to 15 μm diameter) are oval with a large nucleus with prominent chromatin and a blue cytoplasm. Parabasal cells in a vaginal smear imply the absence of estrogen or progesterone influence.

TABLE 26-2	MATURATION INDEX[a] IN VARIOUS CLINICAL SITUATIONS		
	SSC	ISC	PBC
Normal nonpregnant adult woman	70	30	0
Estrogen tumor or therapy Polycystic ovarian syndrome	100	0	0
Pregnant woman Prepubescent girl	0	100	0
Menopausal woman	0	0	100

SSC, superficial squamous cells; ISC, intermediate squamous cells; PBC, parabasal cells.
[a]Maturation index is based on the morphology of 100 observed cells.

B. The **lamina propria** is composed of connective tissue and contains a rich network of blood vessels that is thought to help moisten the vagina.

C. The **muscularis layer** consists of ill-defined bundles of **smooth muscle** and a rich network of **elastic fibers** that are responsible for the great distensibility of the vagina during childbirth.

D. The **adventitia** consists of connective tissue.

IX **Histopathology of the Vagina.** Vaginitis is a chronic infection most often caused by *Trichomonas vaginalis* (15% of cases), *Candida albicans* (25%), or *Gardnerella vaginalis* (30%). The vaginal epithelium is resistant to bacterial, fungal, and protozoan invasion so that the pathogens remain within the lumen of the vagina.

A. ***TRICHOMONAS VAGINALIS*** is a **flagellated protozoan** that is sexually transmitted. It produces a vaginitis characterized by an inflammatory vaginal smear with numerous neutrophils, fiery-red appearance of the vaginal and cervical mucosa ("strawberry mucosa"), and a **thin, gray-white, frothy, purulent, malodorous discharge (pH >4.5)**. Postcoital bleeding is a common complaint. The organism is best seen in fresh preparations diluted with warm saline where the tumbling motility of the organism can be observed.

B. ***CANDIDA ALBICANS*** is yeast that produces pseudohyphae and true hyphae in tissues. It produces superficial white patches or large fluffy membranes that easily detach leaving a red, irritated underlying surface and a **thick, white, "cottage cheese" discharge (pH <4.5)**. The organism can be observed on KOH preparations of the discharge.

C. ***GARDNERELLA VAGINALIS* (A GRAM-NEGATIVE BACILLUS)** is a bacterial infection generally called **bacterial vaginosis** where higher levels than normal of the bacteria are present. It is not sexually transmitted. It produces a vaginitis characterized by no inflammatory vaginal smear, no changes in the mucosa, and a **thin, homogenous, somewhat adherent, fishy-odor discharge (pH >4.5).** The discharge gives a positive amine test ("whiff test"; fishy amine smell) when mixed with KOH. A vaginal smear will show increased number of bacteria and "clue cells," which are squamous cells with a clumped nucleus and a folded cytoplasm covered with bacteria.

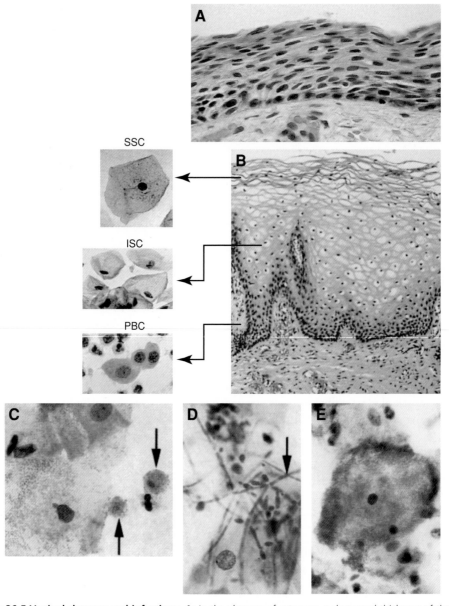

● **Figure 26-5 Vaginal changes and infections. A:** In the absence of estrogen, a decreased thickness of the vaginal epithelium is observed. **B:** In the presence of estrogen, an increased thickness of the vaginal epithelium is observed. A vaginal smear contains three basic cell types from various levels of the vaginal epithelium: superficial squamous cells (SSC), intermediate squamous cells (ISC), and parabasal cells (PBC). **C:** *Trichomonas vaginalis.* The presence of the flagellated protozoan is shown in a vaginal smear. **D:** *Candida albicans.* The presence of the yeast is shown in a vaginal smear. **E:** *Gardnerella vaginalis.* A "clue cell," which is a squamous cell with a clumped nucleus and folded cytoplasm covered with bacteria, is shown.

Breast. The breast lies in the superficial fascia of the anterior chest wall overlying the **pectoralis major** and **serratus anterior muscles** and extends into the **superior lateral quadrant** of the axilla as the **axillary tail** where a high percentage of tumors occur. The breast is covered by **skin** (epidermis and dermis), which is modified at the nipple and areola and contains **suspensory (Cooper) ligaments, adipose tissue** (which contributes to size and contour), and **mammary gland tissue.**

A. NIPPLE AND AREOLA

    1. The nipple is a round, raised area of modified skin in the center of the **areola.** The skin has a lightly **keratinized stratified squamous epithelium** and a dermis of **connective tissue with elastic fibers and smooth muscle fibers** arranged circularly around the base of the nipple and longitudinally that parallel the lactiferous ducts. Contraction of the smooth muscles due to cold, tactile, or emotional stimulation results in **erection of the nipple.** The base of the epithelium is invaded by deep dermal papillae containing numerous capillaries that bring blood close to the surface and impart a **pinkish color** to the nipple in children and blonde individuals. At puberty, the epithelium becomes pigmented (melanin) and changes the color to **light → dark brown.**

    2. The skin around the nipple is called the **areola,** which is modified skin that contains large sebaceous glands that form small nodular elevations in the areola called **Montgomery tubercles.** The color of the areola is initially pinkish (like the nipple), but during pregnancy the color changes to light → dark brown as a result of increased pigmentation (melanin). After delivery, the areola may lighten in color but rarely returns to its original shade. The **sensory innervation** of the nipple and areola are important because stimulation of the nipple and areola by the suckling infant triggers a sequence of neurohormonal events that result in **ejection of milk (oxytocin)** and **production of milk (prolactin).**

    3. Clinical considerations. Nipple secretion typically contains exfoliated duct cells, α-lactalbumin, immunoglobulins, lactose, cholesterol, steroids, and fatty acids, along with ethanol, caffeine, nicotine, barbiturates, pesticides, and technetium.

        a. A nipple discharge that is green, milky, yellow, or brown; not spontaneous; and bilateral and affects multiple ducts is usually a **benign situation.**

        b. A milky discharge (galactorrhea) along with a headache and peripheral vision loss may indicate a **pituitary adenoma (prolactinoma).**

        c. A nipple discharge that is bloody or clear (serous), spontaneous, or unilateral and affects a single duct usually indicates a **malignant situation.**

B. MAMMARY GLAND (FIGURE 26-6). In general, the mammary gland is a compound, tubuloalveolar gland that develops as downgrowths of the epidermis along the **milk line,** which runs from the axilla to the groin on each side. The mammary gland consists of **alveoli,** which are ultimately drained by **15 to 20 lactiferous ducts** that open onto the tip of the **nipple arranged in a ring.** Just deep to the surface of the nipple, each lactiferous duct expands into a **lactiferous sinus,** which serves as a reservoir for milk during lactation. The histology of the mammary gland changes as the female progresses through prepuberty, puberty, pregnancy, and lactation.

    1. Prepuberty. At birth and prepuberty, the nipple and a simple system of ducts (or epithelial downgrowths) embedded in connective tissue are present. The full development of epithelial downgrowths begins at puberty.

    2. At Puberty. The development of breasts at puberty is one of the secondary sex characteristics of women. Under the influence of **estrogen** from the ovary, the breast accumulates **adipose tissue,** which is largely responsible for variations in breast size. In addition, epithelial downgrowths begin in earnest and branch into the connective tissue to form a system of ducts. There are no alveoli present, only **solid masses of epithelial cells.**

3. **During Pregnancy.** Under the influence of estrogen and progesterone, the duct system grows prolifically in length and branching. Eventually, the characteristic structure of the mammary gland takes shape: **15 to 20 lobules** drained by **intralobular ducts** that empty into **interlobular ducts** and eventually into the **lactiferous ducts.** In addition, the solid masses of epithelial cells grow and form **alveoli,** which are surrounded by **myoepithelial cells.** Ducts and alveoli distend as alveoli secrete **colostrum.** This proliferation of glandular tissue takes place at the expense of the adipose tissue, which concurrently decreases as glandular tissue increases.

4. **During Lactation.** The epithelial cells of the alveoli become active in **milk production.** Numerous fat droplets and secretory vacuoles containing dense aggregates of milk proteins can be observed ultrastructurally at the apical end of the alveolar epithelial cells. Human breast milk is produced 1 to 3 days after childbirth. Breast milk contains a substantial amount of lipid, protein, lactose, vitamins, and secretory immunoglobulin A (IgA; which affords temporary enteric passive immunity). Although milk is produced continuously by the alveoli (milk production), it is delivered only in response to suckling **(milk letdown).** Suckling stimulates afferent neurons, which relay the information to the hypothalamus such that the following actions occur: (a) **oxytocin** is released from the posterior hypophysis, which causes the contraction of myoepithelial cells and mild letdown, and (b) **prolactin-inhibiting hormone (PIH; dopamine)** is inhibited, which causes the release of **prolactin** from the adenohypophysis and further milk production.

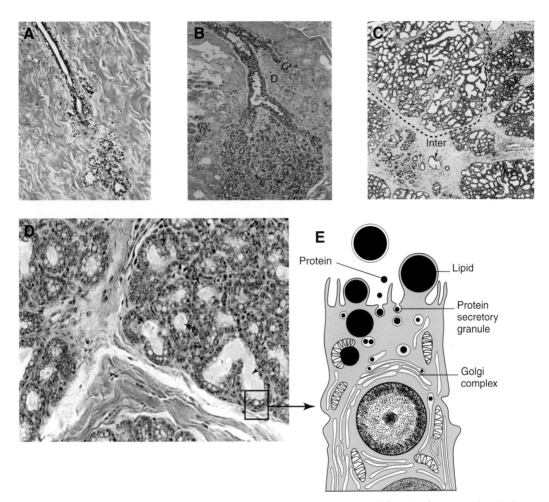

● **Figure 26-6 Mammary gland. A:** Prepuberty. Breast tissue from a 4-month-old female infant. Note the simple system of ducts or epithelial downgrowths (D). **B:** At puberty. Breast tissue from an 11-year-old girl. Note the elongation and branching system of ducts (D) and the early formation of epithelial buds from the small terminal ducts. **C:** During pregnancy. Breast tissue taken from a pregnant woman. Note the lobule (*dotted line*; L) consisting of alveoli distended with colostrum. An interlobular duct (inter) is shown. **D:** During lactation. Breast tissue taken from a lactating woman. Note that the alveoli of the mammary glands (*arrows*) are filled with milk. The cellsin the boxed area are shown in E. **E:** Diagram of an alveolar epithelial cell from an alveolus of a breast during lactation. Note that the alveolar epithelial cell secretes both a lipid product and protein product as components of the milk.

XI **Selected Photomicrographs**

    A. Cervical biopsy of cervical intraepithelial neoplasia (CIN I, CIN II, CIN III), Pap smears of cervical intraepithelial neoplasia (CIN I, CIN II, CIN III), human papilloma virus (HPV), and squamous cell carcinoma (Figure 26-7)

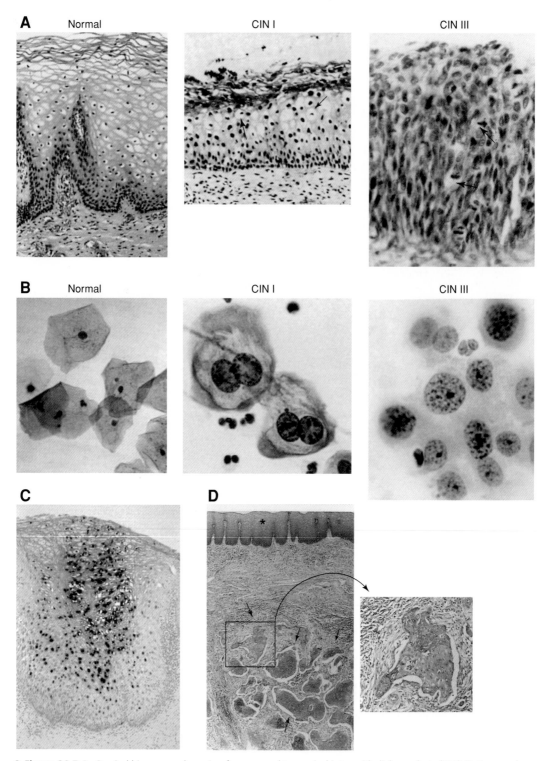

● **Figure 26-7 A:** Cervical biopsy panel ranging from normal to cervical intraepithelial neoplasia (CIN) III. A normal cervical biopsy shows a typical appearance of stratified squamous epithelium. CIN I shows superficial keratinization and koilocytotic atypia as evidenced by prominent perinuclear halos (*small arrows*). CIN III shows atypical oblong nuclei, vertical orientation of epithelial cells, and mitotic figures near the surface (*arrows*). **B:** Pap smear panel ranging from normal to CIN III. A normal Pap smear shows typical superficial squamous epithelial cells with a relatively small nucleus and with a large cytoplasmic area. Progression from CIN I → CIN III is generally reflected in a reduction in the amount of cytoplasm and an increase in the nucleus:cytoplasm ratio. CIN I shows nuclear enlargement, hyperchromatism, and binucleation disproportionate to cytoplasmic maturity. CIN III shows nuclei that vary in size and shape. The chromatin material is coarse and granular. **C:** Human papilloma virus (HPV) localized in cervical biopsy by in situ hybridization for DNA sequences specific for HPV. **D:** Squamous cell carcinoma of the cervix. CIN I → CIN III usually precedes the appearance of squamous cell carcinoma. Stratified squamous epithelium (*asterisk*) in the transformation zone has invaded the underlying stroma, forming nests of malignant cells (*arrows*). High magnification of the nests (*boxed area*) is shown.

B. Fibroadenoma of the breast, infiltrating duct carcinoma of the breast (Figure 26-8)

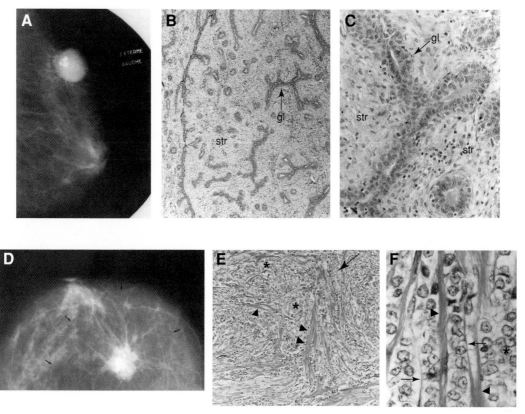

● **Figure 26-8 Breast pathology. A–C:** Fibroadenoma of the breast. **A:** A mediolateral oblique mammogram. A benign mass is shown. A benign mass has the following characteristics: **shape** is round/oval, **margins** are well circumscribed, **density** is low-medium contrast, it becomes smaller over time, and **calcifications** are large, smooth, and uniform. **B, C:** Light micrograph (LM) of a fibroadenoma, which is a benign proliferation of the connective tissue stroma (str). As a consequence, the glands (gl) are compressed into cords of epithelium with slitlike spaces. A fibroadenoma presents clinically as a sharply circumscribed, spherical nodule that is freely movable. **D–F:** Infiltrating duct carcinoma. **D:** A craniocaudal mammogram. A malignant mass is shown. A malignant mass has the following characteristics: **shape** is irregular with many lobulations, **margins** are irregular or spiculated, **density** is medium-high, breast architecture may be distorted, it becomes larger over time, and **calcifications** (not shown) are small, irregular, variable, and found within ducts (ductal casts). *Arrows* indicate a clear zone around the tumor with spicules. **E, F:** LM of infiltrating duct carcinoma of the breast. The tumor cells are arranged in cell nests (*), cell cords (*arrows*), anastomosing masses, or a mixture of all of these. The cells are surrounded by fairly thick bands of connective tissue stroma (*arrowheads*). This is the most common type of breast cancer, accounting for 65% to 80% of all breast cancers. Some features that are common to all infiltrative breast carcinomas include fixed in position, retraction and dimpling of the skin, thickening of the skin (peau d'orange), and retraction of the nipple. The presence of estrogen receptors or progesterone receptors within the carcinoma cells indicates a good prognosis for treatment. Tamoxifen is an estrogen receptor blocker and is the drug of choice for treatment. The presence of the c-erb B2 oncoprotein (similar to the epidermal growth factor receptor) on the surface of the carcinoma cells indicates a poor prognosis for treatment. *BRCA1* gene (breast cancer susceptibility gene) is an antioncogene (tumor suppressor gene) located on chromosome 17q21 that encodes for **BRCA protein** (a zinc finger gene-regulatory protein) containing phosphotyrosine, which will suppress the cell cycle. A mutation of the *BRCA1* gene is present in 5% to 10% of women with breast cancer and confers a very high lifetime risk of breast and ovarian cancer.

Case Study 26-1

A 55-year-old woman comes to your office complaining that "I'm having real bad pains in my stomach. I feel bloated and uncomfortable even though I've lost a few pounds recently." She also tells you that "I've got to pee a lot more often lately." After some discussion, she informs you that she has never been pregnant and her menstrual periods have always been regular. Her mother and sister both died of breast cancer. The woman does not seem to be very concerned about her condition as she says, "Doc, I've had regular breast exams ever since my mom died and they have always been negative, thank God. You know, my mother and sister got a bad break with breast cancer and I'm very lonely without them. I really feel lucky that I only have a little stomach ache to deal with." What is the most likely diagnosis?

Differentials

- Cancer metastasis to the ovary, endometrial carcinoma

Relevant Physical Examination Findings

- Mass in the pelvis
- Ascites in the abdomen
- No vaginal discharge

Relevant Lab Findings

- Blood chemistry: serum CA-125 high
- Computed tomography (CT) scan: 7-cm right ovarian mass; 5-cm left ovarian mass
- Biopsy: extensive network of papillae projecting from the wall of the mass along with invasion of the stroma and capsule; many laminated calcified concretions (psammoma bodies) are observed.

Diagnosis: Ovarian Serous Cystadenocarcinoma

- Ovarian serous cystadenocarcinoma (OS) is the most common ovarian neoplasm ($\approx$50% of ovarian cancers) and is commonly bilateral. OS is a multiloculated tumor with soft, delicate papillae lining the entire surface. Solid areas with necrosis and hemorrhage are commonly present. The majority of ovarian tumors do not secrete hormone but are associated with serum CA-125 antigen. Risk factors for ovarian cancer are nulliparity and a family history of cancer associated with the *BRCA1* mutation. Clinical findings of ovarian tumors include abdominal distention, lower abdominal pain, pelvic pressure, compression of regional organs, ascites, increased urinary frequency, and weight loss.
- The most common cancer metastasis to the ovary occurs from tumors of the uterus, uterine tubes, contralateral ovary, breast, and gastrointestinal tract. The Krukenberg tumor describes stomach cancer that metastasizes to the ovaries.
- Endometrial carcinoma is the most common gynecologic malignancy in the United States and has been linked to prolonged estrogen stimulation of the endometrium (e.g., estrogen replacement therapy during menopause). Endometrial carcinoma often presents with vaginal bleeding. Risk factors for endometrial carcinoma are nulliparity, obesity, diabetes, late menopause, early menarche, and unopposed estrogen stimulation.

Chapter 27

Male Reproductive System

Testes. The testes (plural) are paired, ovoid organs located in the scrotum. Each mature adult testis (singular) is 4 to 5 cm in length, 2.5 cm in width, and 3 cm in thickness and weighs about 11 to 17 g. The right testis is commonly slightly larger and heavier than the left. The testes are surrounded incompletely (medially, laterally, and anteriorly, but not posteriorly) by a sac of peritoneum called the **tunica vaginalis.** Beneath the tunica vaginalis, the testes are surrounded by a thick connective tissue capsule called the **tunica albuginea** because of its whitish color. Beneath the tunica albuginea, the testes are surrounded by a highly vascular layer of connective tissue called the **tunica vasculosa.** The tunica albuginea projects connective tissue **septae** inward toward the mediastinum, which divides the testis into about **250 lobules,** each of which contains **one to four highly coiled seminiferous tubules.** These septae converge toward the midline on the posterior surface where they meet to form a ridge-like thickening called the mediastinum. The septae are continuous with the **interstitial connective tissue** that contains the Leydig (interstitial) cells that secrete testosterone. The testes contain the **seminiferous tubules, straight tubules, rete testes** and **Leydig (interstitial) cells.**

A. **SEMINIFEROUS TUBULES (FIGURES 27-1 AND 27-2 AND TABLE 27-1).** In a sexually mature male, a seminiferous tubule is about 30 to 80 cm in length, is 150 μm in diameter, and has a lumen. (In a sexually immature boy, the seminiferous "tubules" have no lumen and are therefore more appropriately referred to as **seminiferous cords.**) The combined total length of all the seminiferous tubules in each testis is about 300 to 900 m. The seminiferous tubules are lined by a complex stratified epithelium (**germinal epithelium**) consisting of two basic cell types: **Sertoli cells** and **spermatogenic cells.**

   1. **Sertoli cells.** Sertoli cells are columnar cells with unusually ruffled apical and lateral surfaces due to the fact that these surfaces surround the developing spermatogenic cells. Sertoli cells extend the full thickness of the germinal epithelium. Sertoli cells have the following functions:

      a. Provide mechanical and nutritional support for developing spermatogenic cells

      b. Phagocytose excess cytoplasm discarded by spermatids

      c. Form the **blood-testes barrier** through **tight junctions** on their lateral surfaces

      d. Secrete **inhibin** that inhibits release of follicle-stimulating hormone (FSH) from adenohypophysis

      e. Secrete **müllerian inhibitory factor (MIF)** during fetal development that inhibits development of the paramesonephric duct in a genotypic XY fetus

      f. Synthesize **androgen-binding protein (ABP)** that binds testosterone so that high levels of testosterone are present in the seminiferous tubules, which is necessary for spermatogenesis to occur

      g. Possess **FSH receptors** (G protein–linked receptors) so that FSH from the adenohypophysis stimulates spermatogenesis and synthesis of ABP

   2. **SPERMATOGENIC CELLS.** Spermatogenic cells are the "male germ cells" that are undergoing the transformation from type A spermatogonia → sperm. This transformation is called **spermatogenesis.** As the spermatogenic cells undergo spermatogenesis,

they migrate from the basal layer to the luminal layer of the germinal epithelium and consist of the following cell types: **type A spermatogonia (dark type A and pale type A), type B spermatogonia, primary spermatocytes, secondary spermatocytes, spermatids (early and late stages), and spermatozoa (sperm).** Spermatogenesis is divided into three stages: **spermatocytogenesis, meiosis, and spermiogenesis.**

a. **Spermatocytogenesis.** Dark type A spermatogonia undergo <u>mitosis</u> to provide a continuous supply of stem cells throughout the reproductive life of the male. Then, pale type A spermatogonia undergo mitosis and differentiate to form **type B spermatogonia.** Type B spermatogonia may also undergo mitosis to produce more type B spermatogonia. Type B spermatocytes then enter meiosis.

b. **Meiosis.** Meiosis is a cell division process that occurs only in the production of the male and female gametes (do not confuse meiosis with mitosis). **MEIOSIS OCCURS ONLY IN THE OVARY AND TESTES.** Meiosis consists of two cell divisions (**meiosis I and meiosis II**) and results in the formation of four gametes containing 23 chromosomes and 1N amount of DNA. Meiosis does three important things: (**i**) reduces the number of chromosomes within the gametes to ensure that the human species number of chromosomes (46) can be maintained from generation to generation, (**ii**) redistributes maternal and paternal chromosomes to ensure genetic variability, and (**iii**) promotes the exchange of small amounts of maternal and paternal DNA via crossover during meiosis I.

c. **Spermiogenesis.** Spermiogenesis is a **postmeiotic** series of <u>morphologic</u> changes by which spermatids (round-shaped cells) are transformed into sperm ("sleek swimmers"). The transformation is divided into four phases.

   i. **Golgi Phase.** Numerous **proacrosomal granules** appear in the Golgi vesicles and coalesce to form a single **acrosomal granule** within the **acrosomal vesicle.** The centrioles migrate to the posterior pole of the spermatid and initiate assembly of the 9 + 2 microtubule arrangement of the axoneme (i.e., cilium) of the sperm tail.

   ii. **Cap Phase.** The acrosomal vesicle flattens and spreads over the anterior two thirds of the nucleus and is now called the **acrosomal cap.**

   iii. **Acrosome Phase.** The large acrosome granule diffuses throughout the acrosomal vesicle, thereby forming the **acrosome.** The nuclear chromatin begins to condense as the nucleus begins to elongate. Cytoplasmic microtubules organize into a cylindrical sheet called the **manchette,** which assists in the elongation of the spermatid and extends from the posterior rim of the acrosome toward the developing tail. Centrioles migrate to the posterior pole of the spermatid and initiate the formation of the **outer dense fibers** around the axoneme. Cytoplasmic mitochondria migrate to form a **helical sheath** around the outer dense fibers. The spermatid rotates so that the acrosomal cap orientates toward the basal lamina of the seminiferous tubule and the tail orientates toward the lumen.

● **Figure 27-1 General features of the testes. A:** Diagram of the testis and duct system. **B:** Light micrograph of a seminiferous tubule within the testis. The seminiferous tubule contains spermatogonia (1), primary spermatocytes (2), secondary spermatocytes (3), early spermatids (4), late spermatids (5), and Sertoli cells (6). In addition, the three stages of spermatogenesis (spermatocytogenesis, meiosis, and spermiogenesis) are indicated by the brackets (correlate with Table 27-1). The level of the blood-testes barrier is indicated by the *dotted line.* **C:** Diagram of the Sertoli cell. Note the close relationship of the Sertoli cell and spermatogenic cells (*arrows*), whereby the spermatogenic cells indent the surface of the Sertoli cell so that the cell border of the Sertoli is quite irregular. **D–G:** Diagram of the four phases of spermiogenesis. **D:** Golgi phase. 1, Golgi; 2, Golgi vesicles; 3, acrosomal granule with the acrosomal vesicle; 4, nucleus; 5, centrioles and developing axoneme (cilium). **E:** Cap phase. 1, Golgi; 2, acrosomal cap; 3, centrioles and developing axoneme (cilium). **F:** Acrosome phase. 1, acrosome; 2, nucleus; 3, manchette; 4, Golgi. **G:** Maturation phase. 1, nucleus; 2, mitochondrial sheath; 3, annulus (a dense ring that separates the middle piece from the principal piece); 4, principal piece; 5, excess cytoplasm.

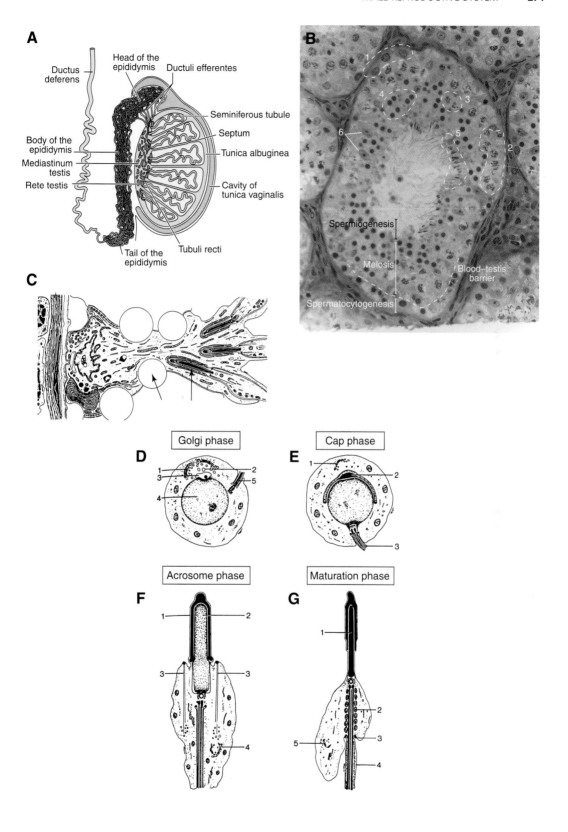

A

Ductus deferens

Head of the epididymis

Ductuli efferentes

Seminiferous tubule

Septum

Tunica albuginea

Body of the epididymis

Mediastinum testis

Rete testis

Cavity of tunica vaginalis

Tail of the epididymis

Tubuli recti

B

Spermiogenesis

Meiosis

Spermatocytogenesis

Blood–testis barrier

C

Golgi phase

D

Cap phase

E

Acrosome phase

F

Maturation phase

G

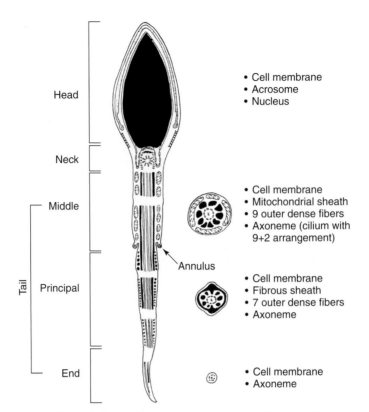

Head
• Cell membrane
• Acrosome
• Nucleus

Neck

Middle
• Cell membrane
• Mitochondrial sheath
• 9 outer dense fibers
• Axoneme (cilium with 9+2 arrangement)

Annulus

Tail

Principal
• Cell membrane
• Fibrous sheath
• 7 outer dense fibers
• Axoneme

End
• Cell membrane
• Axoneme

● **Figure 27-2 Ultrastructural morphology of a mature spermatozoon.** The spermatozoon consists of a **head region, neck region,** and **tail region** (which is further divided into the **middle piece, principal piece,** and **end piece**). Cross sections of the middle piece, principal piece, and end piece are shown. Note the list of components from outside to inside. The annulus is a dense ring that separates the middle piece from the principal piece. Newly ejaculated sperm are incapable of fertilization until they undergo capacitation. Capacitation is a reversible process whereby freshly ejaculated sperm develop the capacity to fertilize a secondary oocyte. Capacitation normally occurs in the female reproductive tract and takes 7 hours. It involves the following: unmasking of glycosyltransferases on the sperm cell membrane and removal of surface-coating proteins derived from seminal fluid.

iv. **Maturation Phase.** The nucleus acquires its final elongated and condensed state. Excess spermatid cytoplasm is discarded and phagocytosed by Sertoli cells. The manchette disassembles. Intercellular bridges are lost.

B. **STRAIGHT TUBULES.** Toward the terminal portion of each seminiferous tubule, the spermatogenic cells disappear such that the germinal epithelium lining the seminiferous tubule consists solely of Sertoli cells. At the end of the each seminiferous tubule, there is an abrupt narrowing or transition to the **straight tubules** (also called **tubuli recti**), which are lined by **simple cuboidal epithelium.**

C. **RETE TESTES.** The straight tubules empty into an anastomosing labyrinth of channels located at the mediastinum called the rete testes. The rete testes are lined by **simple cuboidal epithelium.**

D. **LEYDIG CELLS (FIGURE 27-3).** The Leydig cells (or interstitial cells) of the testes are located in the loose connective tissue between the seminiferous tubules. Leydig cells are large, irregularly shaped, polygonal, acidophilic cells. Leydig cells have an elaborate smooth endoplasmic reticulum (sER), lipid droplets, mitochondria with tubular cristae, and highly refractive, rod-shaped crystals called crystals of Reinke. Leydig cells are steroid-secreting cells (i.e., testosterone) and therefore have all the cell organelles that are typically found in steroid-secreting cells. The functions of the Leydig cells include:

1. Possess **leuteinizing hormone (LH) receptors** (G protein–linked receptors) so that LH from the adenohypophysis stimulates testosterone secretion

TABLE 27-1   **SUMMARY OF SPERMATOGENESIS**

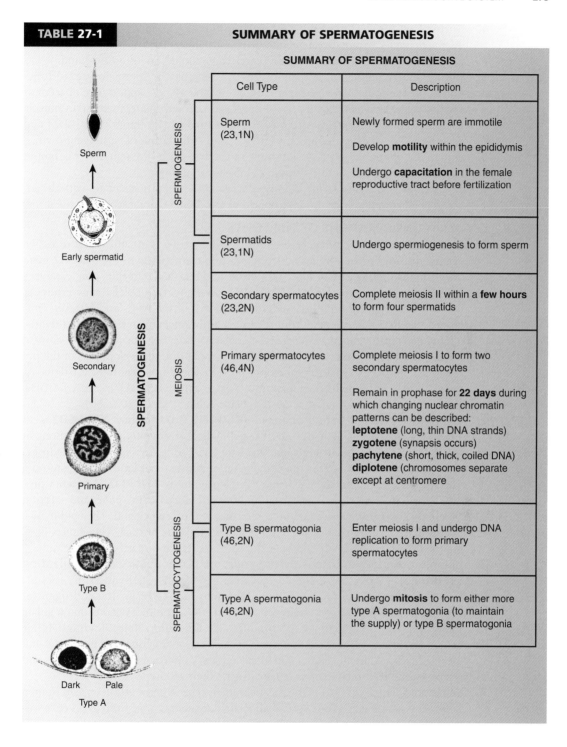

SUMMARY OF SPERMATOGENESIS

Cell Type	Description
Sperm (23,1N)	Newly formed sperm are immotile Develop **motility** within the epididymis Undergo **capacitation** in the female reproductive tract before fertilization
Spermatids (23,1N)	Undergo spermiogenesis to form sperm
Secondary spermatocytes (23,2N)	Complete meiosis II within a **few hours** to form four spermatids
Primary spermatocytes (46,4N)	Complete meiosis I to form two secondary spermatocytes Remain in prophase for **22 days** during which changing nuclear chromatin patterns can be described: **leptotene** (long, thin DNA strands) **zygotene** (synapsis occurs) **pachytene** (short, thick, coiled DNA) **diplotene** (chromosomes separate except at centromere
Type B spermatogonia (46,2N)	Enter meiosis I and undergo DNA replication to form primary spermatocytes
Type A spermatogonia (46,2N)	Undergo **mitosis** to form either more type A spermatogonia (to maintain the supply) or type B spermatogonia

2. Secrete **testosterone**. Testosterone gives rise to two other potent androgens via the following pathways:

$$\text{Testosterone} \xrightarrow{\text{5}\alpha\text{-reductase}} \textbf{dihydrotestosterone (DHT)}$$

$$\text{Testosterone} \xrightarrow{\text{3}\alpha\text{-reductase}} \textbf{5}\alpha\text{-androstanediol}$$

3. Aromatization of testosterone and androstenedione within the liver and adipose tissue by P_{450} **aromatase** produces significant amounts of estradiol and estrone in males.

4. During fetal life, testosterone is essential in the development of the epididymis, ductus deferens, seminal vesicle, and ejaculatory duct. DHT is essential in the development of the penis and scrotum (external genitalia) and prostate gland.

5. During puberty and adult life, androgens are essential for spermatogenesis; function of prostate, seminal vesicle, and bulbourethral glands; appearance of secondary sex characteristics; closure of the epiphyseal growth plate; increase in muscle mass; lipid metabolism (testosterone increases low-density lipoprotein [LDL] and decreases high-density lipoprotein [HDL]); and stimulation of cartilage growth.

6. One to 2% of circulating testosterone is in the free form; the remainder is bound to a liver-derived **sex steroid–binding globulin** or **albumin**.

7. Testosterone is degraded in the liver by conversion to various metabolites with the addition of glucuronide (e.g., 3α-androstanediol glucuronide) and excreted in the urine.

E. CLINICAL CONSIDERATIONS OF THE TESTES

1. **5α-Reductase 2 Deficiency.** 5α-Reductase 2 deficiency is an autosomal recessive genetic disorder caused by loss-of-function point mutations in the *SRD5A2* **gene** on **chromosome 2p23** for the **5α-steroid reductase 2** enzyme that catalyzes the conversion of **testosterone (T) → DHT**. 5α-Reductase 2 deficiency produces the following clinical findings: underdevelopment of the penis and scrotum (microphallus, hypospadias, and bifid scrotum) and prostate gland. The epididymis, ductus deferens, seminal vesicle, and ejaculatory duct are normal. These clinical findings have led to inference that DHT is essential in the development of the penis and scrotum (external genitalia) and prostate gland in a genotypic XY fetus. At puberty, these individuals demonstrate a striking virilization. An increased T:DHT ratio is diagnostic (normal = 5; 5α-reductase 2 deficiency = 20 to 60).

2. **17β-Hydroxysteroid Dehydrogenase 3 (17βHSD3) Deficiency.** 17β-HSD3 is an autosomal recessive genetic disorder caused by loss-of-function point mutations in the *HSD17B3* **gene** on **chromosome 9q22** for the **17β-hydroxysteroid dehydrogenase 3** enzyme that catalyzes the conversion of **androstenedione → testosterone**. This is the most common defect in androgen biosynthesis. 17β-HSD3 deficiency produces the following clinical findings: underdevelopment of the penis and scrotum (microphallus, hypospadias, and bifid scrotum) and prostate gland. The epididymis, ductus deferens, seminal vesicle, and ejaculatory duct are normal. The clinical findings in 17β-HSD deficiency and 5α-reductase 2 deficiency are very similar.

3. **Complete Androgen Insensitivity Syndrome (CAIS; Testicular Feminization Syndrome).** CAIS is an X-linked recessive genetic disorder caused by loss-of-function mutations in the *AR* **gene** on **chromosome Xq12** for the **androgen receptor**, which is activated by androgens to bind DNA promoter regions that regulate transcription of other genes. CAIS produces the following clinical findings: 46,XY genotype; testes; and normal-appearing female external genitalia. The uterus and uterine tubes are absent. These individuals present as normal-appearing females and their psychosocial orientation is female despite their genotype.

4. **Seminoma** (Figure 27-4A) is the most common type of germ cell neoplasm in men 20 to 40 years of age. About 90% of all testicular cancers arise from germ cells. Almost all germ cell neoplasms involve the isochromosome of the short arm of chromosome 12 [i(12p)], which is virtually diagnostic. Seminoma causes either a painless testicular mass (usually on the right side) or a diffuse nodularity throughout the testis. Seminoma is associated with **elevated human chorionic gonadotropin (hCG) levels**.

5. **Testicular teratocarcinoma** (Figure 27-4B) is a germ cell neoplasm. In its early histologic stages, a testicular teratocarcinoma resembles a blastocyst (!!!) with three primary germ layers and may be loosely referred to as a "male pregnancy." Later, the tumor is composed of well-differentiated cells and structures from each of the three primary germ layers: colon glandular tissue (endoderm), cartilage (mesoderm), and squamous epithelium (ectoderm). Testicular teratocarcinoma is associated with elevated hCG and α-fetoprotein (AFP) levels.

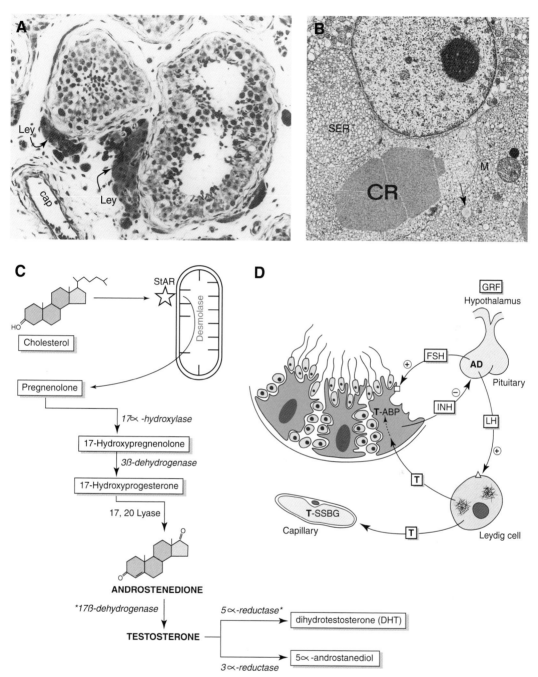

● **Figure 27-3 Histology and functional aspects of the Leydig cell. A:** Light micrograph of Leydig cells (Ley) found in the connective tissue between the seminiferous tubules (SEM) near capillaries (cap). **B:** Electron micrograph of Leydig cells. Smooth endoplasmic reticulum (SER), mitochondria with tubular cristae (M), and lipid droplets (*arrows*) are typically found in a steroid-secreting cell. CR, crystals of Reinke. **C:** Flow chart of androgen biosynthesis. Deficiencies of enzymes with an *asterisk* are clinically important. StAR, steroidgenic acute regulatory protein. **D:** Diagram of hormonal control of the male reproductive system. Gonadotropin-releasing factor (GRF) from the hypothalamus stimulates the adenohypophysis. In response to GRF, the adenohypophysis (AD) secretes follicle-stimulating hormone (FSH) and leuteinizing hormone (LH). FSH binds to FSH receptors (□) on the Sertoli cells, which stimulates the synthesis of androgen-binding protein (ABP). The Sertoli cells secrete inhibin (INH) that inhibits FSH secretion (a feedback loop). LH binds to LH receptors (∇) on the Leydig cells, which stimulates the secretion of testosterone (T). T circulates in the blood bound to sex steroid–binding globulin (SSBG). T binds to ABP within Sertoli cells to maintain high levels of T necessary for spermatogenesis.

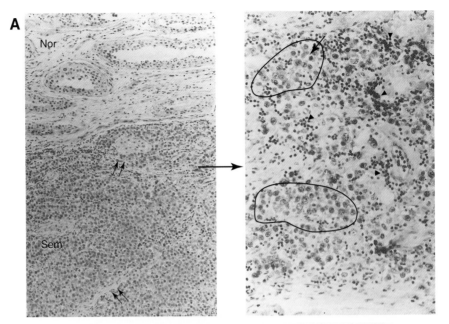

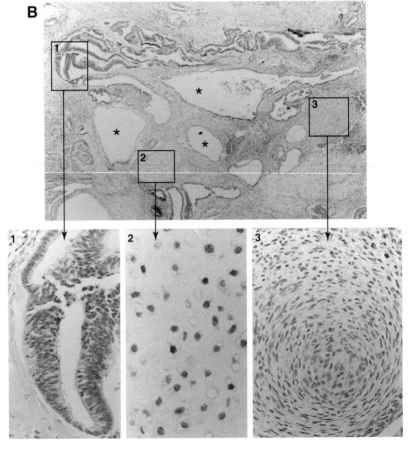

● **Figure 27-4 Testicular neoplasms. A:** Light micrograph (LM) of seminoma. About 95% of testicular neoplasms arise from germ cells. Almost all germ cell neoplasms involve the isochromosome of the short arm of chromosome 12 [i(12p)], which is virtually diagnostic. Seminoma is the most common type of germ cell neoplasm. Low magnification LM of a seminoma showing normal testicular tissue at the periphery (Nor) with typical seminiferous tubules and seminoma (Sem). High magnification LM of a seminoma, which consists of clusters of moderately sized round cells with large centrally located nuclei with prominent nucleoli (*outlined areas*). Mitotic figures can be observed (*arrow*). The cell clusters are separated by fibrous cords (*double arrows*). The fibrous cords are heavily infiltrated with lymphocytes (*arrowhead*), which may play a role in the immune rejection of seminomas and contribute to the favorable prognosis these neoplasms. **B:** LM of testicular teratocarcinoma (TC). TC is another type of germ cell neoplasm that is composed of a collection of well-differentiated cells or structures from each of the three primary germ layers. TC is composed of a fibrous stroma with many cystlike structures (*). In addition, well-differentiated glandular structures resembling colon glandular epithelium (endoderm; *box 1*), cartilage (mesoderm; *box 2*), and squamous epithelium (ectoderm; *box 3*) are shown.

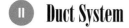 **Duct System**

A. EFFERENT DUCTULES. About 15 efferent ductules leave the testis by penetrating the tunica albuginea and connect the rete testis to the proximal portion of the epididymis. The efferent ductules are lined by a **simple columnar epithelium** that contains both **tall columnar cells** and **short columnar cells,** which give the luminal surface a saw-toothed appearance. The tall columnar cells are **ciliated** and have a role in the movement of sperm through the ductule. The short columnar cells are not ciliated but have numerous **microvilli, apical invaginations, and numerous pinocytotic vesicles** (indicating intense endocytotic activity). Eighty percent of the testicular fluid secreted in the seminiferous tubules is reabsorbed in the efferent ductules. The efferent ductules also have a thin **circular layer of smooth muscle** that aids in the movement of sperm.

B. EPIDIDYMIS. The epididymis is a very long (6 meters) and highly coiled duct that is described as having a **head region, body region,** and **tail region. Sperm maturation (i.e., motility) and storage** occur in the epididymis. Histologically, the epididymis has an epithelial lining and muscular coat.
   1. **Epithelium.** The epididymis is lined by a **pseudostratified columnar epithelium** consisting of tall columnar **principal cells** and **basal cells.** The epididymis has a **smooth luminal surface** (in contrast to the saw-toothed pattern of the efferent ductules).
      a. **The principal cells** are characterized by **stereocilia,** apical invaginations, numerous pinocytotic vesicles, coated vesicle, lysosomes, well-developed rough endoplasmic reticulum (rER), and Golgi. The principal cells have the following functions: resorption of testicular fluid begun in the efferent ductules; phagocytosis of degenerating sperm or spermatid residual bodies not phagocytosed by the Sertoli cells; and secretion of glycoproteins, which bind to the surface of the cell membrane of the sperm, sialic acid, and glycerophosphocholine (which inhibits capacitation, thus preventing sperm from fertilizing a secondary oocyte until the sperm enter the female reproductive tract).
      b. **The basal cells** act as a stem cell population to resupply the principal cells.
   2. **Muscular coat.** In the head and body region of the epididymis, the muscular coat consists of a **circular layer of smooth muscle** that aids in the movement of sperm. In the tail region of the epididymis, the muscular coat consists of an **inner longitudinal layer, middle circular layer,** and **outer longitudinal layer of smooth muscle.** These three layers contract due to neural stimulation during sexual excitation and force sperm from the tail of the epididymis to the ductus deferens. This is the initial muscular component that contributes to the force of ejaculation.

C. DUCTUS DEFERENS. The ductus deferens begins at the inferior pole of the testis, ascends to enter the spermatic cord, transits the inguinal canal, and enters the abdominal cavity by passing through the deep inguinal ring. The distal end of the ductus deferens enlarges to form the **ampulla** where it is joined by a short duct from the seminal vesicle and then continues as the ejaculatory duct. The epithelium is similar to the epididymis (i.e., **pseudostratified columnar epithelium with principal cells and basal cells**). The smooth muscular coat is similar to the tail region of the epididymis (i.e., **inner longitudinal layer, middle circular layer, and outer longitudinal layer of smooth muscle**) and contributes to the force of ejaculation.

D. EJACULATORY DUCT. The ejaculatory duct passes through the prostate gland and opens into the prostatic urethra at the **seminal colliculus** of the urethral crest. The epithelium is similar to the epididymis and ductus deferens. However, the ejaculatory duct has no smooth muscular coat. The force for ejaculation is derived primarily by the smooth muscular coat of the tail region of the epididymis and ductus deferens.

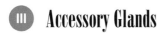

Accessory Glands

- **A. SEMINAL VESICLE.** The seminal vesicles are highly coiled tubular diverticula that originate as evaginations of the ductus deferens distal to the ampulla. The mucosa (epithelium and lamina propria) is thrown into highly convoluted folds forming labyrinthlike cul-de-sacs, all of which open into a central lumen. The **lamina propria** consists of connective tissue. The **muscular coat** consists of an inner circular layer and outer longitudinal layer. Contraction of the smooth muscle during ejaculation discharges the secretory product (seminal fluid) into the ejaculatory duct. The **adventitia** consists of connective tissue. The seminal vesicles are lined by a **pseudostratified columnar epithelium** consisting of **columnar cells** and **basal cells.**

  1. **Columnar cells** have numerous microvilli, rER, Golgi, lipid droplets, secretory granules, and lipochrome pigment. These are characteristics of cells active in secretion. The secretion product is a whitish yellow viscous material that contains fructose (the principal metabolic substrate for sperm) and other sugars, choline, proteins, amino acids, ascorbic acid, citric acid, and prostaglandins. Seminal vesicle secretion (i.e., seminal fluid) accounts for 70% of the volume of the ejaculated semen. The characteristic pale yellow color of semen is due to the lipochrome pigment secreted by the columnar cells. In forensic medicine, the presence of fructose (which is not produced elsewhere in the body) and choline crystals is used to determine the presence of semen.

  2. **Basal cells.** The basal cells are stem cells.

- **B. BULBOURETHRAL (BU) GLANDS OF COWPER.** The BU glands are located in the deep perineal space embedded in the skeletal muscles of the urogenital diaphragm (i.e., deep transverse perineal muscle and sphincter urethrae muscle) and adjacent to the membranous urethrae. The ducts of the BU glands open into the penile urethra. The BU glands are compound tubuloalveolar glands (resemble mucus-secreting glands) surrounded by a connective tissue capsule that extends septae that divide the BU gland into many lobules. The compound tubuloalveolar glands are lined by a simple cuboidal epithelium. The epithelium produces a clear, mucuslike, slippery fluid that contains galactose, galactosamine, galacturonic acid, sialic acid, and methylpentose. This fluid makes up a major portion of the preseminal fluid (or pre-ejaculate fluid) and probably serves to lubricate the penile urethra.

- **C. PROSTATE GLAND (FIGURE 27-5)**

  1. **General Features.** The prostate gland is located between the base of the urinary bladder and the urogenital diaphragm. The anterior surface of the prostate is related to the retropubic space. The posterior surface of the prostate is related to the seminal vesicles and rectum. The prostate gland can be easily palpated by a digital examination via the rectum. The prostate gland consists of five lobes: **right and left lateral lobes, right and left posterior lobes, and a middle lobe.** The prostate gland is a collection of 30 to 50 compound tubuloalveolar glands that are arranged in three zones: the **peripheral zone** (contains the largest glands and highest number of glands), **central zone,** and **periurethral zone.** The compound tubuloalveolar glands are lined by a simple columnar epithelium (however, it may vary from pseudostratified to cuboidal epithelium). The prostatic epithelium contains **basal cells, secretory cells,** and **endocrine cells.** The **basal cells** are the stem cell or proliferative compartment of the prostatic epithelium normally dividing and maturing into secretory cells. The **secretory cells** contain rER, Golgi, small clear secretory vacuoles, and lysosomes. The epithelium produces the prostatic fluid, which contains citric acid, prostatic acid phosphatase (PAP), prostaglandins, fibrinogen, and prostate-specific antigen (PSA). Serum levels of **PSA** and **PAP** are used as a diagnostic tool for prostatic carcinoma. PSA is a serine protease that liquifies semen after

ejaculation. The **endocrine cells** are randomly scattered and contain serotonin, somatostatin, calcitonin, and bombesin. The lumen of the glands contains **corpora amylacea (or prostatic concretions)**, which are calcified or precipitated prostatic fluid, the significance of which is not understood. The number of prostatic concretions increases with age. The prostate gland is surrounded by a **capsule** consisting of connective tissue and smooth muscle. The capsule is highly vascularized (important in carcinoma metastasis). The capsule (both connective tissue and smooth muscle) extends into the prostate gland, forming the **stroma**.

2. **Clinical Considerations of the Prostate Gland**

   a. **Benign Prostatic Hyperplasia (BPH)** (Figure 27-6). BPH is characterized by hypertrophy of the **transitional (periurethral) zone**, which generally involves the lateral and middle lobes. BPH compresses the prostatic urethra and obstructs urine flow. The hypertrophy may be due to increased sensitivity of prostate to **DHT**. BPH is NOT premalignant. Clinical features include: increased frequency of urination, nocturia, difficulty starting and stopping urination, and sense of incomplete emptying of bladder. Treatment may include 5α-reductase inhibitors (e.g., **finasteride [Proscar]**) to block conversion of $T \rightarrow DHT$ and/or α-adrenergic antagonists (e.g., **terazosin, prazosin, doxazosin**) to inhibit prostate gland secretion.

   b. **Prostatic carcinoma (PC)** (Figure 27-7). PC is most commonly found in the **peripheral zone**, which generally involves the posterior lobes (which can be palpated upon a digital rectal examination). Since PC begins in the peripheral zone, by the time urethral blockage occurs (i.e., patient complains of difficulty in urination), the carcinoma is in an advanced stage. **Prostatic intraepithelial neoplasia (PIN)** is frequently associated with PC. Serum **PSA levels** are diagnostic. Metastasis to bone (e.g., lumbar vertebrae, pelvis) is frequent. Treatment may include **leuprolide (Lupron)**, which is a gonadotropin-releasing hormone (GnRH) agonist that inhibits the release of FSH and LH when administered in a continuous fashion, thereby inhibiting secretion of testosterone; **cyproterone (Androcur)** or **flutamide (Eulexin)**, which are androgen receptor antagonists; radiation; and/or prostatectomy.

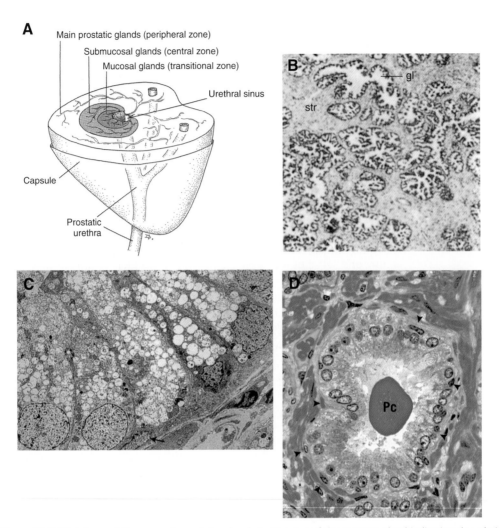

● **Figure 27-5 Histology of the normal prostate gland. A:** Diagram of the prostate gland indicating the relationship of the peripheral zone, central zone, and periurethral zone to the prostatic urethra. **B:** Light micrograph (LM) of prostate gland. Note the network tubuloalveolar glands (gl) surrounded by a connective tissue stroma (str). **C:** Electron micrograph of prostatic epithelium. The secretory cells show an abundance of closely packed, small, clear secretory vacuoles within the cytoplasm. Note the basal cell nucleus (*arrow*). **D:** LM of the lumen of a tubuloalveolar gland within the prostate. Note the corpora amylacea or prostatic concretions (PC) within the lumen, which is a distinguishing characteristic. The simple columnar epithelium consists of numerous secretory cells and basal cells (*arrowheads*).

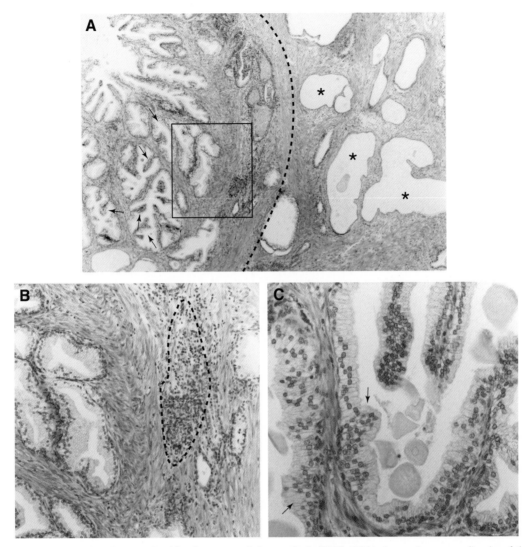

● **Figure 27-6 Light micrograph of benign prostatic hyperplasia (BPH).** BPH is the most common disorder of the prostate gland and generally occurs in elderly men. The glands in the periurethral zone and central zone (close to the urethra) are characteristically enlarged so that compression of the urethra occurs with resulting **difficulty in urination. A:** Low magnification shows a proliferation of both glands within a fairly well-defined nodule (*dotted lines*) and the connective tissue stroma. The epithelium of the glands characteristically forms papillary buds or infoldings (*arrows*), which are much more prominent than in the normal prostate. Other glands are cystically dilated (*). **B:** High magnification of the *boxed area* in A shows a hyperplastic glands and stroma infiltrated by lymphocytes (*dotted area*). **C:** High magnification of hyperplastic glands lined by a conspicuous epithelium of tall columnar cells that appear multilayered in some locations (*arrows*). Within the lumen, corpus amylacea and papillary buds or infoldings can be seen.

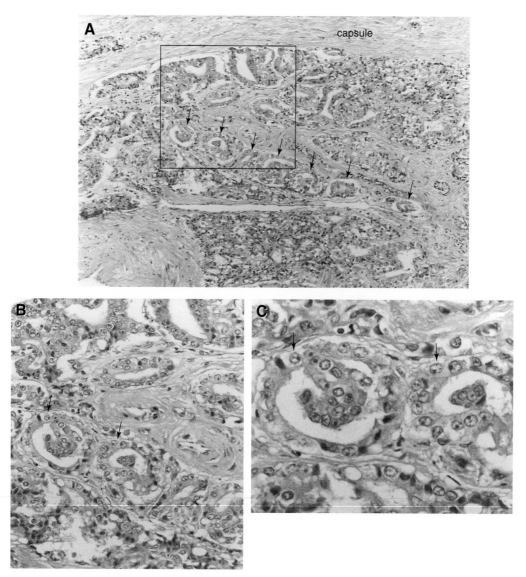

Figure 27-7 Light micrograph of prostatic carcinoma (PC). PC generally starts in the glands of the peripheral zone near the capsule. Hence, by the time blockage of the urethra occurs, PC is already in an advanced state. The most reliable sign of malignancy is the invasion of the capsule that contains lymphatics, blood vessels, and nerves. The finding of osteoblastic metastasis in bone, particularly lumbar vertebral bodies, is diagnostic of PC. **A:** Low magnification of PC showing the main glands of the prostate near the capsule. Numerous small malignant alveoli can be observed lying side by side to each other (*arrows*). **B, C:** High magnification of the *boxed area* in A shows malignant alveoli lined by simple cuboidal epithelium (*arrows*). The alveoli may be filled with cell nests. In a poorly differentiated PC alveoli are not apparent; instead, cords of neoplastic cells will invade the stroma.

Case Study 27-1

A 28-year-old married man comes to your office complaining that "I have a lump on my right testicle. It doesn't hurt, but I'm sure worried about it." He also tells you that "It can't be a venereal disease, because I swear to you that I have never cheated on my wife." After some discussion, he informs you that he cannot recall any incident where he received trauma to the groin area (e.g., a straddle injury during bicycle riding or a kick to the groin). The man has an obvious grave look of foreboding on his face and says, "Doc, my wife and I want to have children but this lump is getting bigger. Am I going to lose my testicle and be sterile?" Which of the following is the most likely diagnosis?

Differentials

- Epididymitis, hydrocele, mumps, orchitis, spermatocele, testicular torsion

Relevant Physical Examination Findings

- Nodular enlargement of the right testicle
- Normal left testicle

Relevant Lab Findings

- Blood chemistry: β-hCG levels = high; AFP levels = normal
- Computed tomography (CT) scans: no metastatic lesions in the abdomen or pelvis
- Ultrasound reveals a solid mass (not fluid filled).
- Nodular biopsy: sheet of moderately sized cells with copious cytoplasm and large centrally placed nuclei with prominent nucleoli

Diagnosis: Seminoma

- **Seminoma.** Seminoma is the most common type of germ cell neoplasm in men 20 to 40 years of age. About 90% of all testicular cancers arise from germ cells. Almost all germ cell neoplasms involve the isochromosome of the short arm of chromosome 12 [i(12p)], which is virtually diagnostic. Clinical findings of seminoma include either a painless testicular mass (usually on the right side) or a diffuse nodularity throughout the testis. Seminoma is associated with elevated β-hCG levels.
- Epididymitis is usually caused by *Chlamydia trachomatis* or *Neisseria gonorrhoeae*. Clinical findings of epididymitis include epididymal pain, swelling, and fever.
- Hydrocele of the testes occurs when a small patency of the processus vaginalis remains so that peritoneal fluid can flow into the processus vaginalis, which results in a fluid-filled cyst near the testes.
- Mumps viral infection in postpubertal males may result in mumps orchitis, where both testes becomes swollen and tender (rarely causes sterility). Clinical findings of mumps viral infection include malaise, fever, and shaking chills.
- A spermatocele is a cystic, fluid-filled mass containing sperm.
- Testicular torsion is the rotation of the testes about the spermatic cord, usually toward the penis (i.e., medial rotation). The incidence is increased when the testes are positioned horizontally and the tunica vaginalis is attached high on the spermatic cord ("bell clapper deformity"). Because the pampiniform venous plexus collapses more easily than the testicular artery, the testis becomes distended with blood and very painful. This is a medical emergency since compression of the testicular vessels results in ischemic necrosis with 6 hours.

Chapter 28

Skin

① **General Features.** Skin is the largest organ in the body. Skin consists of three layers: the outer **epidermis**, the middle **dermis**, and the deep **hypodermis** (or **subcutaneous layer**) that corresponds to the superficial fascia in gross anatomy. Skin is classified as **thick skin** (>5 mm; covering the palms of the hand and soles of the feet) and **thin skin** (1 to 2 mm; covering the rest of the body). In addition, skin has a number of epidermal derivatives (or skin appendages), namely, **hair, nails, eccrine sweat glands, apocrine sweat glands, and sebaceous glands.** Skin has the following functions: regulation of body temperature, a water barrier, nonspecific barrier to microorganisms, excretion of salt, **synthesis of vitamin D**, and a sensory organ.

② **Epidermis (Figure 28-1).** This layer is classified as **stratified squamous keratinized epithelium.** A number of different cell types can be found in this epithelium as indicated here.

A. KERATINOCYTES are so named because their major product is **keratin (an intermediate filament).** Keratinocytes are arranged in five strata: **basale, spinosum, granulosum, lucidum, and corneum.**

B. NONKERATINOCYTES
1. **Melanocytes** are **clear cells** that have long, branching cytoplasmic processes and are found in the **stratum basale.**
   a. They are derived from **neural crest cells.**
   b. They synthesize **melanin** pigment in organelles called **melanosomes.** Melanosomes contain **tyrosinase,** which catalyzes the conversion of tyrosine → 3,4,dihydroxyphenylalanin (DOPA) → dopaquinone → melanin. When melanin synthesis is completed, the melanosome loses its tyrosinase activity and the melanosome is then called a **melanin granule.** Melanin granules are transferred to neighboring keratinocytes within the stratum basale and spinosum via cytoplasmic processes.
2. **Merkel Cells** are **mechanoreceptor cells** found in the **stratum basale.**
   a. They are derived from **neural crest cells.**
   b. They contain many **dense-core granules,** presumably containing neurotransmitters.
   c. They are in contact with sensory nerve fibers that project from the dermis into the epidermis and terminate in a platelike ending called the **nerve plate.**
3. **Langerhans Cells** are **antigen-presenting cells** that have long, branching cytoplasmic processes and are found mainly in the **stratum spinosum.**
   a. They originate in the bone marrow (mesoderm) and participate in **type IV delayed-type reactions.**
   b. They phagocytose antigens, leave the epidermis to enter the lymphatic system, enter a regional lymph node where they become **dendritic cells** that express major histocompatibility complex (MHC) class I, MHC class II, and B7 molecules and activate T cells.
   c. They contain **Birbeck granules.**

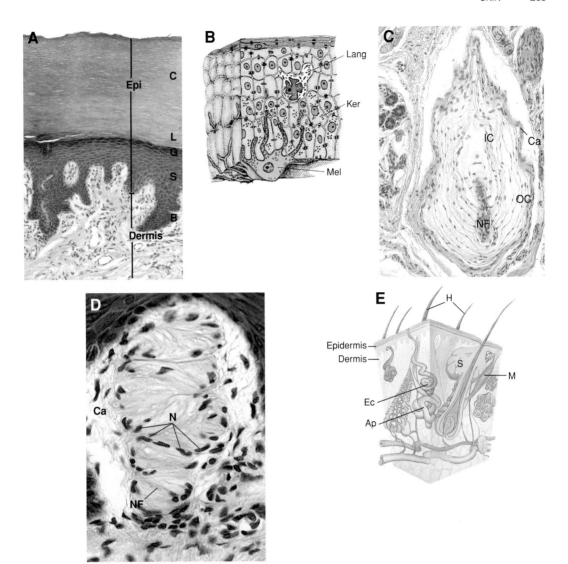

● **Figure 28-1 General features of the skin. A:** Table of characteristics of keratinocytes within various strata of the epidermis. Light micrograph (LM) of thick skin indicating the various strata of the epidermis (Epi) and dermis (Derm). B, stratum basale; S, stratum spinosum; G, stratum granulosum; L, stratum lucidum; not shown in this section, C, stratum corneum. **B:** Diagram of a melanocyte (Mel), Langerhans cell (Lang), and keratinocyte (Ker). **C:** LM of a Pacinian corpuscle within the dermis. A Pacinian corpuscle consists of inner core cells (IC) and outer core cells (OC) surrounded by a capsule (Ca). The inner core cells invest an unmyelinated axon (NF) surrounded by 20 to 29 concentric layers of cells forming the characteristic appearance of the cut surface of an onion. **D:** LM of a Meissner corpuscle within the dermis. A Meissner corpuscle consists of flattened, disc-shaped epithelial cells (N) surrounded by a capsule (Ca). An unmyelinated axon (NF) penetrates the capsule and pursues a zigzag course among the disc-shaped epithelial cells. **E:** Diagram of skin appendages showing an eccrine sweat gland (Ec), apocrine sweat gland (Ap), sebaceous gland (S), and hair (H) with its associated arrector pili muscle (M).

Dermis. The dermis consists of connective tissue composed of fibroblasts, type I collagen, and elastic fibers. The epidermal–dermal junction is stabilized by **hemidesmosomes** between the keratinocytes of the stratum basale and the **basement membrane.**

IV Glands

A. **ECCRINE SWEAT GLANDS** are widely distributed throughout the skin and are active throughout life.
   1. The **secretory portion** contains **clear cells** that secrete a product composed of H_2O, Na^+, Cl^-, K^+, urea, and NH_4^+. **Dark cells** secrete a glycoprotein by **merocrine** secretion (i.e., the cell remains intact during the secretory process).
   2. The **excretory portion (duct)** consists of **cuboidal cells** that reabsorb H_2O, Na^+, and Cl^- under the influence of **aldosterone** and open onto the skin surface as **sweat pores.**
   3. They **regulate body temperature** via postganglionic sympathetic neurons that use acetylcholine (cholinergic). Note: As a rule, postganglionic sympathetic neurons use norepinephrine as their neurotransmitter. However, there is an exception to the rule in the regulation of body temperature.
   4. They **regulate emotional sweating** via postganglionic sympathetic neurons that use norepinephrine (adrenergic).

B. **APOCRINE SWEAT GLANDS** are found in the axilla, mons pubis, and anal regions and are active at puberty.
   1. The **secretory portion** contains cells that secrete a viscous product via **merocrine** secretion.
   2. The **excretory portion (duct)** opens into the pilosebaceous canal of a hair shaft.
   3. Apocrine sweat glands are under the influence of **androgens** and **estrogens.**
   4. Modified apocrine sweat glands are found in the eyelids (**glands of Moll**) and external auditory meatus (**ceruminous glands**, which produce cerumen, i.e., ear wax).
   5. They **produce a malodorous body scent** (pheromones; for sexual attraction) via postganglionic sympathetic neurons that use norepinephrine (adrenergic).

C. **SEBACEOUS GLANDS** are widely distributed throughout the skin (except palms of the hands and soles of the feet) and are very active during puberty.
   1. The **secretory portion** contains cells with numerous lipid droplets that secrete **sebum** (composed of triglycerides, wax esters, squalene, and cholesterol) via **holocrine** secretion (i.e., the cell breaks down during the secretory process).
   2. The **excretory portion (duct)** opens into the pilosebaceous canal of a hair shaft.
   3. Sebaceous glands are under the influence of **androgens** (increase activity) and **estrogens** (decrease activity).
   4. Hair-independent sebaceous glands are found on the lips, areolae of the nipple, labia minora, and prepuce of the penis.
   5. They lubricate the skin and play a role in **acne.**

V Nerves

A. **MOTOR NERVES.** Postganglionic sympathetic neurons activate glands, contract arrector pili muscle, and control blood flow.

B. **SENSORY NERVES AND RECEPTORS**
   1. **Free Nerve Endings.** Unmyelinated axons enter the epidermis and terminate in the stratum granulosum. They function in **pain and temperature sensation.**
   2. **Merkel Endings (mechanoreceptor).** Myelinated axons terminate in a platelike ending called the **nerve plate** that contacts Merkel cells in the stratum basale. They function in **tactile sensation (high resolution).**

3. **Meissner corpuscles (mechanoreceptor).** A myelinated axon loses its myelin sheath, enters a connective tissue capsule within the dermal papillae, and pursues a zigzag course among disc-shaped epithelial cells. They function in **tactile two-point discrimination.**

4. **Pacinian Corpuscles (mechanoreceptor).** A myelinated axon loses its myelin sheath in the dermis and enters a connective tissue capsule within the dermis and hypodermis. The unmyelinated axon is surrounded by 20 to 60 concentric layers of cells and gelatinous material ("onion appearance"). They function in **touch, vibration, and pressure sensation.**

Ⓥ **Clinical Considerations (Figure 28-2)**

A. **MALIGNANT MELANOMA** is a skin lesion with irregular borders and striking variations in pigmentation. Melanomas involve the transformation of melanocytes with long, branching cytoplasmic processes to oval cells that breach the basement membrane and grow in nests within the dermis. **Dysplastic nevi** are precursors of malignant melanoma.

B. **PSORIASIS** is a chronic disease that presents as recurrent eruptions of **red or silvery plaques.** Psoriasis is characterized by epidermal hyperplasia (acanthosis) due to abnormal cell proliferation, retention of nuclei in keratinized surface cells (parakeratosis), and elongation of dermal papillae.

C. **VITILIGO** is an autoimmune disorder characterized by the **loss of melanocytes** resulting in patches of hypopigmented skin most noticeable in darkly pigmented individuals. This disorder contrasts with **albinism**, where melanocytes are present but lack the enzyme tyrosinase so no melanin pigment is produced.

D. **PIEBALDISM** is a rare autosomal dominant disorder caused by mutations in the *KIT* gene (proto-oncogene) on **chromosome 4q11** for the **steel factor (an embryonic growth factor) receptor** (a receptor tyrosine kinase). This results in defective cell proliferation and migration of neural crest–derived melanocytes finally leads to an abnormal distribution of melanocytes during embryogenesis. Clinical features include: congenital white forelock and congenital depigmented patches of skin. The white hair and depigmented patches of skin are completely formed at birth and usually do not expand. Piebaldism is one of the cutaneous signs of Waardenburg syndrome, and patients with piebaldism are generally otherwise healthy and have normal life spans.

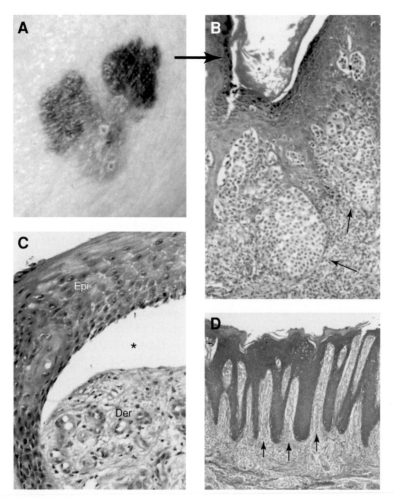

● **Figure 28-2 Skin pathology. A, B:** Malignant melanoma. **A:** Photograph of a malignant melanoma showing the clinical warning signs: asymmetry, border irregularity, color variation, and diameter greater than 6 mm. **B:** Light micrograph (LM) of malignant melanoma shows the invasion of melanocytes into the dermis forming cell nests (*arrow*). **C:** LM of bullous pemphigoid shows the separation of the epidermis (Epi) from the dermis (Der) forming a subepidermal blister (*). Bullous pemphigoid presents clinically as prominent skin blisters usually found on the inner thigh, flexor surface of the arm, and oral mucosa. **D:** LM of psoriasis showing the characteristic elongation of the dermal papillae (*arrows*). Psoriasis presents clinically as red or silvery plaques usually found on the elbows, knees, buttocks, or scalp.

Case Study 28-1

A 40-year-old man with freckles, a light complexion, and naturally blonde hair comes to your office complaining that "I have a pink bump on my nose. I can tell that people are starting to stare at it because it looks funny." He also tells you that "the bump bleeds sometimes, but it heals pretty quickly." After some discussion, he informs you that he has been a professional golfer since he was 20 years old and he first noticed something on his nose about 1 year ago but it was "just a shiny, pearl-like bump and didn't look too bad so I ignored it." Although the man expressed concern only over his cosmetic appearance, his real worry becomes apparent when he says to you, "Doc, a few of my golfing buddies got skin cancer and they died pretty quick. Do you think I'm next?" What is the most likely diagnosis?

Differentials

- Actinic keratosis, malignant melanoma, squamous cell carcinoma

Relevant Physical Examination Findings

- A firm, nontender nodule on the nose
- No other skin lesions found

Relevant Lab Findings

- Skin biopsy: multiple nests of deeply basophilic epithelial cells that protrude into the dermis and are attached to the epidermis; the periphery of the nests is composed of an organized layer of polarized, columnar keratinocytes with the long axis of each cell perpendicular to the surrounding basement membrane (i.e., palisading).

Diagnosis: Basal Cell Carcinoma

- Basal cell carcinoma (BCC) is a locally invasive tumor that derives its name from the histologic similarity of the tumor cells to basal layer keratinocytes. BCC is the most common malignant skin neoplasm in persons with pale skin over 40 years of age with excessive exposure to sunlight. Although BCC is aggressive, it rarely metastasizes.
- Actinic keratosis (AK) presents as a rough, scaly, keratotic patch (wartlike appearance) on the face, neck, upper trunk, or extremities. AK is a premalignant lesion that may eventually develop into squamous cell carcinoma.
- A melanoma presents as a flat, dark brown or black lesion with irregular borders and alternating hypopigmentation. The most important clinical characteristic of a melanoma is a new or preexisting lesion that enlarges or changes pigmentation. Melanomas involve the transformation of melanocytes with long, branching cytoplasmic processes to oval cells that breach the basement membrane and grow in nests in the dermis. Melanomas that demonstrate an aggressive vertical growth pattern will readily metastasize.
- Squamous cell carcinoma (SCC) presents as an ulcerating, scaling nodule on the back of hands, face, lips, and ears. SCC is the second most common malignant skin neoplasm and may be caused by sun exposure, ionizing radiation, chemical carcinogens, or human papilloma virus. SCC may begin as actinic keratosis. SCC rarely metastasizes. SCC is composed of cells that resemble the stratum spinosum and extend into the dermis with whorls of keratin present.

Chapter 29

Eye

I **General Features (Figure 29-1).** The eye consists of three concentric tunics that make up the wall of the eye. The **corneoscleral tunic** (outermost fibrous tunic) consists of the white, opaque **sclera** and transparent **cornea**. The **uveal tunic** (middle vascular tunic) consists of the **choroid**, and **stroma of the ciliary body and iris**. The **retinal tunic** (innermost tunic) consists of the **pigment epithelium and neural retina (posteriorly)** and **epithelium of the ciliary body and iris (anteriorly)**. The **lens** is suspended by **zonular fibers** (forming the suspensory ligament) from the ciliary body behind the iris. The **posterior chamber** and **anterior chamber** of the eye are filled with **aqueous humor,** which is a clear fluid secreted by the ciliary body epithelium. The **vitreous cavity** is filled with the **vitreous body,** which is a transparent gelatinous substance.

II **Cornea** is a transparent structure composed of five layers (Table 29-1). The central portion of the cornea receives nutrients from the **aqueous humor** within the anterior chamber of the eye, whereas the peripheral portion receives nutrients from **blood vessels of the limbus**. The cornea is an **avascular** structure, but is **highly innervated** by branches of CN V_1 (ophthalmic division of trigeminal nerve).

TABLE 29-1	LAYERS OF THE CORNEA
Layers	**Characteristics**
Corneal epithelium	Anterior aspect of cornea (exposed to air) Nonkeratinized stratified squamous epithelium Many free nerve endings (CN V_1) High capacity for repair (regeneration) Continuous with the conjunctiva at the limbus
Bowman layer	A distinctive portion of the corneal stroma Contains type I collagen Not a true basement membrane
Stroma	Connective tissue Contains type I and V collagen Thickest layer of the cornea
Descemet membrane	A basement membrane
Corneal endothelium	Posterior aspect of cornea (exposed to aqueous humor) Simple squamous epithelium Participates in active transport of nutrients into the stroma

CN, cranial nerve.

III **Sclera** is a thick, opaque layer of collagen and elastic fibers produced by fibroblasts. The tendons of the extraocular muscles attach to the sclera.

IV **Limbus** (**corneoscleral junction**) is the junction of the transparent cornea and the opaque sclera. The limbus contains a **trabecular network** and the **canal of Schlemm**, which are involved in the flow of aqueous humor. The flow of aqueous humor follows this route: **posterior chamber → anterior chamber → trabecular network → canal of Schlemm → aqueous veins → episcleral veins**. The drainage rate of aqueous humor is balanced by the secretion rate of aqueous humor from the ciliary epithelium, thus maintaining a constant **intraocular pressure of 23 mm Hg**. An obstruction of aqueous humor flow will increase intraocular pressure, causing a condition called **glaucoma**, which may lead to blindness if untreated. There are two types of glaucoma.

A. OPEN-ANGLE GLAUCOMA (most common) occurs when the trabecular network is open but the canal of Schlemm is obstructed.

B. CLOSED-ANGLE GLAUCOMA occurs when the trabecular network is closed usually due to an inflammatory process of the uvea (uveitis; e.g., infection by cytomegalovirus).

V **Iris.** The posterior surface is lined by two layers of simple columnar epithelium. The anterior surface of the iris lacks an epithelial covering and consists of the stroma. The stroma contains the dilator pupillae muscle and sphincter pupillae muscle.

A. DILATOR PUPILLAE MUSCLE is radially arranged around the entire circumference of the iris and is innervated by the sympathetic nervous system. Preganglionic sympathetic neurons project to the sympathetic trunk and ascend to the superior cervical ganglion. The superior cervical ganglion projects postganglionic sympathetic neurons through the perivascular plexus of the carotid system entering the orbit through the superior orbital fissure. The postganglionic sympathetic neurons release **norepinephrine**, which stimulates contraction (i.e., **pupil dilation or mydriasis**) via **α-adrenergic receptors**. Any pathology that compromises this sympathetic pathway will result in **Horner syndrome**, which causes **miosis** (constriction of pupil due to paralysis of dilator pupillae muscle), **ptosis** (drooping of eyelid due to paralysis of superior tarsal muscle), and **hemi-anhydrosis** (loss of sweating on one side).

B. SPHINCTER PUPILLAE MUSCLE is circularly arranged around the entire circumference of the iris and is innervated by the parasympathetic nervous system. Preganglionic parasympathetic neurons from the **Edinger-Westphal nucleus of cranial nerve (CN) III** project to the ciliary ganglion. The **ciliary ganglion** projects postganglionic parasympathetic neurons to the sphincter pupillae muscle. The postganglionic parasympathetic neurons release **acetylcholine (ACh)**, which stimulates contraction (i.e., **pupil constriction or miosis**) via **muscarinic acetylcholine receptors (mAChRs)**. Lesions involving **CN III** (oculomotor nerve) will result in a **fixed and dilated pupil**.

Ciliary Body.   The ciliary body is lined by two layers of simple columnar epithelium called the **ciliary epithelium**. The ciliary epithelium **secretes aqueous humor** and **produces the zonular fibers** that attach to the lens. The stroma contains the **ciliary muscle**. The ciliary muscle is circularly arranged around the entire circumference of the ciliary body and is innervated by the parasympathetic nervous system. Preganglionic parasympathetic neurons from the **Edinger-Westphal nucleus of CN III** project to the **ciliary ganglion**. The ciliary ganglion projects postganglionic parasympathetic neurons to the ciliary muscle. The postganglionic parasympathetic neurons release **ACh**, which stimulates contraction (i.e., **accommodation**) via **mAChRs**.

A. **ACCOMMODATION** is the process by which the lens becomes **rounder to focus a nearby object** or flatter to focus a distant object.

B. **FOR CLOSE VISION (e.g., READING),** the ciliary muscle contracts, which **reduces tension on the zonular fibers** attached to the lens and thereby allows the lens to take a **rounded shape**.

C. **FOR DISTANT VISION,** the ciliary muscle relaxes, which **increases tension on the zonular fibers** attached to the lens and thereby allows the lens to take a **flattened shaped**.

 Lens.   The lens is a biconvex, transparent, and avascular structure that receives its nutrients from the aqueous humor. It consists of the following components:

A. **LENS CAPSULE** is a thick basement membrane that completely surrounds the lens.

B. **LENS EPITHELIUM** is a simple cuboidal epithelium located beneath the lens capsule only on the anterior surface (i.e., no epithelium is found on the posterior surface). The lens epithelium is mitotically active and migrates to the equatorial region of the lens where the cells elongate and rotate so that they are parallel to the lens surface.

C. **LENS FIBERS** are prismatic remnants of the elongated lens epithelium that lose their nuclei and organelles. They are filled with cytoskeletal proteins called **filensin** and **α,β,γ-crystallin**, which maintain the conformation and transparency of the lens. The older lens fibers are displaced to the center of the lens, whereas the newer lens fibers are found at the periphery.

D. **CATARACTS** are an opacity of the lens due to a change in the solubility of lens proteins, filensin, and α,β,γ-crystallin. This causes light scattering and impairs accurate vision. Cataracts are observed in elderly persons and associated with diabetes. Glucose is the major metabolite of the lens. When glucose levels are high (diabetes), the byproduct sorbitol is formed in high concentration, which reduces the solubility of α,β,γ-crystallin, leading to lens opacity (cataracts).

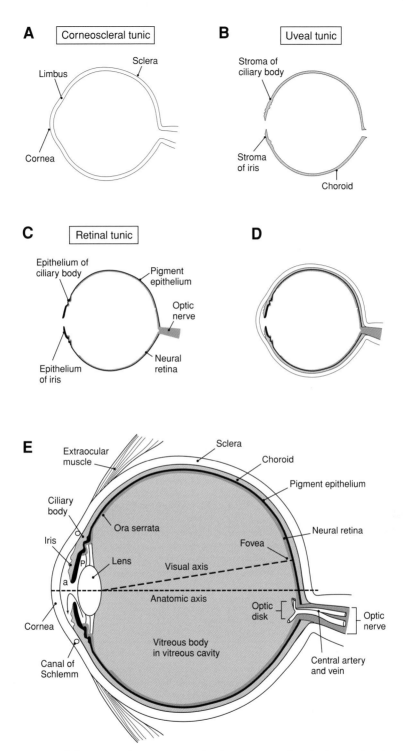

● **Figure 29-1 Diagram of the eye tunics. A:** Corneoscleral tunic. **B:** Uveal tunic. **C:** Retinal tunic. **D:** This diagram shows all three tunics combined into the adult structure of the eye. **E:** Adult eye with its various components. The *curved arrow* indicates the flow of aqueous humor. a, anterior chamber; p, posterior chamber.

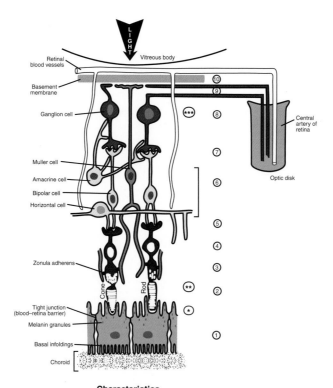

Layers		Characteristics
10	Inner limiting membrane	Termination of Müller cells and their basement membrane
9	Optic nerve fibers	Unmyelinated axons of ganglion cells
8	Ganglion cells	Nuclei of ganglion cells
		Site of action potential generation
7	Inner plexiform layer	Synapses between bipolar and amacrine cells with ganglion cells
6	Inner nuclear layer	Nuclei of horizontal, bipolar, amacrine, and Müller cells
5	Outer plexiform layer	Synapses between bipolar and horizontal cells with rods and cones
		Retinal blood vessels may extend to this layer
4	Outer nuclear layer	Nuclei of rods and cones
3	Outer limiting membrane	Zonula adherens between rods/cones and Müller cells
2	Photoreceptor layer	Outer segment with membrane disks containing **Na^+ ion channels,** connecting cilium, and inner segment of rods and cones
		Location of intraretinal space; detached retina occurs between 1 and 2
1	Pigment epithelium	Has tight junctions at apical border to form blood–retinal barrier, basal infoldings, and contains melanin
		Converts 11-trans retinal → 11-cis retinal
		Phagocytoses shed tips of rod outer segments
		Transports nutrients from choroid capillaries up to layer 4

● **Figure 29-2 Diagram of the retina.** Tight junctions between the pigment epithelial cells establish a **blood-retinal barrier.** Therefore, blood supply to most of the retina (up to layer 5, outer plexiform layer) is from retinal blood vessels via the central artery of the retina (a branch of the ophthalmic artery). Retinal blood vessels are visible by ophthalmoscopic examination where visible changes may be observed in hypertension or diabetic retinopathy. The central artery of the retina leaves the optic disc and travels between layer 10 (inner limiting membrane) and the vitreous body. Other layers of the retina (layers 1 through 4) are supplied by choroid capillaries. Muller cells act as supporting glial-type cells. Note the direction of the incident light and that it must pass through many layers of the retina before reaching the rods and cones. The asterisk indicates the site of retinal detachment; the double asterisk indicates the presence of Na^+ ion channels; the triple asterisk indicates the site of action potential generation.

 Retina (Figure 29-2). The posterior two thirds of the retina is a light-sensitive area (**pars optica**) and the anterior one third is a light-insensitive area (**par ciliaris and iridis**); these two areas are separated by the **ora serrata**. The 10 layers that constitute the retina are described and illustrated in Figure 29-2. The retina has a number of specialized areas, which include the following:

A. **OPTIC DISC.** The optic disc is the site where axons of the ganglion cells converge to form the optic nerve (CN II) by penetrating the sclera forming the **lamina cribrosa**. The optic disc lacks rods and cones and is therefore a **blind spot**. The central artery and vein of the retina pass through the optic disc.

B. **FOVEA.** The fovea is a shallow depression of the retina located 3 mm lateral (temporal side) to the optic disc along the visual axis. The **fovea centralis** is located at the center of the fovea and is the area of highest visual acuity and color vision. The fovea centralis contains **only cones (no rods or capillaries)** that are arranged **at an angle** so that light directly impinges on the cones without passing through other layers of the retina and are linked to a single ganglion, both of which contribute to visual acuity. The **macula lutea** is a yellowish area (due to xanthophyll pigment accumulation in ganglion cells) surrounding the fovea centralis.

IX Clinical Considerations

A. **RETINITIS PIGMENTOSA (RP)** is a complex group of genetic disorders that demonstrate autosomal dominant inheritance, autosomal recessive inheritance, or X-linked inheritance, or may occur spontaneously. The three most common genes involved in RP are the *RHO* gene on **chromosome 3q21.3** for rhodopsin; *USH2A* gene on **chromosome 1q41** for **usherin**, which has been localized to the connecting cilia that connect inner and outer photoreceptor segments; and the *RPGR* gene on **chromosome Xp21** for **retinitis pigmentosa guanosine triphosphatase (GTPase) regulator.** RP is characterized by progressive degeneration and dysfunction of the retina primarily affecting photoreceptor and pigment epithelium function. Clinical findings include degeneration of rods and cones, night blindness (nyctalopia), and "gun barrel" vision. RP may be caused by abetalipoproteinemia (Bassen-Kornzweig syndrome) and may be arrested by massive doses of vitamin A. In RP, blood supply to the retina is reduced and a pigment is observed on the surface of the retina (hence the name).

B. **DIABETIC RETINOPATHY.** In patients with diabetes, retinal blood vessels frequently become leaky and exude fluid into the retina (particularly in the fovea), leading to loss of visual acuity. It is the leading cause of blindness in the developed world and may be reduced by strict regulation of blood glucose levels.

C. **PAPILLEDEMA (CHOKED DISC)** is a noninflammatory edema of the optic disc (papilla) due to increased intracranial pressure usually caused by brain tumors, subdural hematoma, or hydrocephalus. It usually does not alter visual acuity, but may cause bilateral **enlarged blind spots**.

D. **NIGHT BLINDNESS (NYCTALOPIA)** is a condition in which vision in poor illumination is defective due to vitamin A (retinol) deficiency. An aldehyde of vitamin A (retinol) called **retinal** is the chromophore component of rhodopsin.

E. **RETINOBLASTOMA (RB)** is a tumor of the retina that occurs in childhood and develops from precursor cells in the immature retina. The *RB* gene is located on chromosome 13 and encodes for RB protein, which binds to a gene regulatory protein and causes suppression of the cell cycle (i.e., the *RB* gene is a tumor suppressor gene [also called an antioncogene]). A mutation in the *RB* gene encodes an abnormal RB protein such that there is no suppression of the cell cycle. This leads to the formation of retinoblastoma. Hereditary retinoblastoma causes multiple tumors in both eyes. Nonhereditary retinoblastoma causes one tumor in one eye.

X Selected Photomicrographs

A. **CORNEA, RETINA, IRIS, AND CILIARY BODY (FIGURE 29-3)**

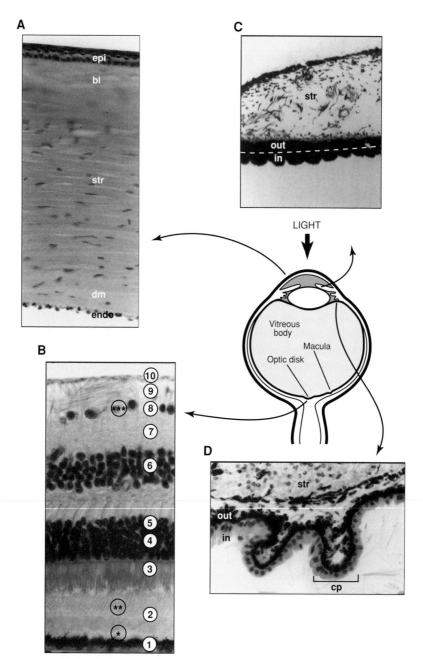

● **Figure 29-3 General features of the eye. A:** Light micrograph (LM) of cornea. The five layers of the cornea are indicated. epi, corneal epithelium; bl, Bowman layer; str, stroma; dm, Descemet membrane; endo, corneal endothelium. **B:** LM of retina. The 10 layers of the retina are indicated. The asterisk indicates the site of retinal detachment; the double asterisk indicates the presence of Na$^+$ ion channels; the triple asterisk indicates the site of action potential generation. **C:** LM of iris. The posterior surface of the iris is lined by two layers of simple columnar epithelium, which are derived embryologically from the outer pigment layer (out) and inner (in) neural layer of the optic cup. Both of these layers are so highly pigmented that the two cell layers cannot be distinguished (see *dotted line* for boundary). The iris contains the dilator pupillae muscle and sphincter pupillae muscle, which are formed from the epithelium of the outer pigment layer (out) by the transformation of the epithelial cells into contractile cells. The stroma (str) of the iris contains connective tissue, blood vessels, nerves, and melanocytes. **D:** LM of ciliary body. The ciliary body is lined by two layers of simple columnar epithelium, which are derived embryologically for the outer pigment layer (out) and the inner neural layer (in) of the optic cup. The outer pigment layer is pigmented, but the inner neural layer is nonpigmented. The ciliary body is thrown into folds called ciliary processes (cp). Both layers of epithelium are involved in the production of aqueous humor and zonular fibers of the lens. The stroma (str) of the ciliary body contains connective tissue and the ciliary muscle.

B. ROD PHOTORECEPTOR CELL (FIGURE 29-4)

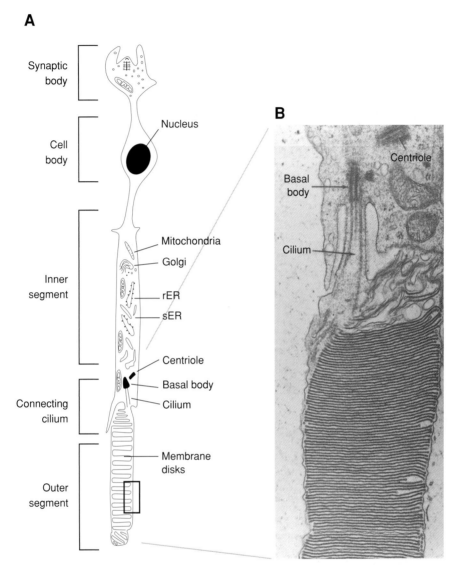

● **Figure 29-4 A:** Diagram of a rod photoreceptor cell. Note the various regions of the rod: outer segment, which contains Na$^+$ ion channels and membrane discs; connecting cilium, which contains the cilium, basal body, and centriole; inner segment, which contains mitochondria, rough endoplasmic reticulum (rER), smooth endoplasmic reticulum (sER), and Golgi; cell body, which contains the nucleus; and synaptic body, which contains synaptic vesicles. **B:** Electron micrograph of the outer segment and connecting cilium regions. Note the cilium, basal body, and centriole.

Chapter 30

Ear

I **General Features.** The ear is the organ of hearing and balance. The ear consists of the external ear, middle ear, and inner ear.

II **External Ear** consists of the following:

A. **EXTERNAL AUDITORY MEATUS** is an air-filled tubular space. The lateral portion is supported by cartilage and lined by skin that contains hair follicles, sebaceous glands, and ceruminous glands (produce ear wax). The medial portion is supported by the temporal bone and is lined by thinner skin. The external auditory meatus develops from the **pharyngeal groove 1**, which becomes filled with ectodermal cells, forming a temporary **meatal plug** that disappears before birth. The external auditory meatus is innervated by **cranial nerve (CN) V$_3$ and CN IX**.

B. **AURICLE** (known as "the ear" by laypeople) is supported by elastic cartilage and covered by skin. The auricle develops from **six auricular hillocks** that surround pharyngeal groove 1. The auricle is innervated by **CN V$_3$, CN VII, CN IX, and CN X** and **cervical nerves C2 and C3.**

III **Middle Ear** consists of the following:

A. **OSSICLES**
1. **Malleus** develops from cartilage of **pharyngeal arch 1** (Meckel cartilage). The malleus is attached to the **tympanic membrane** and is moved by the **tensor tympani muscle**, which is innervated by CN V$_3$.
2. **Incus** develops from the cartilage of **pharyngeal arch 1** (Meckel cartilage). The incus articulates with the malleus and stapes.
3. **Stapes** develops from the cartilage of **pharyngeal arch 2** (Reichert cartilage). The stapes is attached to the **oval window** of the vestibule and is moved by the **stapedius** muscle, which is innervated by CN VII.

B. **AUDITORY TUBE AND MIDDLE EAR CAVITY** develop from **pharyngeal pouch 1.**

C. **TYMPANIC MEMBRANE (EARDRUM)** develops from **pharyngeal membrane 1.** The tympanic membrane separates the middle ear from the external auditory meatus of the external ear, has a conical depression at it center due to the attachment of the malleus, and is innervated (sensory) by CN V$_3$ and CN IX. The tympanic membrane consists of three layers.
1. Keratinized stratified squamous epithelium covers the external surface.
2. Connective tissue, which is vascularized and innervated, constitutes the middle layer.
3. Simple squamous epithelium covers the internal surface.

IV **Internal Ear.** The internal ear consists of the semicircular ducts, utricle, saccule, and cochlear duct, all of which are referred to as the **membranous labyrinth** containing **endolymph**. The membranous labyrinth is initially surrounded by mesoderm that later becomes cartilaginous and ossifies to become the **bony labyrinth** of the temporal bone. The mesoderm closest to the membranous labyrinth degenerates, thus forming the **perilymphatic space** containing **perilymph**. Thereby, the membranous labyrinth is suspended within the bony labyrinth by perilymph. Perilymph, which is similar in composition to **cerebrospinal fluid (CSF)**, communicates with the subarachnoid space via the **perilymphatic duct**.

A. SEMICIRCULAR DUCTS (KINETIC LABYRINTH) (FIGURE 30-1). Type I and type II **hair cells** that cover the **cristae ampullaris** (a prominent ridge within the ampulla) have numerous stereocilia and a single **kinocilium** on their apical border. These cells synapse with bipolar neurons of the vestibular ganglion of CN VIII. The kinetic labyrinth also contains **supporting cells**. Hair cells and supporting cells are covered by a gelatinous mass called by **cupula**. The semicircular ducts respond to **angular acceleration** and **deceleration of the head**.

B. UTRICLE AND SACCULE (STATIC LABYRINTH) (FIGURE 30-1). Type I and type II **hair cells** within **maculae** (a specialized receptor area within the wall) have stereocilia and a single **kinocilium** on their apical border. These cells synapse with bipolar neurons of the vestibular ganglion of CN VIII. The static labyrinth also contains **supporting cells**. Hair cells and supporting cells are covered by a gelatinous mass called the **otolithic membrane**, which contains $CaCO_3$ crystals (**otoliths**). The utricle and saccule respond to the position of the head with respect to **linear acceleration** and **pull of gravity**.

C. COCHLEAR DUCT (FIGURE 30-2). This triangular duct is composed of a **vestibular membrane** (roof), **basilar membrane** (floor), and **stria vascularis** (lateral wall). The stria vascularis participates in the formation of endolymph. The cochlear duct contains the **organ of Corti**. The organ of Corti contains a single row of **inner hair cells** and three rows of **outer hair cells** that have stereocilia (but no kinocilium) on their apical border and synapse with bipolar neurons of the cochlear (spiral) ganglion of CN VIII (90% of these bipolar neurons synapse with inner hair cells). It also contains **pillar** and **phalangeal supporting cells**. The outer hair cells are in contact with a gelatinous mass called the **tectorial membrane** (contains α- and β-tectorin protein). The organ of Corti responds to **sound**.

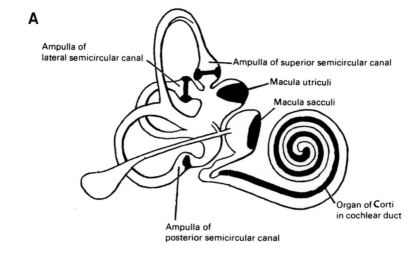

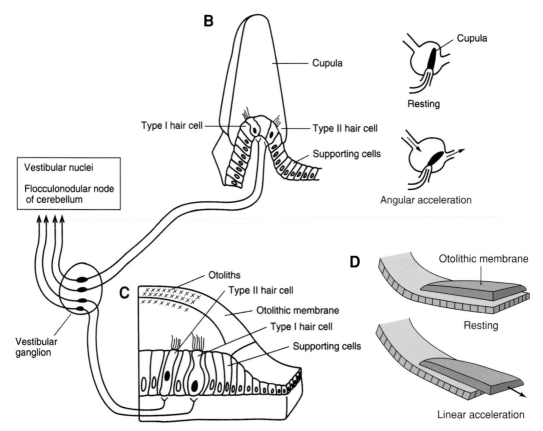

● **Figure 30-1 A:** Diagram of the membranous labyrinth. Note the location of specialized sensory areas (*black color*) for angular acceleration (cristae ampullaris), linear acceleration (maculae), and hearing (organ of Corti). **B: Cristae ampullaris** of the semicircular ducts (kinetic labyrinth). The deflection of the cupula by endolymph movement during angular acceleration stimulates the hair cells. When stereocilia move toward the kinocilium, hair cells are depolarized and afferent nerve fibers are stimulated. When stereocilia move away from the kinocilium, hair cells are hyperpolarized and afferent nerve fibers are not stimulated. **C, D: Macula** of the utricle and saccule (static labyrinth). The displacement of otoliths by endolymph movement during linear acceleration stimulates hair cells.

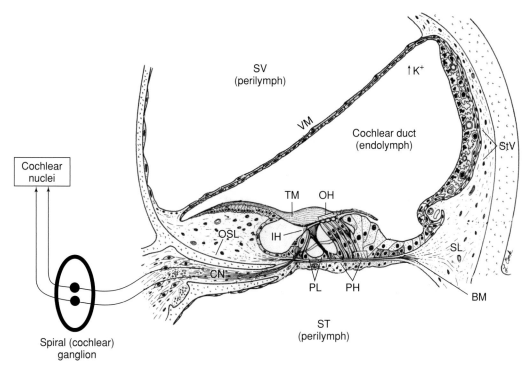

● **Figure 30-2 Organ of Corti of the cochlear duct.** The organ of Corti responds to sound. The hearing process begins when air-borne sound waves cause vibration of the tympanic membrane, which moves the stapes against the oval window. This produces waves of perilymph within the scala vestibuli and scala tympani. The waves of perilymph cause an upward displacement of the basilar membrane such that the stereocilia of the hair cells hit the tectorial membrane. As a result, K$^+$ ion channels open, hair cells are depolarized, and afferent nerve fibers are stimulated. Note that the endolymph has a high K$^+$ concentration, which is maintained by the stria vascularis (StV). Note the vestibular membrane (VM), stria vascularis (StV), basilar membrane (BM), nerve fibers (NF), scala vestibuli (SV) containing perilymph, scala tympani (ST) containing perilymph, cochlear duct containing endolymph, three rows of outer hair cells (OH), one row of inner hair cells (IH), tectorial membrane (TM), spiral ligament (SL), outer phalangeal cells (PH), pillar cells (PL), and osseous spiral lamina (OSL). The basilar membrane extends between the osseous spiral lamina and the spiral ligament.

Clinical Considerations

A. **RUBELLA VIRUS.** The organ of Corti may be damaged by exposure to rubella virus during week 7 and week 8 of embryologic development.

B. **MÉNIÈRE DISEASE** is caused by an increase in endolymph. Clinical findings include vertigo (the illusion of rotational movement), nausea, positional nystagmus (involuntary rhythmic oscillations of the eye), vomiting, and tinnitus (ringing of the ears).

C. **WAARDENBURG SYNDROME** is an autosomal dominant congenital deafness associated with pigment abnormalities resulting from abnormal neural crest cell migration.

Credit List

Chapter 1

Figure 1-1: From Dudek RW. *BRS Genetics*. Philadelphia: Lippincott Williams & Wilkins, 2010:172, Fig 16-2. Original source: Modified from Dudek RW. *High-Yield Cell and Molecular Biology*. Philadelphia: Lippincott Williams & Wilkins, 1999:81, Fig. 15-1.

Figure 1-2: From Dudek RW. *BRS Genetics*. Philadelphia: Lippincott Williams & Wilkins, 2010:178, Fig 16-3. Original source: Dudek RW. *High-Yield Cell and Molecular Biology*. Philadelphia: Lippincott Williams & Wilkins, 1999:75, Fig. 14-1.

Figure 1-3: From Dudek RW. *BRS Genetics*. Philadelphia: Lippincott Williams & Wilkins, 2010:179, Fig. 16-4. Original source: From Dudek RW. *High-Yield Cell and Molecular Biology*. Philadelphia: Lippincott Williams & Wilkins, 1999:76, Fig. 14-2.

Figure 1-4: From Dudek RW. *BRS Genetics*. Philadelphia: Lippincott Williams & Wilkins, 2010:180, Fig. 16-5. Original source: From Dudek RW. *High-Yield Cell and Molecular Biology*. Philadelphia: Lippincott Williams & Wilkins, 1999:78, Fig. 14-3.

Figure 1-5: From Dudek RW. *High-Yield Cell and Molecular Biology*. 2nd Ed. Philadelphia: Lippincott Williams & Wilkins, 2006:22, Fig. 4-2.

Figure 1-6: **A:** From Dudek RW. *High-Yield Histology*. 3rd Ed. Philadelphia: Lippincott Williams & Wilkins, 2004:15, Fig. 1-7A. Original source: Modified from Cormack DH. *Essential Histology*. 2nd Ed. Philadelphia: Lippincott Williams & Wilkins, 2001:26, Fig. 2-2. **B, C:** From Cormack DH. *Essential Histology*. 2nd Ed. Philadelphia: Lippincott Williams & Wilkins, 2001:27–28, Figs. 2-3 and 2-4. **D:** From Dudek RW. *High-Yield Histology*. 3rd Ed. Philadelphia: Lippincott Williams & Wilkins, 2004:15, Fig. 1-7C. Original source: Stafstrom J, Stahelin L. Are annulate lamellae in the Drosophila embryo the result of overproduction of nuclear pore components? *J Cell Biol* 98:699. Copyright 1984 by Rockefeller University Press. Reproduced with permission of Rockefeller University Press in the format Textbook via Copyright Clearance Center. **E:** From Dudek RW. *High-Yield Histology*. 3rd Ed. Philadelphia: Lippincott Williams & Wilkins, 2004, Fig. 1-7B. Original source: Feldherr C, Kallenbach E, Schultz N. Movement of a karyophilic protein through the nuclear pores of oocytes. *J Cell Biol* 99:2216. Copyright 1984 by Rockefeller University Press. Reproduced with permission of Rockefeller University Press in the format Textbook via Copyright Clearance Center. **F, G:** Courtesy of Dr. R.W. Dudek. **H:** Courtesy of Dr. Scott H. Kaufmann, Mayo Clinic.

Table 1-2: Modified from Alberts B, Johnson A, Lweis J, Raff M, et al. *Molecular Biology of the Cell*. 3rd Ed. New York: Garland, 1994:18-1.

Chapter 2

Figure 2-1: Modified from Dudek RW. *High-Yield Cell and Molecular Biology*. Philadelphia: Lippincott Williams & Wilkins, 1999:108, Fig. 19-4.

Figure 2-2: From Dudek RW. *High-Yield Cell and Molecular Biology*. Philadelphia: Lippincott Williams & Wilkins, 1999:45, Fig. 8-3. Original source: Redrawn from Alberts B, Johnson A, Lewis J, Roff M, et al. *Essential Cell Biology*. New York: Garland, 1998:230.

Figure 2-3: **A, B:** From Cormack DH. *Essential Histology*. 2nd Ed. Philadelphia: Lippincott Williams & Wilkins, 2001:65, 67, Figs. 3-6, 3-7. **C, E:** Courtesy of Dr. J. Brinn, East Carolina University, Brody School of Medicine. **Inset:** From Heuser J. Protocol for 3-D visualization of molecules on mica via the quick-freeze, deep-etch technique. *J Electron Microscopy Tech* 13:244, 1989. **D, G:** From Dellmann HD, Eurell J. *Textbook of Veterinary Histology*. 5th Ed. Philadelphia: Lippincott Williams & Wilkins, 1998:8, 10: Figs. 1-12, 1-14. **F:** Modified from Cormack DH. *Essential Histology*. 2nd Ed. Philadelphia: Lippincott Williams & Wilkins, 2001:73, Fig. 3-11.

Figure 2-4: **A:** From Cormack DH. *Essential Histology*. 2nd Ed. Philadelphia: Lippincott Williams & Wilkins, 2001:86, Fig. 3-24. **B:** From Erlandson R. *Diagnostic Transmission Electron Microscopy of Tumors*. Philadelphia: Lippincott Williams & Wilkins, 1993:26, Fig. 1-20G. **C:** From Ross MH, Romrell L. *Histology: A Text and Atlas*. 2nd Ed. Philadelphia: Lippincott Williams & Wilkins, 1992:38, Fig. 2-21. Courtesy of M. McGill, D.P. Highfield, T.M. Monahan, and B. Brinkley.

Figure 2-5: **A:** From Dellmann HD, Eurell J. *Textbook of Veterinary Histology*. 5th Ed. Philadelphia: Lippincott Williams & Wilkins, 1998:9, Fig. 1-13B. **B:** From Damjanov I. *Histopathology: A Color Atlas and Textbook*. Philadelphia: Lippincott Williams & Wilkins, 1996:109, Fig. 5-18. **C:** From Cormack DH. *Essential Histology*. 2nd Ed. Philadelphia: Lippincott Williams & Wilkins, 2001:79, Fig. 3-16.

Figure 2-6: **A:** Courtesy of Dr. J. Brinn, East Carolina University, Brody School of Medicine. **B, inset:** From Dellmann HD, Eurell J. *Textbook of Veterinary Histology*. 5th Ed. Philadelphia: Lippincott Williams & Wilkins, 1998:10–11, Figs. 1-14, 1-16.

Chapter 3

Figures 3-1, 3-2, 3-4: From Dudek RW. *High-Yield Cell and Molecular Biology*. 2nd Ed. Philadelphia: Lippincott Williams & Wilkins, 2007:2, 4, 20, Figs. 1-1, 1-2, 1-4.

Chapter 4

Figure 4-2. **A, B:** From Cormack DH. *Essential Histology*. 2nd Ed. Philadelphia: Lippincott Williams & Wilkins, 2001:101, Figs. 4-5, Fig. 4-6. **C:** From Gartner LP, Hiatt JL. *Color Atlas of Histology*. 4th Ed. Philadelphia: Lippincott Williams & Wilkins, 2006:30, Graphic 2-1. **D:** From Arias IM, Boyer JL, Chisari FV, et al. *The Liver: Biology and Pathobiology*. 4th Ed. Philadelphia: Lippincott Williams & Wilkins, 2001:30, Fig. 3-1C. **E:** From Dellmann HD, Eurell J. *Textbook of Veterinary Histology*. 5th Ed. Philadelphia: Lippincott Williams & Wilkins, 1998:3, Fig. 1-4. **F, G:** From Cormack DH. *Essential Histology*. 2nd Ed. Philadelphia: Lippincott Williams & Wilkins, 2001:83, Fig. 3-22.

Chapter 5

Figure 5-1. **A:** From McMillian JA, DeAngelis CD, Feigin RD, et al. *Oski's Pediatrics*. 3rd Ed. Philadelphia: Lippincott Williams & Wilkins, 1999:2149. **B:** From Rubin R, Strayer DS. *Rubin's Pathology*. 5th Ed. Philadelphia: Lippincott Williams & Wilkins, 2008:712, Fig. 16-32. **C1, D1:** From Cormack DH. *Essential Histology*. 2nd Ed. Philadelphia: Lippincott Williams & Wilkins, 2001:119–120, Figs. 5-4, 5-5. **C2:** From Dudek RW. *High-Yield Embryology*. 2nd Ed. Philadelphia: Lippincott Williams & Wilkins, 2000:94, Fig. 16-1B. Original source: Smith DW, Jones KL. *Recognizable Patterns of Human Malformation*. 3rd Ed. Philadelphia: WB Saunders, 1982:359. **D2:** From Dudek RW. *High-Yield Embryology*. 2nd Ed. Philadelphia: Lippincott Williams & Wilkins, 2000:104, Fig. 17-5B. Original source: Salmon MA, Lindenbaum RH. *Developmental Defects and Syndromes*. Aylesbury, England: HM & M Publishers, 1978:172. **E:** From Gartner L, Hiatt J. *Color Atlas of Histology*. 3rd Ed. Philadelphia: Lippincott Williams & Wilkins, 2000:60, Fig. 1. Original source: Simpson D, Avery B. Pathologically altered fibroblasts within lymphoid cell infiltrates in early gingivitis. *J Periodontol* 45:500–510, 1974. Reprinted with permission from the American Academy of Periodontology. **F:** From Dellmann HD, Eurell J. *Textbook of Veterinary Histology*. 5th Ed. Philadelphia: Lippincott Williams & Wilkins, 1998:36, Fig. 3-8. **G:** From Rubin R, Strayer DS. *Rubin's Pathology*. 5th Ed. Philadelphia: Lippincott Williams & Wilkins, 2008:53, Fig. 2-18D. **(H)** Courtesy of Dr. R.W. Dudek.

Chapter 7

Figure 7-1: **A:** From Rohen JW, Yokochi C, Lutjen-Drecoll E. *Color Atlas of Anatomy*. 4th Ed. Philadelphia: Williams & Wilkins, 1998:9. **B, C:** Courtesy of Dr. R.W. Dudek. **D:** From Cormack DH. *Essential Histology*. 2nd Ed. Philadelphia: Lippincott Williams & Wilkins, 2001, Plate 8-6. **E:** From Cormack DH. *Clinically Integrated Histology*. Philadelphia: Lippincott-Raven, 1998:89, Fig. 4-16.
Figure 7-2: **A–E:** Courtesy of Dr. R.W. Dudek.
Figure 7-3. **A, B:** From Cormack DH. *Clinically Integrated Histology*. Philadelphia: Lippincott-Raven, 1998:73, Figs. 4-5D, 4-5C. **D:** From Damjanov I. *Histopathology: A Color Atlas and Textbook*. Baltimore: Williams & Wilkins, 1996:432, Fig. 17-9.
Figure 7-4: **A, D:** From Damjanov I. *High-Yield Pathology*. Philadelphia: Lippincott Williams & Wilkins, 2000:126, 127, Figs. 17-3, 17-4. **B, E:** From Damjanov I. *Histopathology: A Color Atlas and Textbook*. Baltimore: Williams & Wilkins, 1996:441, 443, Figs. 17-20A, 17-21A. **C:** From Cormack DH. *Clinically Integrated Histology*. Philadelphia: Lippincott-Raven, 1998:74, Fig. 4-6.

Chapter 8

Figure 8-1: **A:** Courtesy of Charles J. Tanner, MA; Joseph A. Houmard, PhD; and Robert Gray, MA.
Figure 8-3: **A, F:** From Cormack D. *Essential Histology*. 2nd Ed. Philadelphia: Lippincott Williams & Wilkins, 2001:240, 251, Figs. 10-2, 10-15. **B, C:** From Dellmann HD, Eurell J. *Textbook of Veterinary Histology*. 5th Ed. Philadelphia: Lippincott Williams & Wilkins, 1998:86, Fig. 5-9.
Figure 8-4: **A:** From Cormack D. *Essential Histology*. 2nd Ed. Philadelphia: Lippincott Williams & Wilkins, 2001:242, Fig. 10-5. **B, C:** From Dudek RW. *High-Yield Histology*. 2nd Ed. Baltimore: Lippincott Williams & Wilkins, 2000:49, Fig. 6-4A, B. Original source: Lindgren CA, Emery DG, Haydon PG. Intracellular acidification reversibly reduces endocytosis at the neuromuscular junction. *J Neurosci* 17:3074, 1997. **D:** Reprinted with permission from Gartner L, Hiatt J. *Color Atlas of Histology*. 3rd Ed. Philadelphia: Lippincott Williams & Wilkins, 2000:117, Fig. 1. Original source: Ovalle W, Dow P. Comparative ultrastructure of the inner capsule of the muscle spindle and the tendon organ. *Am J Anat* 166:343–357, 1983.
Figure 8-5: **A, B:** From Bacha WJ, Bacha LM. *Color Atlas of Veterinary Histology*. 2nd Ed. Hoboken, NJ: Wiley-Blackwell, 2000:44, Figs. 8.8, 8.9. **C, G, H:** From Cormack D. *Essential Histology*. 2nd Ed. Philadelphia: Lippincott Williams & Wilkins, 2001:250, 253, Figs. 10-14, 10-17A,B. **D, J:** From Dellmann HD, Eurell J. *Textbook of Veterinary Histology*. 5th Ed. Philadelphia: Lippincott Williams & Wilkins, 1998:89, 83, Figs. 5-14, 5-3. **E, F, I:** From Gartner L, Hiatt J. *Color Atlas of Histology*. 3rd Ed. Philadelphia: Lippincott Williams & Wilkins, 2000:119,121, Figs. 2, 4, Plate 6-7.

Chapter 9

Figure 9-1: **A, C, D:** From Cormack DH. *Essential Histology*. 2nd Ed. Philadelphia: Lippincott Williams & Wilkins, 2001:212, 213, Figs. 9-2, 9-3, Plate 9-4 (no page number). **B:** From Bacha WJ, Bacha LM. *Color Atlas of Veterinary Histology*. 2nd Ed. Hoboken, NJ: Wiley-Blackwell, 2000:50, Fig. 9.15. **E–J:** From Damjanov I. *Histopathology: A Color Atlas and Textbook*. Baltimore: Williams & Wilkins, 1996:466, 467, 483, Figs. 19-1A, 19-1E, 19-10, 19-25, 19-1C, 19-1F.
Figure 9-2: **A:** Reprinted with permission from Sternberg SS. *Histology for Pathologists*. 2nd Ed. Philadelphia: Lippincott Williams & Wilkins, 1997:290, Fig. 5A. **B:** From Gartner LP, Hiatt JL. *Color Atlas of Histology*. 4th Ed. Philadelphia: Lippincott Williams & Wilkins, 2006:143, Fig. 1b. **C:** From Cormack DH. *Essential Histology*. 2nd Ed. Philadelphia: Lippincott Williams & Wilkins, 2001:228, Fig. 9-23A. **D, E:** From Dudek RW. *High-Yield Histology*. 2nd Ed. Philadelphia: Lippincott Williams & Wilkins, 2000:59, Fig. 7-4; and p. 60, Fig. 7-6. Original source: Peters A, Palay SL, Webster HF. *The Fine Structure of the Nervous System: Neurons and Their Supporting Cells*. 3rd Ed. London: Oxford University Press, 1990. © 1990 by Alan Peters. Reprinted with permission from Oxford University Press, Inc.
Figure 9-3: **A, C–F:** From Cormack DH. *Essential Histology*. 2nd Ed. Philadelphia: Lippincott Williams & Wilkins, 2001:221, Fig. 9-14. **B:** From Dudek RW. *High-Yield Histology*. 2nd Ed. Philadelphia: Lippincott Williams & Wilkins, 2000:58, Fig. 7-3. Original source: Siegel GJ, Agranoff BW, Albers RW, et al. *Basic Neurochemistry*. 6th Ed. Philadelphia: Lippincott-Raven, 1998:22. **G:** Reprinted with permission from Sternberg SS. *Histology for Pathologists*. 2nd Ed. Philadelphia: Lippincott Williams & Wilkins, 1997:272, Fig. 47C.
Figure 9-4: **A, B:** Courtesy of Dr. R.W. Dudek. **C:** From Dudek RW. *High-Yield Histology*. 2nd Ed. Philadelphia: Lippincott Williams & Wilkins, 2000:59, Fig. 7-5. Original source: Chazel G, Baude A, Barbe A, et al. Ultrastructural organization of the interstitial subnucleus of the nucleus of the tractus solitarius in the cat: identification of vagal afferents. *J Neurocytol* 20:859, 1991.
Figure 9-5: **A:** From Dudek RW. *High-Yield Histology*. 2nd Ed. Philadelphia: Lippincott Williams & Wilkins, 2000:61, Fig. 7-7. Courtesy of the East Carolina University School of Medicine, Department of Pathology slide collection. **B:** Courtesy of Dr. R.W. Dudek. **C:** From Troncoso JC, Rubio A, Fowler D. *Essential Forensic Neuropathology*. Philadelphia: Lippincott Williams & Wilkins, 2010:242, Fig. 19.2B. **D:** From Damjanov I. *Histopathology: A Color Atlas and Textbook*. Baltimore: Williams & Wilkins, 1996:483, Fig. 19-27. **E:** From Dudek RW. *High-Yield Histology*. 2nd Ed. Philadelphia: Lippincott Williams & Wilkins, 2000:204, Fig. 29-2. Original source: Siegel GJ, Agranoff BW, Albers RW, et al. *Basic Neurochemistry*. 6th Ed. Philadelphia: Lippincott-Raven, 1999:951. **F:** From Troncoso JC, Rubio A, Fowler D. *Essential Forensic Neuropathology*. Philadelphia: Lippincott Williams & Wilkins,

2010:260, Fig. 20.29B. **G:** From Troncoso JC, Rubio A, Fowler D. *Essential Forensic Neuropathology*. Philadelphia: Lippincott Williams & Wilkins, 2010:253, Fig. 20.12A.

Chapter 10

Figure 10-2: A: Courtesy of Dr. R.W. Dudek.
Figure 10-3: (A) From Damjanov I. *High-Yield Pathology*. Philadelphia: Lippincott Williams & Wilkins, 2000:38, Fig. 7-1. **D:** From Damjanov I. *Histopathology: A Color Atlas and Textbook*. Baltimore: Williams & Wilkins, 1996: 101, Fig. 5-5.
Figure 10-4: A, C, D: Courtesy of Dr. R.W. Dudek. **B:** From Cormack DH. *Clinically Integrated Histology*. Philadelphia: Lippincott-Raven, 1998:134, Fig. 5-16.
Figures 10-5, 10-6: Courtesy of Dr. R.W. Dudek.

Chapter 11

Figure 11-2: A, C, D inset: From Stiene-Martin EA, Lotspeich-Steininger CA, Koepke JA. *Clinical Hematology: Principles, Procedures, Correlations*. 2nd Ed. Philadelphia: Lippincott, 1998:91, 96, 99. **B, D:** Courtesy of Jean Shafer, Department of Medicine, University of Rochester, Rochester, NY, Carden Jennings Publishing Co. Ltd. Charlottesville, VA.
Figure 11-4: A, B, D: From Stiene-Martin EA, Lotspeich-Steininger CA, Koepke JA. *Clinical Hematology: Principles, Procedures, Correlations*. 2nd Ed. Philadelphia: Lippincott, 1998:95, 98, 97. **A inset:** From Carr JH, Rodak BF. *Clinical Hematology Atlas*. Philadelphia: Saunders, 1999:143. **C:** Courtesy of Jean Shafer, Department of Medicine, University of Rochester, Rochester, NY, Carden Jennings Publishing Co. Ltd. Charlottesville, VA.
Figure 11-5: A–D: Reprinted with permission from Stiene-Martin EA, Lotspeich-Steininger CA, Koepke JA. *Clinical Hematology: Principles, Procedures, Correlations*. 2nd Ed. Philadelphia: Lippincott, 1998:92–93.
Figure 11-6: 3–6: From Gartner L, Hiatt J. *Color Atlas of Histology*. 3rd Ed. Philadelphia: Lippincott Williams & Wilkins, 2000:100, Figs. 3-6.
Figure 11-7: From Cormack DH. *Clinically Integrated Histology*. Philadelphia: Lippincott-Raven, 1998:43, Fig. 3-17 J–O.
Figure 11-8: A–I: From Cormack DH. *Clinically Integrated Histology*. Philadelphia: Lippincott-Raven, 1998:37, 43, Figs. 3-11 C, D, F, G, H, K; 3-17 H, I.

Chapter 12

Figure 12-1: A: Modified from Schiffman RJ. *Hematologic Pathophysiology*. Philadelphia: Lippincott-Raven, 1998:16, Fig. 1-18. Redrawn from Weiss L. *Cell and Tissue Biology*. Reprinted with permission from Cormack DH. *Clinically Integrated Histology*. Philadelphia: Lippincott-Raven, 1998:58, Fig. 3-22A. **C, D:** Courtesy of Dr. R.W. Dudek.
Figure 12-2: B: From Cormack DH. *Clinically Integrated Histology*. Philadelphia: Lippincott-Raven, 1998:58, Fig. 3-22A.
Figure 12-3: Courtesy of Dr. R.W. Dudek.

Chapter 13

Figure 13-1: A: Redrawn from Takahashi M. *Color Atlas of Cancer Cytology*. 3rd Ed. Philadelphia: Lippincott Williams & Wilkins, 2000:375, Fig. 17-2A. **B:** Redrawn from Ross MH, Romrell LJ, Kaye GI. *Histology: A Text and Atlas*. 3rd Ed. Philadelphia: Lippincott, Williams & Wilkins, 1995:343, Fig. 13-8. Based on Bloom W, Fawcett DW. *A Textbook of Histology*. 10th Ed. Philadelphia: WB Saunders, 1975. **C:** Cour-

tesy of Dr. R.W. Dudek. **D:** From Cormack DH. *Essential Histology*. 2nd Ed. Philadelphia: Lippincott Williams & Wilkins, 2001:166, Fig. 7-8B.

Chapter 14

Figure 14-1: A: Redrawn from Ross MH, Romrell LJ, Kaye GI. *Histology: A Text and Atlas*. 3rd ed. Philadelphia: Lippincott Williams & Wilkins, 1995:350, Fig. 13-14. Based on Weiss L, Tavossoli M. Anatomical hazards to the passage of erythrocyte through the spleen. *SEM Hematol* 7:372, 1970. **B:** Redrawn from Cormack DH. *Essential Histology*. 2nd Ed. Philadelphia: Lippincott Williams & Wilkins, 2001:169, Fig. 7-11.

Chapter 15

Figure 15-1: Modified from Ross MH, Romrell LJ, Kaye GI. *Histology: A Text and Atlas*. 3rd Ed. Philadelphia: Lippincott Williams & Wilkins, 1995:448–450, Figs. 16-7, 16-8, 16-9. Cell drawings based on Lentz TL. *Cell Fine Structure: An Atlas of Drawings of Whole-Cell Structure*. Philadelphia: WB Saunders, 1971.

Chapter 16

Figure 16-1: Picture of enterocyte courtesy of Dr. R.W. Dudek. Picture of Paneth cell reprinted with permission from Satoh Y. Ultrastructure of Paneth cells in the intestine of various mammals. *J Electron Microsc Tech* 16:69, 1990. John Wiley and Sons, Inc.
Figure 16-2: A: From Fenoglio-Preiser CM. *Gastrointestinal Pathology: A Text and Atlas*. 2nd Ed. Philadelphia: Lippincott Williams & Wilkins, 1999:293, Fig. 8-38. **B:** From Damjanov I. *Histopathology: A Color Atlas and Textbook*. Baltimore: Williams & Wilkins, 1996:197, Fig. 8-16A. **C:** From Yamada T, Alpers DH, Laine L, Owyang C, et al. *Atlas of Gastroenterology*. 2nd Ed. Philadelphia: Lippincott Williams & Wilkins, 1999:334, Fig. 36-10A. **D:** From Yamada T, Alpers DH, Laine L, Owyang C, et al. *Atlas of Gastroenterology*. Vol 1. 3rd Ed. Philadelphia: Lippincott Williams & Wilkins, 1999:1484, Fig. 66-17A.

Chapter 17

Figures 17-1, 17-2: Courtesy of Dr. R.W. Dudek.

Chapter 18

Figure 18-1: Reprinted with permission from Henrikson RC, Kaye GI, Mazurkiewicz JE. *NMS Histology*. 3rd Ed. Philadelphia: Williams & Wilkins, 1997:292, Fig. 26-2.
Figure 18-2: Courtesy of Dr. R.W. Dudek.
Figure 18-3: B–D: From East Carolina University, School of Medicine, Department of Pathology slide collection.
Figure 18-4: B: From East Carolina University, School of Medicine, Department of Pathology slide collection.

Chapter 19

Figure 19-1: Islet figure from Henrikson RC, Kaye GI, Mazurkiewicz JE. *NMS Histology*. 3rd Ed. Philadelphia: Williams & Wilkins, 1997:368, Fig. 33-2.
Figure 19-2: A, B: From Bakerman S, Bakerman P, Strausbach P. *Bakerman's ABC's of Interpretive Laboratory Data*. 4th Ed. Scottsdale, AZ: Intepretive Laboratory Data, Inc., 2002: 403.

Chapter 20

Figure 20-1: B: From Cormack DH. *Essential Histology*. 2nd Ed. Philadelphia: Lippincott Williams & Wilkins, 2001:343, Fig. 14-7A. **C:** From Dellmann HD, Eurell J. *Textbook of Veterinary Histology*. 5th Ed. Philadelphia: Lippincott Williams & Wilkins, 1998:157, Fig. 9-16.

Figure 20-3: B: From Cormack DH. *Essential Histology*. 2nd Ed. Philadelphia: Lippincott Williams & Wilkins, 2001:345, Fig. 14-11. **C:** From Cormack DH. *Clinically Integrated Histology*. Philadelphia: Lippincott-Raven, 1998:156, Fig. 6-13.

Figure 20-4: From East Carolina University, School of Medicine, Department of Pathology slide collection.

Figure 20-5: A, B, C, F: From Damjanov I. *Histopathology: A Color Atlas and Textbook*. Baltimore: Williams & Wilkins, 1996:137, 135, Figs. 6-10, 6-8B, 6-7C, 6-9C, 6-8B. **D:** From Takahashi M. *Color Atlas of Cancer Cytology*. 3rd Ed. Philadelphia: Lippincott Williams & Wilkins, 2000:189, Fig. 8-59.

Chapter 21

Figure 21-1. 2, 3: Drawings of proximal and distal tubules from Henrikson RC, Kaye GI, Mazurkiewicz JE. *NMS Histology*. 3rd Ed. Baltimore: Williams & Wilkins, 1997:331, Fig. 29-6. **4, 5:** Light micrographs of proximal convoluted tubule (PCT), distal straight tubule (DCT), and collecting duct (CD) are courtesy of Dr. R.W. Dudek. **7:** Drawing of kidney, sagittal section from Cormack DH. *Essential Histology*. 2nd Ed. Philadelphia: Lippincott Williams & Wilkins, 2001:351, Fig. 15-1. **9:** Electron micrograph of thin loop of Henle from Jennette JC, Olson JL, Schwartz MM, Silva FG, et al. *Heptinstall's Pathology of the Kidney*. Vol 1. 5th Ed. Philadelphia: Lippincott Williams & Wilkins, 1998:43, Fig. 1-54.

Figure 21-2: A: From Dudek RW. *High-Yield Kidney*. Philadelphia: Lippincott Williams & Wilkins, 2007:52, Fig. 4-3A. Originally modified from *Gray's Anatomy*. 38th Ed. New York: Churchill-Livingston, 1995:1829, Fig. 13-18a. **B:** From Cormack DH. *Essential Histology*. 2nd Ed. Philadelphia: Lippincott Williams & Wilkins, 2001:353, Fig. 15-2.

Figure 21-3: From Dudek RW. *High-Yield Kidney*. Philadelphia: Lippincott Williams & Wilkins, 2007:59, Fig. 4-5.

Figure 21-4: A: From Dudek RW. *High-Yield Kidney*. Philadelphia: Lippincott Williams & Wilkins, 2007:54, Fig. 4-4B. **B:** Courtesy of Dr. R.W. Dudek. **C:** Courtesy of D. Friend, Brigham & Women's Hospital, Boston, MA. **D:** From Sledin DW. *The Kidney: Physiology and Pathophysiology*. Vol 1. 3rd Ed. Philadelphia: Lippincott Williams & Wilkins, 2000:615, Fig. 23-26A.

Figure 21-5: From Dudek RW. *High-Yield Kidney*. Philadelphia: Lippincott Williams & Wilkins, 2007:197, Fig. 8-2.

Figure 21-6: A–D: Courtesy of Dr. R.W. Dudek. **E–H:** From Damjanov I. *Histopathology: A Color Atlas and Textbook*. Baltimore: Williams & Wilkins, 1996:283, 288, 289, 291, Figs. 11-14B, 11-22A, 11-23D, 11-24.

Chapter 22

Figure 22-1: A: From Dudek RW. *High-Yield Histology*. 2nd Ed. Philadelphia: Lippincott Williams & Wilkins, 2000:149, Fig. 20-1. **B–F:** From Sternberg SS. *Histology for Pathologists*. 2nd Ed. Philadelphia: Lippincott Williams & Wilkins, 1997:1060, 1065, Figs. 21B, 23A&B, 28, 29.

Chapter 23

Figure 23-1: From Dudek RW. *High-Yield Histology*. 2nd Ed. Philadelphia: Lippincott Williams & Wilkins, 2000:151, Fig. 21-1.

Figure 23-2: A: From Dudek RW. *High-Yield Histology*. 2nd Ed. Philadelphia: Lippincott Williams & Wilkins, 2000:154, Fig. 21-2B. **B:** From Sternberg SS. *Histology for Pathologists*. 2nd Ed. Philadelphia: Lippincott Williams & Wilkins, 1997:1082, Fig. 9. **C, D:** From East Carolina University, School of Medicine, Department of Pathology slide collection.

Figure 23-3: A, B: From East Carolina University, School of Medicine, Department of Pathology slide collection. **Insets:** From Sternberg SS. *Diagnostic Surgical Pathology*. Vol 1. 3rd Ed. Philadelphia: Lippincott Williams & Wilkins, 1999:536, 551, Figs. 9A and 30A.

Chapter 24

Figure 24-1: From Dudek RW. *High-Yield Histology*. 3rd Ed. Philadelphia: Lippincott Williams & Wilkins, 200:2004, Fig. 24-1.

Figure 24-2: A–D: From Sternberg SS. *Histology for Pathologists*. 2nd Ed. Philadelphia: Lippincott Williams & Wilkins, 1997:1096, 1088, 1100, Figs. 7, 21, 20, 22.

Chapter 25

Figures 25-1, 25-2: From Dudek RW. *High-Yield Histology*. 2nd Ed. Philadelphia: Lippincott Williams & Wilkins, 2000:160, 163, Figs. 23-1, 23-2.

Figure 25-3: A, F, G: From Sternberg SS. *Histology for Pathologists*. 2nd Ed. Philadelphia: Lippincott Williams & Wilkins, 1997:1108, 1114, Figs. 1B, 11, 12. **B:** Reprinted with permission from Copenhaver WM, Bunge RP, Bunge MB. *Bailey's Textbook of Histology*. 16th Ed. Baltimore: Williams & Wilkins, 1978:651, Fig. 21-19. **C–E:** Courtesy of Dr. R.W. Dudek.

Figure 25-4: Courtesy of Dr. R.W. Dudek.

Figure 25-5: A, C: From Sternberg SS. *Diagnostic Surgical Pathology*. Vol 1. 3rd Ed. Philadelphia: Lippincott Williams & Wilkins, 1999:614, 609, Figs. 43, 33. **B, D:** From Dudek RW. *High-Yield Histology*. 2nd Ed. Philadelphia: Lippincott Williams & Wilkins, 2000:166, Figs. 23-4B&C.

Chapter 26

Figure 26-1: 1, 2: Photos of secondary and primary follicles from Sternberg SS. *Histology for Pathologists*. 2nd Ed. Philadelphia: Lippincott Williams & Wilkins, 1997:942, Figs. 23 and 22. **3:** From Bacha WJ, Bacha LM. *Color Atlas of Veterinary Histology*. 2nd Ed. Hoboken, NJ: Wiley-Blackwell, 2000:225, Fig. 18.2. **4, 5:** From Cormack DH. *Clinically Integrated Histology*. Philadelphia: Lippincott Williams & Wilkins, 1998:252, 256, Figs. 9-33, 9-37.

Figure 26-2: A–C: From Sternberg SS. *Histology for Pathologists*. 2nd Ed. Philadelphia: Lippincott Williams & Wilkins, 1997:918, Figs. 46A–C. **D, E:** From Sternberg SS. *Diagnostic Surgical Pathology*. Vol 2. 3rd Ed. Philadelphia: Lippincott Williams & Wilkins, 1999:2396, 2399, Figs. 1, 10.

Figure 26-3: 1: From Cormack DH. *Clinically Integrated Histology*. Philadelphia: Lippincott Williams & Wilkins, 1998:260, Fig. 9-41C. **2, 3:** Courtesy of Dr. R.W. Dudek.

Figure 26-4: 1–3: From Sternberg SS. *Histology for Pathologists*. 2nd Ed. Philadelphia: Lippincott Williams & Wilkins, 1997:886, 888, 885, Figs. 8, 11A, 6. **4:** From Mills SE. *Histology for Pathologists*. 3rd Ed. Philadelphia: Lippincott Williams & Wilkins, 2007:1023, Fig. 41.16. **Figure 26-5. A, B:** From Sternberg SS. *Histology for Pathologists*. 2nd Ed. Philadelphia: Lippincott Williams & Wilkins, 1997:872, 873, Figs. 7, 8. **C–E:** From Damjanov I. *Histopathology: A Color Atlas and Textbook*. Philadelphia: Lippincott Williams & Wilkins, 1996:327, Fig. 13-13, Fig. 13-14, and Fig. 13-2.

1–3: From Koss L, Gompel C, Bergeron C. *Introduction to Gynecologic Cytopathology*. Philadelphia: Lippincott Williams & Wilkins, 1999:39–41 Figs. 6-1, 6-4, 6-7.

Figure 26-6: A, B: From Sternberg SS. *Histology for Pathologists*. 2nd Ed. Philadelphia: Lippincott Williams & Wilkins, 1997:72, 74, Figs. 1, 2. C: From Cormack DH. *Clinically Integrated Histology*. Philadelphia: Lippincott-Raven, 1998:263, Fig. 9-45. D: From Gartner LP, Hiatt JL. *Color Atlas of Histology*. 4th Ed. Philadelphia: Lippincott Williams & Wilkins, 2006:367, Fig. 3. E: From Ross M, Romrell L. *Histology: A Text and Atlas*. 2nd Ed. Baltimore: Williams & Wilkins, 1989:682, Fig. 22-37. Redrawn after Bloom W, Fawcett DW. *A Textbook of Histology*. 10th Ed. Philadelphia: WB Saunders, 1975.

Figure 26-7: A1: From Sternberg SS. *Histology for Pathologists*. 2nd Ed. Philadelphia: Lippincott Williams & Wilkins, 1997:872, Fig. 7. A2: From Koss LG. *Diagnostic Cytology*. 4th Ed. Vol 1. Philadelphia: Lippincott Williams & Wilkins, 1992:397, Fig. 11-21B. B1: From Koss L, Gompel C, Bergeron C. *Introduction to Gynecologic Cytopathology*. Philadelphia: Lippincott Williams & Wilkins, 1999:39, Fig. 6-1. B2, B3: From Takahashi M. *Color Atlas of Cancer Cytology*. 3rd Ed. Philadelphia: Lippincott Williams & Wilkins, 2000:83, 92, Figs. 6-109, 6-126B. C: From Sternberg SS. *Diagnostic Surgical Pathology*. Vol 2, 3rd Ed. Philadelphia: Lippincott Williams & Wilkins, 1999:2156, Fig. 1B. D: Courtesy of Dr. R.W. Dudek.

Figure 26-8: A, D: From Le Treut A, Dilhuydy MH. *Mammography: A Guide to Interpretation*. St. Louis: Mosby-Year Book, 1991:36,103. B, C: From East Carolina University, School of Medicine, Department of Pathology slide collection. E, F: From Dudek RW. *High-Yield Histology*. 2nd Ed. Philadelphia: Lippincott Williams & Wilkins, 2000:177, Figs. 24-6 A&C.

Chapter 27

Figure 27-1: A: From Henrikson R, Kaye G, Mazurkiewicz J. *NMS Histology*. Philadelphia: Lippincott Williams & Wilkins, 1997:393, Fig. 36-2. Originally adapted from Weiss L, ed. *A Textbook of Histology*. 6th Ed. Baltimore: Urban & Schwarzenberg, 1988:932. B: From Dudek RW. *High-Yield Histology*. 2nd Ed. Philadelphia: Lippincott Williams & Wilkins, 2000:183, Fig. 25-3. C–G: From Dellmann HD, Eurell J. *Textbook of Veterinary Histology*. 5th Ed. Philadelphia: Lippincott Williams & Wilkins, 1998:299, 232, Figs. 12-4, 12-6.

Figure 27-2: From Dellmann HD, Eurell J. *Textbook of Veterinary Histology*. 5th Ed. Philadelphia: Lippincott Williams & Wilkins, 1998:233, Fig. 12-7.

Figure 27-3: A, B: From Kerr JB. Ultrastructure of the seminiferous epithelium and intertubular tissue of the human testis. *J Electron Microsc Tech* 19(2):215–240, 1991. D: From Dudek RW. *High-Yield Histology*. 2nd Ed. Philadelphia: Lippincott Williams & Wilkins, 2000:181, Fig. 25-2.

Figure 27-4: From East Carolina University, School of Medicine, Department of Pathology slide collection.

Figure 27-5: A, B: From Cormack DH. *Clinically Integrated Histology*. 2nd Ed. Philadelphia: Lippincott-Raven, 1998:272–

273, Figs. 9-55, 9-56A. C: From Sternberg SS. *Histology for Pathologists*. 2nd Ed. Philadelphia: Lippincott Williams & Wilkins, 1997:1007, Fig. 22. D: From Gartner LP, Hiatt JL. *Color Atlas of Histology*. 4th Ed. Philadelphia: Lippincott Williams & Wilkins, 2006:385, Fig. 2.

Figure 27-6: From East Carolina University, School of Medicine, Department of Pathology slide collection.

Figure 27-7: From East Carolina University, School of Medicine, Department of Pathology slide collection.

Table 27-1. 1, 2: From Dellmann HD, Eurell J. *Textbook of Veterinary Histology*. 5th Ed. Philadelphia: Lippincott Williams & Wilkins, 1998:233, 232, Figs. 17-7, 12-6B. 3–6: From Sternberg SS. *Histology for Pathologists*. 2nd Ed. Philadelphia: Lippincott Williams & Wilkins, 1997:1022, Fig. 7.

Chapter 28

Figure 28-1: A, C, D, E: From Gartner LP, Hiatt JL. *Color Atlas of Histology*. 4th Ed. Philadelphia: Lippincott Williams & Wilkins, 2006:227, Fig. 1; 233, Figs. 3 and 4, 224, top figure. B: From Ross MH, Kaye GI, Pawlina W. *Histology: A Text and Atlas*. 4th Ed. Philadelphia: Lippincott Williams & Wilkins, 2003:408, Fig. 14-7. Originally modified from Weiss L, ed. *Cell and Tissue Biology: A Textbook of Histology*. 6th Ed. Baltimore: Urban & Schwarzenberg, 1988.

Figure 28-2: A, B: From Cormack DH. *Clinically Integrated Histology*. Philadelphia: Lippincott William & Wilkins, 1998:14, Fig. 2-2A. B, C, D: From Damjanov I. *Histopathology: A Color Atlas and Textbook*. Philadelphia: Lippincott Williams & Wilkins, 1996: 405, Figs. 16-3, 16-2.

Chapter 29

Figure 29-1: From Dudek RW. *High-Yield Histology*. 3rd Ed. Philadelphia: Lippincott Williams & Wilkins, 2004:250, Fig. 29-1.

Figure 29-2: From Dudek RW. *High-Yield Histology*. 2nd Ed. Philadelphia: Lippincott Williams & Wilkins, 2000:198, Fig. 28-1.

Figure 29-3: From Dudek RW. *High-Yield Histology*. 2nd Ed. Philadelphia: Lippincott Williams & Wilkins, 2000:200, Fig. 28-2.

Figure 29-4: (A) From Dudek RW. *High-Yield Histology*. 3rd Ed. Philadelphia: Lippincott Williams & Wilkins, 2000:256, Fig. 29-4A. (B) From Fawcett DW. *A Textbook of Histology*. 12th Ed. New York: Chapman and Hall Medical, 1994:902. Courtesy of T. Kuwabara.

Chapter 30

Figure 30-1: A: From Copenhaver WM, Bunge RP, Bunge MB. *Bailey's Textbook of Histology*. 16th Ed. Baltimore: Williams & Wilkins, 1978. B, C left: From Dudek RW. *High-Yield Histology*. 2nd Ed. Philadelphia: Lippincott Williams & Wilkins, 2000:194, Fig. 27-1A, B.

Figure 30-2: From Dellmann HD, Eurell J. *Textbook of Veterinary Histology*. 5th Ed. Philadelphia: Lippincott Williams & Wilkins, 1998:350, Fig. 18-5.

Index

Page numbers followed by f indicate figure; those followed by t indicate table.